Study Guide to Accompany

Brunner and Suddarth's Textbook of Medical-Surgical Nursing

ELEVENTH EDITION

Study Guide to Accompany

Brunner and Suddarth's Textbook of Medical-Surgical Nursing

ELEVENTH EDITION

Mary Jo Boyer, R.N., D.N.Sc.
Coadjutant Nursing Faculty
Former Dean and Professor of Allied Health and Nursing
Delaware County Community College
Media, Pennsylvania

Wolters Kluwer | Lippincott Williams & Wilkins
Health
Philadelphia · Baltimore · New York · London
Buenos Aires · Hong Kong · Sydney · Tokyo

Ancillary Editor: Claudia Vaughn
Composition: Techbooks
Printer/Binder: Victor

11th Edition

ISBN 13: 978-0-7817-6543-5
ISBN 10: 0-7817-6543-9

The material contained in this volume was submitted as previously unpublished material, except in the instances in which credit has been given to the source from which some of the illustrative material was derived.

Any procedure or practice described in this book should be applied by the health care practitioner under appropriate supervision in accordance with professional standards of care used with regard to the unique circumstances that apply in each practice situation. Care has been taken to confirm the accuracy of information presented and to describe generally accepted practices. However, the authors, editors, and publishers cannot accept any responsibility for errors or omissions or for any consequences from application of the information in this book and make no warranty, express or implied, with respect to the contents of the book.

The authors and publisher has exerted every effort to ensure that drug selection and dosage set forth in this text are in accordance with current recommendations and practice at the time of publication. However, in view of ongoing research, changes in government regulations, and the constant flow of information relating to drug therapy and drug reactions, the reader is urged to check the package insert for each drug for any change in indications and dosage and for added warnings and precautions. This is particularly important when the recommended agent is a new or infrequently employed drug.

Materials appearing in this book prepared by individuals as part of their official duties as U.S. Government employees are not covered by the above-mentioned copyright.

9 8 7 6 5 4

This book is dedicated to . . .

. . . My mother, *Eremelina,* who at age 86 continues to be a role model for educated and successful women

. . . My husband *Bill,* a trusted partner who has shared my life for 30 years

. . . My son *Brian,* a teacher, philosopher and musician whose commitment to education and learning has enriched the lives of many

. . . My daughter *Susan,* my beautiful friend, a college student whose happy heart, passionate determination, and athletic talents have and will continue to shape the course of her life and those she touches

Preface

The *Study Guide to Brunner and Suddarth's Textbook of Medical-Surgical Nursing, Eleventh Edition,* was developed as a learning tool to help you, a nursing student, focus on content areas considered essential for understanding the concepts, techniques, and disease processes presented in the textbook. A Critical Thinking approach was used to present facts from a knowledge-based level (using multiple-choice, matching, fill-in and crossword puzzles) to the highest levels of analysis and synthesis (using comparison analysis, pattern identification, contradiction recognition, supportive argumentation, and critical analysis and discussion). The application of theory to practice is tested by having you complete nursing care plans, outline detailed patient teaching guides, and complete decision-making trees and critical clinical pathways. Case studies are offered at the end of most sections.

The answer to every question is presented in the Answer Key at the end of the book. Critical thinking, the nursing process, and a community-based focus to nursing care are incorporated throughout; information is tested from the viewpoint of nursing intervention. Some answers are derived from analysis and are implied. They may not be found specifically in the chapter. Pathophysiologic processes are included only if relevant to specific nursing actions.

It was my intent to present information in a manner that will stimulate critical thinking and promote learning. It is my hope that knowledge gained and reinforced will be used to provide competent nursing care to those in need.

Mary Jo Boyer, R.N., D.N.Sc.

Contents

CHAPTER 1

Health Care Delivery and Nursing Practice

I. Interpretation, Completion, and Comparison

MULTIPLE CHOICE

Read each question carefully. Circle your answer.

1. The definition of nursing has evolved over time. According to the American Nurses Association (ANA), registered nurses can and should:
   a. diagnose health alterations and prescribe specific nursing interventions.
   b. promote optimum levels of wellness and prevent illness.
   c. maintain health and assist patients with the dying process.
   d. do all of the above.

2. An underlying focus in any definition of nursing is the registered nurse's responsibility to:
   a. appraise and enhance an individual's health-seeking perspective.
   b. coordinate a patient's total health management with all disciplines.
   c. diagnose acute pathology.
   d. treat acute clinical reactions to chronic illness.

3. A Jewish patient who adheres to the dietary laws of his faith is in traction and confined to bed. He needs assistance with his evening meal of chicken, rice, beans, a roll, and a carton of milk. Choose the nursing approach that is most representative of promoting wellness.
   a. Nurse "A" removes items from the overbed table to make room for the dinner tray.
   b. Nurse "B" pushes the overbed table toward the bed so that it will be within the patient's reach when the dinner tray arrives.
   c. Nurse "C" asks a family member to assist the patient with the tray and the overbed table while the nurse straightens the area in an attempt to provide a pleasant atmosphere for eating.
   d. Nurse "D" prepares the environment and the overbed table and inspects the contents of the dinner tray. The nurse asks the patient whether he would like to make any substitutions in the foods and fluids he has received.

4. Using the concept of the wellness–illness continuum, a nursing care plan for a chronically ill patient would outline steps to:
   a. educate the patient about every possible complication associated with the specific illness.
   b. encourage positive health characteristics within the limits of the specific illness.
   c. limit all activities because of the progressive deterioration associated with all chronic illnesses.
   d. recommend activity beyond the scope of tolerance to prevent early deterioration.

5. To be responsive to the changing health care needs of our society, registered nurses will need to:

   a. focus their care on the traditional disease-oriented approach to patient care, because hospitalized patients today are more acutely ill than they were 10 years ago.

   b. learn how to delegate discharge planning to ancillary personnel so that RNs can spend their time managing the "high-tech" equipment needed for patient care.

   c. place increasing emphasis on wellness, health promotion, and self-care, because the majority of Americans today suffer from chronic debilitative illness.

   d. stress the curative aspects of illness, especially the acute, infectious disease processes.

6. The diagnosis-related groups (DRG) legislation enacted in 1983 provides for:

   a. a fixed rate of Medicare payment per diagnosis for hospital services.

   b. a retrospective method of reimbursement based on a patient's length of stay.

   c. all hospital and extended-care costs (such as nursing homes and home care) per diagnosis

   if the hospital participates with a peer review organization (PRO).

   d. total reimbursement per diagnosis for as long as the patient requires hospitalization (as long as the patient is eligible for Medicare benefits).

7. Quality assurance programs created in the 1980s required that hospitals be accountable for all of the following *except:*

   a. appropriateness of care related to established standards.

   b. cost of services.

   c. staff-patient ratios for nursing care.

   d. quality delivery of services.

8. The primary focus of the nurse advocacy role in managing a clinical pathway is:

   a. continuity of care.

   b. cost-containment practices.

   c. effective utilization of services.

   d. a patient's progress toward desired outcomes.

9. Nursing practice in the home and community requires competence and experience in the techniques of:

   a. decision making.

   b. health teaching.

   c. physical assessment.

   d. all of the above.

10. Certification for registered nursing practice is:

    a. mandatory for nurses working in specialty areas.

    b. offered by the state boards of nursing at the time a graduate writes for licensure.

    c. required in all states after a nurse has been practicing for 5 years.

    d. suggested by the ANA as a way of validating expertise in clinical practice.

SHORT ANSWER

Read each statement carefully. Write your response in the space provided.

According to the Social Policy Statement of the American Nurses Association (ANA) in 2003, nursing practice involves the diagnosis and treatment of human responses to health and illness.

1. List five phenomena of human responses that can be treated by nursing intervention. An example is given.
   Pain and discomfort (Example) _____

   _____

   _____

   _____

   _____

2. List four major health care concerns that are facing practitioners today in contrast to 10 to 20 years ago.

   _____

   _____

   _____

   _____

3. Choose four health problems and write a human response to each that would require nursing intervention. An example is given.

Health and Illness Problems	*Human Response Requiring Nursing Intervention*
Fractured right arm (Example)_____	Self-care limitations (Example)_____
_____	_____
_____	_____
_____	_____
_____	_____

4. According to Hood and Leddy (2003), wellness involves proactively working toward physical, psychological, and spiritual well-being. Four major concepts supporting wellness are:

   _____, _____,

   _____, and _____.

5. List Maslow's hierarchy of needs, and give an example for each need. The first need is provided as an example.

Need	*Example*
Physiologic (Example)_____	Food and Water (Example)_____
_____	_____
_____	_____
_____	_____
_____	_____
_____	_____

6. Health promotion efforts today target negative lifestyle behaviors such as:

_____	_____
_____	_____
_____	_____

7. Three infectious diseases that seem to be on the rise are: _____, _____ _____, and _____.

8. Define the term *clinical pathway* as it relates to the concept of managed care:

   _____

9. Explain when "care mapping" may be more beneficial than "clinical pathways" for managing care:

_____

_____

10. List five common features of managed care.

_____

_____

_____

_____

_____

11. Managed health care of the 1990s has contributed to: _____,
_____, _____, and _____.

12. List the purpose and goals of case management: _____

_____.

13. List three prominent roles for nurses.

_____

_____

_____

II. Critical Thinking Questions and Exercises

DISCUSSION AND ANALYSIS

Discuss the following topics with your classmates.

1. As of 2001, it became obvious that the United States was entering a decade that would be known as the worst nursing shortage in history. It is predicted that by the year 2010, there will be significantly fewer nurses than needed. Describe three factors that you believe have influenced the nursing shortage.
2. Analyze the benefits and challenges of implementing a primary nursing care approach to patient care.
3. Discuss the primary differences between community-based nursing and community-oriented/public health nursing.
4. Discuss the current and future role of the advanced practice nurse.

SUPPORTING ARGUMENTS

Read the paragraph below. Fill in the space provided with the best response.

Many recent changes in health care have significantly affected nursing care delivery and nursing education, including the aging population, increased cultural diversity, changing patterns of disease, the rising cost of health care, and federally legislated health care reform. Choose one factor that you believe has had the most impact on nursing care in the last 5 years, and support your argument with data.

The most important factor is: _____.

Supporting argument: _____

_____

_____

RECOGNIZING CONTRADICTIONS

Rewrite each statement correctly. Underline the key concepts.

1. The majority of health problems in the United States today are of an infectious and acute nature.

   _____

2. A person with a chronic illness can never attain a high level of wellness, because part of his or her health potential will never be reached.

   _____

3. The World Health Organization's definition of health is accurate, current, and comprehensive.

   _____

4. It is predicted that by the year 2030, people older than 65 years of age in the United States will constitute about 35% of the total population; racial and minority groups will constitute 60% of the population.

   _____

5. The Prospective Payment System legislation in 1983 created a tiered level of payment, per diagnosis (DRG), allowing hospitals to extend days of care to the most needy.

   _____

6. The main focus of continuous quality improvement (CQI) is on incidents and errors.

   _____

7. Health care costs average about 11% of the U.S. gross domestic product (GDP).

   _____

8. Home health care nursing is a major component of public health nursing.

   _____

EXAMINING ASSOCIATIONS

Answer the following.

1. Examine the progression of Maslow's hierarchy of needs in the accompanying figure. Consider a recent clinical situation. Explain symptoms your patient exhibited that reflect one or more of these needs.

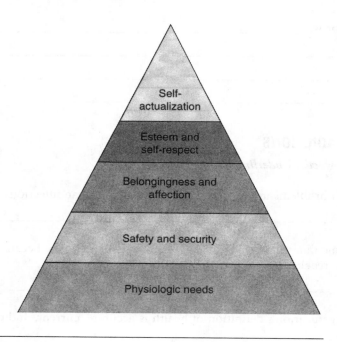

_____

_____

2. Using Figure 1-2 in the text, examine and explain the expected behaviors among the physician, patient, nurse, and ancillary personnel in the collaborative practice model.

_____

_____

CLINICAL SITUATIONS

Complete the following flow charts.

1. Kinsman (2004) affirms the value of clinical pathway mapping as a tool to effectively chart a patient's response to illness or injury. Complete this clinical pathway to illustrate how one lifestyle habit (smoking) can result in illness.

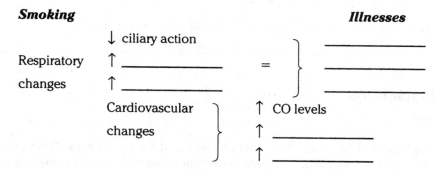

2. Continuous quality improvement (CQI) mandates the standardization of processes that are implemented and improved on a continuous basis. Complete the blank lines on the flow chart for the process of radial pulse assessment.

Radial Pulse Assessment

1.0	*2.0*	*3.0*	*4.0*	*5.0*
Patient ID	Explain Procedure	Identify Site	Palpate Pulse	Document Results

1.1 <u>ID Patient</u>
1.2 _____
   _____
1.3 _____
   _____

2.1 <u>Give instruction at level of patient's learning.</u>

3.1 <u>Extend patient's forearm</u>
3.2 _____
   _____
   _____
   _____

4.1 <u>Place pads of index and middle fingers over radial artery.</u>
4.2 _____
   _____
4.3 _____
   _____
   _____
   _____
4.4 _____
   _____
   _____

5.1 <u>Note rate and character.</u>
5.2 _____
   _____
   _____
5.3 _____
   _____
   _____

3. The Joint Commission on Accreditation of Healthcare Organizations (JCAHO) mandated in 1992 that health care organizations move toward implementation of CQI. Recent amendments to JCAHO standards affirmed the patient's right to quality care (Krozo & Scoggins, 2001) based on analysis of processes that affect patient care outcomes. A cause-and-effect diagram can illustrate potential causes of a process so that the cause can be examined and corrected and patient care improved. Complete the following diagram.

CQI Cause and Effect Diagram: Delayed Medication

Possible Causes

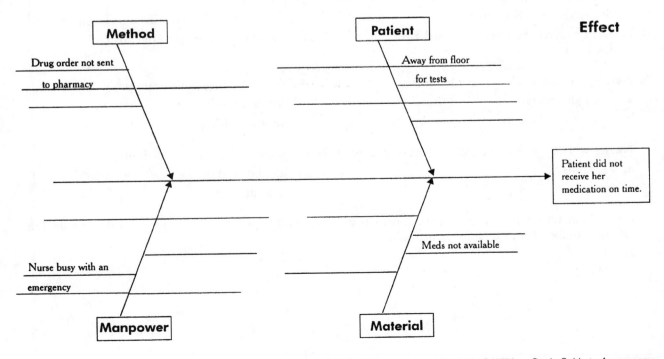

CHAPTER 2

Community-Based Nursing Practice

I. Interpretation, Completion, and Comparison

MULTIPLE CHOICE

Read each question carefully. Circle your answer.

1. The shift in health care delivery from acute care to community-based care is primarily the result of:
   a. alternative health care delivery systems.
   b. changes in federal legislation.
   c. tighter insurance regulations.
   d. the interfacing of all three conditions.

2. Choose an alternative health care delivery system that has dramatically reduced patient-care days in acute care settings.
   a. Health Maintenance Organizations
   b. Managed Health Care Systems
   c. Preferred Provider Organizations
   d. Each of the three is equally significant.

3. The most frequent users of home health services are:
   a. children with chronic, debilitating disorders.
   b. newborns who are sent home with apnea monitors.
   c. the frail and elderly who need skilled care.
   d. young adults on prolonged intravenous therapy.

4. Discharge planning from the hospital to home care begins when the:
   a. discharge order is written.
   b. nurse receives the physician's order for discharge.
   c. physician notifies the insurance company.
   d. patient is admitted to the hospital.

5. Nurses working in elementary schools are trained to deal with the leading health care problem of:
   a. eating disorders.
   b. emotional problems.
   c. infections.
   d. sports injuries.

6. Nurses working in high schools expect to deal with the common health care problem of:
   a. infections.
   b. cancer.
   c. alcohol and drug abuse.
   d. malnutrition.

7. It is estimated that, in any given year, approximately 3.5 million people in the United States are homeless. Of that number, about how many are children?
   a. 10%
   b. 30%
   c. 50%
   d. 60%

SHORT ANSWER

Read each statement carefully. Write your response in the space provided.

1. Name three chronic conditions that are increasing in prevalence and causing an increased need for community health services.

   _____

   _____

   _____

2. List four factors that have affected the shift of health care delivery from the hospital to the home.

   _____

   _____

   _____

   _____

3. List specific skills a nurse will need to function in community-based care: _____

   _____

4. Community-based nursing practice focuses on three primary goals:

   _____

   _____

   _____

5. List the four primary concepts supporting community-based nursing care:

   _____

   _____

   _____

   _____

6. List several examples of "skilled" nursing services provided by home care: _____

   _____

7. The first step in preparing for a home visit is for the nurse to: _____

   _____

8. Explain the purpose of the initial home visit: _____

   _____

9. List some examples of ambulatory health care settings: _____

   _____

10. The homeless have high rates of health care problems such as: _____

    _____

II. Critical Thinking Questions and Exercises

DISCUSSION AND ANALYSIS

Discuss the following topics with your classmates.

1. Explain the concept of "telehealth" and its implications for nursing care. Refer to the book, *Community and Public Health Nursing*, by Stanhope and Lancaster, 2004.
2. Distinguish among primary, secondary, and tertiary levels of preventive care and cite a clinical case example of each level.
3. Describe a common clinical care situation for a patient outside the hospital. Determine whether the role, responsibilities, and suggested scope of practice are within the realm of community-based nursing or community health nursing.

CLINICAL SITUATION

Read the following case study and assess the patients' need for a home visit.

Mrs. Flynn is an 85-year-old who suffered a stroke on December 28. She was admitted to the emergency room and suffered another stroke on December 30. The left occipital area and the cerebellum were affected, resulting in loss of 50% of vision (right half of each eye) and loss of balance. After 2 weeks in the hospital and 10 days in a rehabilitation treatment center, Mrs. Flynn will be discharged to her one-floor home where she lives alone. Her son and daughter both live an hour away. She is capable of walking with a walker. Before the stroke, Mrs. Flynn was independent, was an active member of several citizen groups, and participated in water walking at the YMCA three times a week. Her driver's license has been revoked. Using Chart 2-2, complete the outline to assess Mrs. Flynn's need for a home visit. Create your own answers to several of the questions so you can complete the assessment.

Current Health Status

1. How well is the patient progressing?
2. How serious are the present signs and symptoms?
3. Has the patient shown signs of progressing as expected, or does it seem that recovery will be delayed?

Home Environment

1. Are worrisome safety factors apparent?
2. Are family or friends available to provide care, or is the patient alone?

Level of Self-Care Ability

1. Is the patient capable of self-care?
2. What is the patient's level of independence?
3. Is the patient ambulatory or bedridden?
4. Does the patient have sufficient energy or is he or she frail and easily fatigued?

Level of Nursing Care Needed

1. What level of nursing care does the patient require?
2. Does the care require basic skills or more complex interventions?

Prognosis

1. What is the expectation for recovery in this particular instance?
2. What are the chances that complications may develop if nursing care is not provided?

Educational Needs

1. How well has the patient or family grasped the teaching points made?
2. Is there a need for further follow-up and retraining?
3. What level of proficiency does the patient or family show in carrying out the necessary care?

Mental Status

1. How alert is the patient?
2. Are there signs of confusion or thinking difficulties?

Level of Adherence

1. Is the patient following the instructions provided?
2. Does the patient seem capable of following the instructions?
3. Are the family members helpful, or are they unwilling or unable to assist in caring for the patient as expected?

CHAPTER 3

Critical Thinking, Ethical Decision Making, and the Nursing Process

I. Interpretation, Completion, and Comparison

MULTIPLE CHOICE

Read each question carefully. Circle your answer.

1. The least effective decision-making process used in critical thinking is:
   a. analyzing data.
   b. establishing assumptions.
   c. formulating conclusions.
   d. synthesizing information.

2. The term *metacognition* refers to the critical-thinking skill of:
   a. consultation.
   b. data analysis.
   c. self-reasoning.
   d. validation.

3. Morality is defined as:
   a. adherence to specific codes of conduct.
   b. commitment to informal, personal values.
   c. dependence on specified principles of behavior.
   d. an understanding of defined rules of behavior.

4. When an ethical decision is made based on the reasoning of the "greatest good for the greatest number," the nurse is following the:
   a. deontological theory.
   b. formalist theory.
   c. moral-justification theory.
   d. utilitarian theory.

5. Individual patient rights regarding freedom of choice and the right to privacy are subsumed under the ethical principal of:
   a. autonomy.
   b. beneficence.
   c. fidelity.
   d. paternalism.

6. Consider the ethical situation in which a nurse moves a confused, disruptive patient to a private room at the end of the hall so that other patients can rest, even though the confused patient becomes more agitated. The nurse's judgment is consistent with reasoning based on:
   a. "consequentialism," by which good consequences for the greatest number are maximized.
   b. "duty of obligation," by which an action, regardless of its results, is justified if the decision making was based on moral principles.
   c. "prima facie" duty, by which an action is justified if it does not conflict with a stronger duty.
   d. the "categorical imperative," by which the results of an action are deemed less important than the means to the end.

7. A hospital board of directors decided to close a pediatric burn treatment center (BTC) that annually admits 50 patients and to open a treatment center for terminally ill AIDS patients (with an expected annual admission of 200). This decision meant that the nearest BTC for children was 300 miles away. The board's decision was an example of ethical reasoning consistent with:

   a. a formalist approach.

   b. obligation or duty.

   c. "the means justifies the end."

   d. utilitarianism.

8. A terminally ill patient asks the nurse whether she is dying. The nurse's response is influenced by the moral obligation to:

   a. communicate the patient's wishes to the family.

   b. consult with the physician.

   c. provide correct information to the patient.

   d. consider all of the above measures before disclosing specific information.

9. A patient with a "Do Not Resuscitate" order requires large doses of a narcotic (which may significantly reduce respiratory function) for excruciating pain. After the patient requests pain medication, the nurse assesses a respiratory rate of 12 breaths/min. The nurse's ethical decision should be to:

   a. ask the patient to wait 20 minutes and reassess.

   b. give half of the prescribed dose.

   c. give the pain medication without fear of respiratory depression.

   d. withhold the pain medication and contact the physician.

10. Choose the situation that most accurately represents a moral problem in contrast to a moral dilemma.

    a. Three days after surgery, a patient requests narcotic pain medication every 3 hours. The nurse administers a placebo that reduces pain.

    b. A 32-year-old father of three with advanced cancer of the lungs asks that everything be done to prolong his life, even though his chemotherapy treatments are no longer effective.

    c. A confused 80-year-old needs restraints for protection from injury, even though the restraints increase agitation.

    d. A young patient with AIDS has asked not to receive tube feedings to prolong life because of intense pain.

11. Assessment begins with initial patient contact. Nursing activities during this component of the nursing process include:

    a. interviewing and obtaining a nursing history.

    b. observing for altered symptomatology.

    c. collecting and analyzing data.

    d. all of the above.

12. The end result of data analysis is:

    a. actualization of the plan of care.

    b. determination of the patient's responses to care.

    c. collection and analysis of data.

    d. identification of actual or potential health problems.

13. A therapeutic communication technique that validates what the nurse believes to be the main idea of an interaction is known as:

    a. acknowledgment.

    b. focusing.

    c. restating.

    d. summarizing.

14. An example of a medical diagnosis, in contrast to a nursing diagnosis, is:

    a. fever of unknown origin.

    b. fluid volume excess.

    c. risk for falls.

    d. sleep-pattern disturbances.

15. In choosing the nursing action that illustrates planned nursing care prioritized according to Maslow's hierarchy of needs, a nurse would:

    a. administer pain medication to an orthopedic patient 30 minutes before transportation to physical therapy for crutch-walking exercises.

    b. discourage a terminally ill patient from participating in a plan of care, to minimize fears about death.

    c. help a patient walk to the shower while the breakfast tray waits on the overbed table, because the shower area is vacant at this time.

    d. interrupt a family's visit with a depressed patient to assess blood pressure, because it is time to take the scheduled vital signs.

16. Consider the following nursing diagnosis: "Imbalanced nutrition, less than body requirements, related to inability to feed self." An example of an immediate nursing goal is that the patient will:

    a. acquire competence in managing cookware designed for handicapped people.

    b. assume independent responsibility for meeting self-nutrition needs.

    c. learn about food products that require minimal preparation yet meet individual needs for a balanced diet.

    d. master the use of special eating utensils to feed self.

17. Registered nurses are responsible for delegating patient care responsibilities to licensed practical nurses (LPNs) and ancillary personnel. The most appropriate task to delegate to a nurse aide is:

    a. assessing the degree of lower leg edema in a patient on bed rest.

    b. making the bed of an ambulatory patient.

    c. measuring the circumference of a patient's calf for edema.

    d. recording the size and appearance of a bed sore.

SHORT ANSWER

Read each statement carefully. Write your response in the space provided.

1. List 10 characteristics of critical thinkers as identified by Alfaro-Le Fevre (2003).

    _____
    _____
    _____
    _____
    _____
    _____
    _____
    _____
    _____
    _____

2. List six skills that are needed for critical thinking.

    _____
    _____
    _____
    _____
    _____
    _____

3. Explain this statement: How a nurse perceives a situation and employs critical thinking skills depends on the "lens" through which she sees the situation.

_____

4. Explain the term *moral distress:* _____

_____

5. Write the definition of nursing as proposed in the Nursing Social Policy Statement (ANA, 2003):

_____

_____

6. List two types of "advance directives," or legal documents that specify a patient's wishes before hospitalization.

_____

_____

7. Explain the merit of having an "advanced directive":

_____

_____

8. Suggest an opening statement that a nurse can use during the interview process: _____

_____

9. Discuss how formulation of a nursing diagnosis and identification of collaborative problems differs from making a medical diagnosis: _____

_____

10. Discuss the significance of establishing expected outcomes during the evaluation phase of the nursing process: _____

_____

NURSING OR COLLABORATIVE PROBLEM

Read each statement below. Put "N" in front of every nursing diagnosis and "C" in front of every collaborative problem.

1. _____ Anxiety related to impending surgery

2. _____ Constipation related to altered nutrition

3. _____ Potential complication: paralytic ileus secondary to postoperative inactivity

4. _____ Potential complication: sacral decubiti secondary to bed rest

5. _____ Risk for impaired skin integrity related to prolonged bed rest

6. _____ Ineffective breast-feeding related to fear of discomfort

7. _____ Potential complication: hypoglycemia related to inadequate food intake

8. _____ Potential complication: phlebitis related to intravenous therapy

9. _____ Risk for posttraumatic syndrome related to accident

10. _____ Potential complication: oral lesions related to chemotherapy

MATCHING

Match the critical-thinking strategy in column II with its associated nursing action listed in column I.

Column I

1. _____ Categorize information
2. _____ Design a plan of care
3. _____ Determine assessment processes
4. _____ Evaluate outcomes
5. _____ Implement a standard plan
6. _____ Make a nursing diagnosis
7. _____ Manage collaborative problems

Column II

a. Assert a practice role
b. Formulate a relationship
c. Generate a hypothesis
d. Provide an explanation
e. Recognize a pattern
f. Search for information
g. Set priorities

Match the definitions of ethical principles listed in column II with their associated terms listed in column I.

Column I

1. _____ Autonomy
2. _____ Beneficence
3. _____ Justice
4. _____ Nonmaleficence
5. _____ Paternalism
6. _____ Veracity

Column II

a. Limiting one's autonomy based on the welfare of another
b. Similar cases should be treated the same
c. The commitment to not deceive
d. Freedom of choice
e. The duty to do good and not inflict harm
f. The expectation that harm will not be done

II. Critical Thinking Questions and Exercises

DISCUSSION AND ANALYSIS

Discuss the following topics with your classmates.

Planning nursing care involves setting priorities and distinguishing problems that need urgent attention from those that can be deferred to a later time or referred to a physician. For each of the following patient care problems, circle the *initial priority of nursing care* from among the choices provided and write a rationale for your choice. Standardized interventions from the Nursing Interventions Classification (NIC) (Dochterman & Bulechek, 2004) may be used.

1. Activity intolerance, related to inadequate oxygenation
   a. dyspnea
   b. fatigue
   c. hypotension

Rationale for choice: _____

_____

2. Alterations in bowel elimination: constipation, related to prolonged bed rest
   a. abdominal pressure and bloating
   b. palpable impaction
   c. straining at stool

   Rationale for choice: _____

   _____

3. Altered oral mucous membrane, related to stomatitis
   a. erythema of oral mucosa
   b. intolerance to hot foods
   c. oral pain

   Rationale for choice: _____

   _____

RECOGNIZING CONTRADICTIONS

Rewrite each statement correctly. Underline the key concepts.

1. Nursing ethics is considered an applied form of medical ethics because nurses work only under physician direction.

   _____

2. A moral dilemma, in contrast to a moral problem, infers no conflict of moral principle.

   _____

3. A nurse experiences moral uncertainty when he or she is prevented from doing what he or she believes is the correct action.

   _____

4. A nurse should always honor a terminally ill patient's request to withhold food and hydration if the patient is competent.

   _____

5. By design, living wills are very prescriptive and are always honored as legally binding documents.

   _____

SUPPORTING ARGUMENTS

Read the paragraph below. Fill in the space provided with the best response.

1. In vitro fertilization, based on sophisticated technology, has resulted in women in their 50s and 60s giving birth. Physicians argue that this is ethically sound if the woman meets the criteria that she is healthy and should live another 25 years. List three rationales to support this argument.

   _____

   _____

   _____

2. You are asked to defend the statement that "life support measures should never be used for anyone with a terminal illness." Develop three supporting arguments.

   _____

   _____

   _____

3. List two rationales to support the argument that age should be used as a criterion for determining the allocation of health care resources.

   _____

   _____

CLINICAL SITUATIONS

Read each nursing diagnosis. Write a specific outcome.

The planning phase of the nursing process incorporates documented expected patient outcomes for specific nursing diagnoses (ND). Resources include the Nursing-Sensitive Outcomes Classification (NOC) (see Chart 3-8 in the text). Write one outcome that indicates an improvement for each diagnosis.

1. ND: Activity intolerance, related to dyspnea

Outcome: _____

2. ND: Impaired physical mobility, related to total hip replacement

Outcome: _____

3. ND: Fluid volume excess, related to compromised cardiac output

Outcome: _____

4. ND: Altered nutrition: less than body requirements, related to anorexia

Outcome: _____

5. ND: Sleep-pattern disturbance, related to pain

Outcome: _____

CASE STUDY: Ethical Analysis

Read the following case study. Fill in the blanks below.

You are an RN and a board member of American Red Cross Disaster Relief Services. When a smallpox epidemic erupted among thousands in Washington, D.C., as a result of terrorist activity, the board was asked by the Office of Homeland Security to allocate limited resources. The board decided that those with the greatest chance of survival and those working for the government would be treated. Those individuals with preexisting or terminal conditions would not be treated. The decision resulted in multiple deaths while preserving the lives of those most likely to survive. The framework for decision making followed the utilitarian approach.

Assessment

Write your response in the space provided.

1. List two possible conflicts between ethical principles and professional obligations.

    a. _____   b. _____

2. People involved in the decision:

    a. _____   c. _____

    b. _____

3. Those affected by the decision:

    a. _____   c. _____

    b. _____

Planning

1. Treatment options:

    a. _____   b. _____

2. Medical facts:

    a. _____   b. _____

3. Influencing information:

    a. _____   b. _____

4. Ethical/moral issues:

    a. _____   b. _____

5. Competing claims:

    a. _____   b. _____

Implementation

Compare the Utilitarian and the Deontological approaches.

Utilitarian	*Deontological*

1. Basis of ethical principles:

    a. _____   a. _____

    b. _____   b. _____

2. Predict consequences of actions:

    a. _____   a. _____

    b. _____   b. _____

3. Assign a positive or negative value to each consequence:

    a. _____   a. _____

    b. _____   b. _____

4. Choose the consequence, decision, or action that predicts the highest positive value:

    a. _____   a. _____

    b. _____   b. _____

Evaluation

Finish the following statements.

1. The best, morally correct action is to: _____

_____

2. This decision is based on the ethical reasoning that: _____

_____

3. The decision can be defended based on the following arguments:

    a. _____

    b. _____

    c. _____

CHAPTER 4

Health Education and Health Promotion

I. Interpretation, Completion, and Comparison

MULTIPLE CHOICE

Read each question carefully. Circle your answer.

1. Health education is:
   a. a primary nursing responsibility.
   b. an essential component of nursing care.
   c. an independent nursing function.
   d. consistent with all of the above.

2. Nursing responsibilities associated with patient teaching include:
   a. determining individual needs for teaching.
   b. motivating each person to learn.
   c. presenting information at the level of the learner.
   d. all of the above.

3. A nurse assesses that a patient is emotionally ready to learn when the patient:
   a. has accepted the therapeutic regimen.
   b. is motivated.
   c. recognizes the need to learn.
   d. demonstrates all of the above.

4. Nursing actions that can be used to motivate a patient to learn include all of the following except:
   a. feedback in the form of constructive encouragement when a person has been unsuccessful in the learning process.
   b. negative criticism when the patient is unsuccessful, so that inappropriate behavior patterns will not be learned.
   c. the creation of a positive atmosphere in which the patient is encouraged to express anxiety.
   d. the establishment of realistic learning goals based on individual needs.

5. Normal aging results in changes in cognition. Therefore, when teaching an elderly patient how to administer insulin, the nurse should:
   a. repeat the information frequently for reinforcement.
   b. present all the information at one time so that the patient is not confused by pieces of information.
   c. speed up the demonstration because the patient will tire easily.
   d. do all of the above.

6. The nurse reviews a medication administration calendar with an elderly patient. Being aware of sensory changes associated with aging, the nurse should:
   a. print directions in large, bold type, preferably using black ink.
   b. highlight or shade important dates and times with contrasting colors.
   c. use several different colors to emphasize special dates.
   d. do all of the above.

7. A nursing action that involves modifying a teaching program because a learner is not experientially ready is:

a. changing the wording in a teaching pamphlet so that a patient with a fourth-grade reading level can understand it.

b. contacting family members to assist in goal development to help stimulate motivation.

c. postponing a teaching session with a patient until pain has subsided.

d. all of the above.

8. A nurse identifies a patient's inability to pour a liquid medication into a measuring spoon. This diagnosis is part of the nursing process known as:

a. assessment.

b. planning.

c. implementation.

d. evaluation.

9. A nurse develops a program of increased ambulation for a patient with an orthopedic disorder. This goal setting is a component of the nursing process known as:

a. assessment.

b. planning.

c. implementation.

d. evaluation.

10. Outcome criteria are expressed as expected outcomes of patient behavior resulting from teaching strategies. An example is:

a. ability to climb a flight of stairs without experiencing difficulty in breathing.

b. altered lifestyle resulting from inadequate lung expansion.

c. inadequate ventilation associated with pulmonary congestion.

d. potential oxygenation deficit related to ventilatory insufficiency.

11. Identify the health promotion model that identifies why some people choose actions to foster health and others refuse to participate:

a. Health Belief Model

b. Resource Model of Preventive Health

c. Achieving Health for All Model

d. Social Learning Theory Model

SHORT ANSWER

Read each statement carefully. Write your response in the space provided.

1. List three significant factors for a nurse to consider when planning patient education:

_____

_____

_____

2. Explain why health education is so essential for those with chronic illness: _____

_____

3. Common examples of specific activities that promote and maintain health are:

_____, _____, _____,

_____, and _____.

4. Define the term *adherence* as it relates to a person's therapeutic regimen: _____

_____

5. Name several variables (factors) that influence a person's ability to adhere to a program of care:

_____

_____

_____

6. There is a positive correlation between behavioral changes from patient education and

_____, _____, and _____.

7. Describe the nature of the teaching–learning process: _____

_____

8. List at least six variables that make adherence to a therapeutic regimen difficult for the elderly.

_____

_____

_____

_____

_____

_____

9. Increased age affects cognition by decreasing: _____,

_____, and _____.

10. Discuss how learner readiness affects a learner and the learning situation: _____

_____

_____

11. Identify six teaching techniques that nurses frequently use:

_____

_____

_____

_____

_____

_____

12. Two major goals from the Healthy People 2010 report are:

_____ and _____.

13. Health promotion activities are grounded in four active processes:

_____, _____,

_____, and _____.

II. Critical Thinking Questions and Exercises

DISCUSSION AND ANALYSIS

Discuss the following topics with your classmates.

1. Using Table 4-1 in the text, design two teaching plans: one for a teenage diabetic who has an emotional disability and another for a 70-year-old stroke victim with a visual impairment.
2. Discuss the positive relationship between health and physical fitness. Explain at least five ways that exercise can promote health.

RECOGNIZING CONTRADICTIONS

Rewrite each statement correctly. Underline the key concepts.

1. Health education is a dependent function of nursing practice that requires physician approval.

   _____

2. The largest groups of people in need of health education today are children and those with infectious diseases.

   _____

3. Patients are encouraged to evidence compliance with their therapeutic regimen.

   _____

4. Evaluation, the final step in the teaching process, should be summative (done at the end of the teaching process).

   _____

5. Elderly persons rarely experience significant improvement from health promotion activities.

   _____

6. About 50% of elderly persons have one or more chronic illnesses.

   _____

EXAMINING ASSOCIATIONS

The health status of residents of the United States is a serious concern to individuals, health care practitioners, and health-promotion groups. A nation's health status can be measured by evaluating certain indicators. After reading *Healthy People 2010* (U.S. Department of Health and Human Services, 2000), complete the following chart. For each indicator listed, assign a rating score (1 = not relevant, 2 = important, 3 = very significant) reflecting the degree to which the indicator affects an individual's health, list the rationale for the score, and describe an activity to improve the score. The first row has been filled in as an example.

Indicator	Rating Score	Rationale	Improvement Strategy
Physical activity	3	Research has shown an increased percentage of inactivity among young adults over the last 10 years.	Increase time for physical activity in K–12 schools. Limit TV, video games, and computer time in the home.
Obesity			
Tobacco use			
Substance abuse			
Sexual behavior			
Mental illness			
Violent behavior			
Environmental pollution			
Lack of access to health care			

CHAPTER 5

Health Assessment

I. Interpretation, Completion, and Comparison

MULTIPLE CHOICE

Read each question carefully. Circle your answer.

1. The health history obtained by the nurse should focus on nursing's concern about:
   a. a comprehensive body systems review.
   b. current and past health problems.
   c. family history.
   d. all of the above.

2. A patient has certain rights concerning data collection, such as the right to know:
   a. how information will be used.
   b. that selected information will be held confidential.
   c. why information is sought.
   d. all of the above.

3. Open-ended questions help patients describe their chief complaint. Choose the sentence that is *not* an open-ended question.
   a. "Describe the pain."
   b. "Tell me more about your feelings."
   c. "How did the accident happen?"
   d. "Is the pain sharp and piercing?"

4. The single most important factor in helping the nurse and physician arrive at a diagnosis is the:
   a. family history.
   b. history of the present illness.
   c. past health history.
   d. results of the systems review.

5. Choose the best question an interviewer would use to obtain educational or occupational information.
   a. "Are you a blue-collar worker?"
   b. "Do you have difficulty meeting your financial commitments?"
   c. "Is your income more than $20,000 per year?"
   d. "What college did you attend?"

6. Which of the following is an *inappropriate* interviewer response to the patient statement, "I will not take pain medication when I am in pain"?
   a. "Is there another way you have learned to lessen pain when you experience it?"
   b. "Let a nurse know when you are in pain so you can be helped to decrease stimuli that may exaggerate your pain experience."
   c. "Refusing medication can only hurt you by increasing your awareness of the pain experience."
   d. "You have the right to make that decision. How can the nurses help you cope with your pain?"

7. All of the following are questions that will provide information about a person's lifestyle *except*:
   a. "Do you have any food preferences?"
   b. "Have you always lived in this geographic area?"
   c. "How many hours of sleep do you require each day?"
   d. "What type of exercise do you prefer?"

8. When obtaining a health history from an elderly patient, the nurse must remember to:
   a. ask questions slowly, directly, and in a voice loud enough to be heard by those who are hearing-impaired.
   b. clarify the frequency, severity, and history of signs and symptoms of the present illness.
   c. conduct the interview in a calm, unrushed manner using eye-to-eye contact.
   d. do all of the above.

9. On initial impression, the nurse assesses a patient's posture, stature, and body movements. This assessment is part of the physical examination process known as:
   a. auscultation.
   b. inspection.
   c. palpation.
   d. percussion.

10. An examiner needs to determine the upper border of a patient's liver. With the patient in the recumbent position, the examiner would percuss for a:
    a. dull sound.
    b. flat sound.
    c. resonant sound.
    d. tympanic sound.

11. During a physical examination, the nurse noted hyperresonance over inflated lung tissue in a patient with emphysema. The process used for this assessment was:
    a. auscultation.
    b. inspection.
    c. palpation.
    d. percussion.

12. A heart murmur was detected during a physical examination. The process used to obtain this information was:
    a. auscultation.
    b. inspection.
    c. palpation.
    d. percussion.

13. A waist circumference measurement can be useful in assessing excess abdominal fat. Women should try to maintain a waist circumference of how many inches to remain healthy?
    a. 30 to 34 inches
    b. 35 inches
    c. 36 to 38 inches
    d. 39 to 41 inches

14. A serum albumin level of 2.50 g/dL indicates:
    a. moderate depletion.
    b. low levels of serum protein.
    c. an acceptable amount of protein.
    d. an extremely high measurement of protein.

15. Several factors contribute to the altered nutritional status of the elderly. A primary nutritional nursing consideration during physical assessment is:
    a. altered metabolism and nutrient use secondary to an acute or chronic illness.
    b. decreased appetite related to loneliness.
    c. limited financial resources.
    d. the patient's ability to shop for and prepare food.

SHORT ANSWER

Read each statement carefully. Write your response in the space provided.

1. The role of the nurse in assessment includes two primary responsibilities:

_____

_____

2. Describe five basic guidelines that a nurse should use while conducting a health assessment:

   _____

   _____

   _____

   _____

   _____

3. Explain how mutual trust and confidence between the interviewer and the patient facilitate the communication process: _____

   _____

4. Define the term *chief complaint:* _____

   _____

5. A number of diseases of first- or second-order relatives are significant when a nurse takes a patient's family history. List six diseases that are considered significant.

   _____

   _____

   _____

   _____

   _____

   _____

6. When questioning a patient about lifestyle and health-related behaviors, the nurse should ask about

   _____, _____, _____,

   _____, and _____.

7. The three leading causes of death in the United States that are related in part to poor nutrition are:

   _____, _____, and _____.

8. The body mass index (BMI), a number based on a weight-to-height ratio, provides a quick reference to a person's nutritional status. A score of _____ is considered overweight; a score of _____ is considered obese; and a score greater than _____ is considered extremely obese. Those with a score lower than _____ are at risk for poor nutritional status.

9. In addition to BMI, waist circumference is an indication of weight problems. Men are at risk for obesity with a waist circumference of _____ inches; women at _____ inches.

10. Explain the concept of negative nitrogen balance: _____

    _____

11. Adolescent girls are particularly at risk for nutritional deficits in minerals, such as:

    _____, _____, and

    _____.

12. Which of the following assessments was most likely used to obtain the data for each statement below? Write the word on the line provided.

Inspection
Palpation
Percussion
Auscultation

a. _____ Asymmetry of movement is associated with a central nervous system disorder.

b. _____ Clubbing of the fingers is a diagnostic symptom of chronic pulmonary disorders.

c. _____ Tenderness is present in the area of the thyroid isthmus.

d. _____ Tactile fremitus is diagnostic of lung consolidation.

e. _____ Tympanic or drumlike sounds are produced by pneumothorax.

f. _____ The first heart sound is created by the simultaneous closure of the mitral and tricuspid valves.

g. _____ A friction rub is present with pericarditis.

h. _____ Nodules present with gout lie adjacent to the joint capsule.

MATCHING

Match the body area listed in column II with the descriptive sign of poor nutrition listed in column I.

Column I

1. _____ Atrophic papillae
2. _____ Brittle, dull, depigmented
3. _____ Cheilosis
4. _____ Flaccid, underdeveloped
5. _____ Fluorosis
6. _____ Xerophthalmia

Column II

a. Abdomen
b. Eyes
c. Hair
d. Lips
e. Muscles
f. Skeleton
g. Teeth
h. Tongue

II. Critical Thinking Questions and Exercises

CLINICAL SITUATIONS

Read the following case study. Fill in the blanks below.

CASE STUDY: Calculating a Healthy Diet

Mrs. Allred is a 40-year-old Hispanic woman, 5 feet 5 inches tall, with three children younger than 5 years of age. She weighs 175 lb. She had no known history of any physical illness before experiencing fatigue and irritability that she believed was the result of her parenting responsibilities. Mrs. Allred does not exercise regularly, eats snack foods while watching television with her children, and is too tired to prepare balanced meals for her family. She orders fast food or pizza for dinner at least three times a week.

Part I: Estimate ideal body weight

1. Calculate Mrs. Allred's frame size based on a wrist circumference of 16 cm.
   a. small frame   c. large frame
   b. medium frame

2. Mrs. Allred's ideal body weight (IBW) is _____ lb. Therefore, she needs to _____ (gain/lose) approximately _____ lb.
3. Her body mass index (BMI) is _____, which is considered _____ (ideal, overweight, obese).

Part II: Calculate a balanced diet for Mrs. Allred's ideal body weight, as determined in Part I. Use Chart 5-6 in the text as a guide.

1. Convert IBW in pounds to kilograms: _____
2. Determine basal energy needs (1 kcal/kg/hr): _____ calories
3. Increase activity by 40% (moderate activity): _____ calories
4. Divide calories into carbohydrates (50%) _____, fats (30%) _____, and proteins (20%) _____.
5. Estimate grams for carbohydrates _____, fats _____, and proteins _____.

Part III: Using the USDA's Food Pyramid Guide (Figure 5-7 in the text) design a 2000-calorie diet for Mrs. Allred.

1. The majority of calories should come from two food groups: _____ and _____.
2. The majority of grains should be composed of: _____
3. Mrs. Allred should be advised to eat about _____ of vegetables daily.
4. The least amount of calories should come from two food groups: _____ and _____.
5. Milk products should always be: _____.
6. Mrs. Allred should eat about _____ of fruit daily.

CHAPTER 6

Homeostasis, Stress, and Adaptation

I. Interpretation, Completion, and Comparison

MULTIPLE CHOICE

Read each question carefully. Circle your answer.

1. Stress is a change in the environment that is perceived as:
   a. challenging.
   b. damaging.
   c. threatening.
   d. having all of the above characteristics.

2. An individual's adaptation to stress is influenced by the stressor's:
   a. frequency and duration.
   b. number of occurrences and magnitude.
   c. sequencing (intermittent or enduring).
   d. combined characteristics as listed above.

3. An example of a functional, yet maladaptive, response of the body to a threat is:
   a. collateral circulation subsequent to diminished tissue perfusion.
   b. decreased cardiac output subsequent to cardiomegaly.
   c. increased pulmonary ventilation subsequent to increased levels of carbon dioxide.
   d. muscle atrophy subsequent to disuse.

4. Health promotion should be initiated before compensatory processes become maladaptive. Preventive nursing measures include all of the following *except*:
   a. demonstrating wound cleansing to a patient who has a necrotic leg ulcer resulting from vascular disease.
   b. showing a patient with a casted extremity how to perform isometric exercises.
   c. suggesting stress-reducing measures for a patient with a diagnosis of angina pectoris.
   d. teaching weight management to a patient who has a family history of obesity and a blood pressure reading of 125/90 mm Hg.

5. Maladaptive compensatory mechanisms result in disease processes in which cells may be:
   a. dead.
   b. diseased.
   c. injured.
   d. affected in all of the above ways.

6. Adaptation to a stressor is positively correlated with:
   a. previous coping mechanisms.
   b. the duration of the stressor.
   c. the severity of the stressor.
   d. all of the above.

7. During the initial stress response, primary appraisal refers to:
   a. evaluating the effectiveness of several coping mechanisms.
   b. organizing all available resources to deal with the stressor.
   c. identifying support services needed for coping.
   d. weighing the significance of the stressful event.

8. Helen, age 48, is diagnosed with pneumonia. She has been paralyzed from the chest down for 7 years. The nurse realizes that Helen needs additional support to cope with her infection because:

   a. coping measures become less effective with advancing age.

   b. the patient's available coping resources are already being used to manage the problems of immobility.

   c. an acute infectious process requires more adaptive mechanisms than a chronic stressor does.

   d. this additional physical stressor places unmanageable demands on the patient's internal and external resources.

9. Helen cooperates and willingly follows the treatment regimen. The nurse wonders how Helen can project such a positive outlook and cope with additional stress. Helen's ability to cope is probably due to all of the following *except:*

   a. acceptance that "life is not fair" and that people have limited control over their health.

   b. adoption of the problem-focused method of coping.

   c. her ability to draw on past coping behaviors and apply them to new situations.

   d. the support of family and friends who call and visit frequently

10. The neural and hormonal activities that respond to stress and maintain homeostasis are located in the:

   a. cerebral cortex.

   b. hypothalamus.

   c. medulla oblongata.

   d. pituitary gland.

11. Elizabeth is newly admitted to the medical unit. She has periodic episodes of shortness of breath and tightness in her throat. She is crying. To evaluate the impact of physiologic and psychological components on her illness, the nurse should:

   a. perform a thorough physical examination and include subjective patient statements as well as objective laboratory data.

   b. focus primary attention on the respiratory system, because this is the patient's chief complaint.

   c. determine that the patient is not in acute distress, and then perform a complete physical examination and include data about the patient's lifestyle and social relationships.

   d. attempt to discover the reasons behind the patient's anxieties, because stress can cause breathing difficulties.

12. During the nursing interview, a patient with shortness of breath reveals that she is in the process of getting a divorce. This information alerts the nurse to initially:

   a. try to determine whether there is a psychological basis for the patient's physical symptoms.

   b. restrict family members from visiting, because their presence may aggravate the patient's symptoms.

   c. teach the patient specific breathing exercises that can be used to manage symptoms.

   d. request that the physician recommend counseling services.

13. A patient is admitted to the emergency department for observation after a minor automobile accident. Based on an understanding of the sympathetic nervous system's response to stress, the nurse would expect to find all of the following during assessment *except:*

   a. cold, clammy skin.

   b. decreased heart rate.

   c. rapid respirations.

   d. skeletal muscle tension.

14. Physiologically, the sympathetic-adrenal-medullary response results in all of the following *except:*

   a. decreased blood flow to the abdominal viscera.

   b. decreased peripheral vasoconstriction.

   c. increased myocardial contractility.

   d. increased secretion of serum glucose.

15. The hypothalamic-pituitary response is a long-acting physiologic response to stress that involves:

a. stimulation of the anterior pituitary to produce adrenocorticotropic hormone (ACTH).

b. the production of cortisol from the adrenal cortex.

c. protein catabolism and gluconeogenesis.

d. all of the above mechanisms.

16. An example of a negative feedback process is increased:

a. aldosterone secretion in burn trauma, resulting in excess sodium retention.

b. cardiac output in hemorrhage, resulting in increased blood loss.

c. secretion of antidiuretic hormone (ADH) in congestive heart failure, causing increased fluid retention.

d. secretion of thyroid-stimulating factor (TSF), which stops when circulating thyroxin levels reach normal.

17. A patient experiences lower leg pain associated with lactic acid accumulation (an example of a local response involving a feedback loop). The nurse expects the pain to lessen after:

a. aerobic metabolism is reinstated.

b. anaerobic metabolism becomes the major pathway for energy release.

c. muscle use and subsequent glucose catabolism increase.

d. vasoconstriction diminishes blood flow, thereby slowing the removal of waste products.

18. A patient has a diagnosis of hypertrophy of the heart muscle (an example of cellular adaptation to injury). The nurse expects all of the following *except*:

a. compromised cardiac output.

b. muscle mass changes evident on radiologic examinations.

c. cellular alteration compensatory to some stimulus.

d. decreased cell size, leading to more effective ventricular contractions.

19. Breast changes in a pregnant woman are an example of cellular adaptation to stress known as:

a. dysplasia.

b. hyperplasia.

c. hypertrophy.

d. metaplasia.

20. Cell injury results when stressors interfere with the body's optimal balance by altering cellular ability to:

a. grow and reproduce.

b. synthesize enzymes.

c. transform energy.

d. do all of the above.

21. An adult patient's hemoglobin is 7g/dL. This should alert the nurse to assess for signs and symptoms associated with:

a. hyperemia.

b. hypertension.

c. hypoglycemia.

d. hypoxia.

22. A diabetic is admitted to the hospital with a blood sugar level of 320 mg/dL. The nurse decides to monitor fluid intake and output because:

a. decreased blood osmolarity causes fluid to shift into the interstitial spaces, resulting in polydipsia.

b. polydipsia occurs when glucose catabolism is accelerated, thereby increasing the body's need for fluids.

c. polyuria results from osmotic diuresis, which is compensatory to hyperglycemia.

d. the blood's hypotonicity will result in tissue fluid retention and weight gain.

23. Nursing care for a patient with a fever is based on all of the following body responses *except*:
    a. diaphoresis, which is a compensatory mechanism that cools the body.
    b. increased heart rate, which helps to meet increased metabolic demands.
    c. increased nutrient catabolism, which influences the body's caloric needs.
    d. vasodilation of surface blood vessels, which prevents excessive heat loss.

24. Anti-infective drugs are not useful against biologic agents known as:
    a. bacteria.
    b. fungi.
    c. mycoplasmas.
    d. viruses.

25. Viruses are infectious agents that:
    a. burst out of invaded cells to enter other cells.
    b. infect specific cells.
    c. replicate within invaded cells.
    d. do all of the above.

26. Genetic disorders arising from inherited traits include all of the following *except*:
    a. hemophilia.
    b. meningitis.
    c. phenylketonuria
    d. sickle cell anemia.

27. A nurse who is caring for a patient with a localized response to a bee sting expects symptoms to include all of the following *except*:
    a. blanching due to compensatory vasoconstriction.
    b. hyperemia due to increased blood flow.
    c. pain due to pressure on the nerve endings.
    d. swelling due to increased vascular permeability.

28. While caring for a patient with an infected surgical incision, the nurse observes for signs of a systemic response. These include all of the following *except*:
    a. leukopenia owing to increased white blood cell production.
    b. a febrile state caused by the release of pyrogens.
    c. anorexia, malaise, and weakness.
    d. loss of appetite and complaints of aching.

29. Research has shown that the single most important factor influencing an individual's health is:
    a. health insurance coverage.
    b. income.
    c. level of education.
    d. social relationships.

30. Nursing assessment to determine individual social support systems includes obtaining information about the person's:
    a. belief that he or she belongs to a group that is mutually dependent and communicative.
    b. concept of being cared for and loved.
    c. impression of being esteemed and valued.
    d. perception of all of the above.

31. Mrs. Talbot is scheduled for a breast biopsy in the morning. There is a history of breast malignancy in her family. While caring for her on the evening before surgery, the most appropriate nursing action would be to:
    a. administer a soothing back massage to promote relaxation and decrease stress.
    b. make sure she eats all of her evening meal, because she will be NPO after midnight.
    c. minimize the emotional impact of surgery by encouraging her to socialize with other patients.
    d. sit with her and provide an opportunity for her to talk about her concerns.

MATCHING

Match the primary category of stressors listed in column II with its associated stressors listed in column I.

Column I

1. _____ Anxieties

2. _____ Genetic disorders

3. _____ Hypoxia

4. _____ Infectious agents

5. _____ Life changes

6. _____ Nutritional imbalance

7. _____ Social relationships

8. _____ Trauma

Column II

a. Physiologic

b. Psychosocial

SHORT ANSWER

Read each statement carefully. Write your response in the space provided.

1. List the four concepts that are key to understanding a steady state of balance:

   _____

   _____

   _____

   _____

2. Define a maladaptive response to a stressor:

   _____

   _____

3. Explain why hyperpnea, after intense exercise, is considered an adaptive response to a physiologic stressor:

   _____

   _____

4. Give an example of an acute, time-limited stressor versus a chronic, enduring stressor:

   _____

5. Psychosocial stressors are classified as day-to-day occurrences (daily hassles), major events that affect large groups, and those infrequently occurring situations that directly affect a person. List two examples from your personal experiences that could be included under each classification.

   a. Day-to-day occurrences:

   _____

   _____

   b. Major events that affect large groups of people

   _____

   _____

c. Infrequently occurring major stressors

_____

_____

6. Discuss the linkage between illness and critical life events: _____

_____

7. Discuss how internal cognitive processes and external resources are used by an individual to manage stress:_____

_____

8. Define stress according to Hans Selye: _____

_____

9. List five bodily functions that are regulated by negative feedback mechanisms:

_____

_____

_____

_____

_____

10. List the five cardinal signs of inflammation:

_____

_____

_____

_____

_____

11. List four possible nursing diagnoses for individuals suffering from stress:

_____

_____

_____

_____

II. Critical Thinking Questions and Exercises

DISCUSSION AND ANALYSIS

Discuss the following topics with your classmates.

1. Compare and contrast the three historical theories of balance and a steady state according to Claude Bernard, Walter Cannon, and René Dubos.
2. Distinguish between physical, physiologic, and psychosocial stressors. Cite an example for each and explain how you were able to adapt or not adapt to the stressor.

3. Compare and contrast the stress impact you have felt during a day-to-day stressor (e.g., traffic jam, argument with parent) with the stress experienced around a major life event (e.g., marriage, retirement).
4. Discuss the correlation between stress and illness and recent life events/stressors as proposed by Holmes and Rahe (1967).
5. Discuss the cognitive process and emotional responses that you would experience in appraising a stressful event. Mention the steps involved in primary appraisal, secondary appraisal, and reappraisal.
6. Explain Hans Selye's Theory of Adaptation, both general and local.

CLINICAL SITUATIONS

Complete the flow chart. Fill in the physiologic reactions of the body that represent the sympathetic-adrenal-medullary response to stress. Provide the rationale for each reaction.

General body arousal	*Physiologic Reaction*	*Rationale*
↑ Norepinephrine and epinephrine	↑ _____	↑ _____
	↑ _____	↑ _____
	↑ _____	↑ _____
	↑ _____	↑ _____
Effects on:		
Skeletal muscles	_____	↑ _____
Pupils	_____	_____
Ventilation	_____	_____

CASE STUDY: Hypertensive Heart Disease

Read the following case study. Fill in the blanks below.

The body is capable of integrated responses to stress mediated by the sympathetic nervous system and the hypothalamic-pituitary-adrenocortical axis (see Fig. 6–2). Use the clinical diagnosis of hypertensive heart disease as an example of the body's response to stress.

Renin secretion is compensatory to decreased renal blood flow. Renin indirectly leads to sodium and water retention by stimulating the release of aldosterone. This mechanism initially results in increased cardiac output. For the compensatory mechanism shown, list nursing implications (assessment, nursing diagnoses/collaborative problems, planning, implementation, and evaluation) and give a rationale.

Selected Compensatory Mechanisms	**Nursing Implications**	**Rationale**
Renal blood flow is decreased as a result of hypertensive heart disease.	Assessment _____ _____ _____	_____ _____ _____
	Nursing Diagnoses _____ _____	_____ _____
	Collaborative Problems _____ _____	_____ _____
	Planning _____ Implementation _____ Evaluation _____	_____ _____ _____

IDENTIFYING PATTERNS

The sympathetic-adrenal-medullary response and the hypothalamic-pituitary response to stressors are adaptive and protective mechanisms that maintain homeostasis in the body. Based on the information provided in the text, please complete the following flow chart. The ovals represent the beginning of the process. Fill in the rectangles, as appropriate, with the steps in the process. Fill in the triangles with the physiologic end responses. Use Figure 6-2 in the text as a guide.

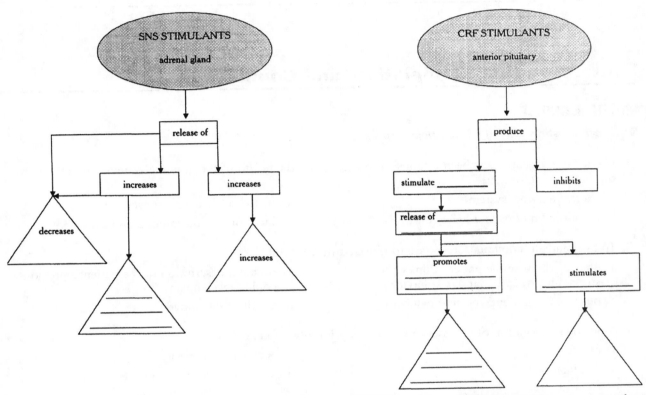

Legend: A ⬭ represents the beginning of the process, a ▭ represents the steps in the process, and a △ represents the physiologic end responses.

CHAPTER 7

Individual and Family Considerations Related to Illness

I. Interpretation, Completion, and Comparison

MULTIPLE CHOICE

Read each question carefully. Circle your answer.

1. Compelling research has been established to show that the health of the immune system is correlated to the functioning of the:
   a. central nervous system.
   b. emotional moods and behavior.
   c. neuroendocrine responses.
   d. interconnections among all of the above.

2. To examine an individual's response to illness, a nurse should:
   a. analyze the way the patient thinks about stress, illness, and adaptive behavior.
   b. observe the patient's present behavior.
   c. obtain a description of the patient's previous coping mechanisms
   d. do all of the above.

3. A person's perception of illness as a stressor is primarily influenced by:
   a. finances.
   b. intelligence.
   c. occupational status.
   d. previous coping experiences.

4. The basic system disturbance believed to be responsible for the symptoms of posttraumatic stress disorder (PTSD) is in the:
   a. cardiopulmonary system.
   b. neurologic system.
   c. renal system.
   d. respiratory system.

5. The incidence of PTSD in high-risk groups is approximately:
   a. 10% to 15%.
   b. 30%.
   c. 50%.
   d. 75% or greater.

6. In the United States, approximately what percentage of clinically depressed individuals commit suicide?
   a. 5%
   b. 15%
   c. 25%
   d. 40%

7. Which of the following is not considered a risk for suicide?
   a. altered body image.
   b. family history.
   c. female gender.
   d. age 25 to 35 years.

8. It took Mr. A 3 months to admit that he was sick and in need of medical and nursing care and to accept his diagnosis of adenocarcinoma of the right kidney. An initial emotional response the nurse would expect to see associated with loss and grief is:

   a. shame.

   b. denial.

   c. guilt and shame.

   d. regression.

9. Nursing interventions to help a patient deal with denial include:

   a. allowing the patient to use denial when it serves an immediate purpose and is not harmful.

   b. challenging the patient's use of denial as a defense mechanism.

   c. encouraging the use of denial as a satisfactory method of dealing with illness.

   d. supporting the denial behavior, knowing that the patient needs this coping mechanism.

10. A communication breakdown will most probably occur if a nurse:

    a. anticipates barriers to communication and works out solutions in advance.

    b. clarifies facts about an illness with the patient during the patient's denial of that illness.

    c. plans a teaching session for a time when the patient is free from pain.

    d. presents a teaching program when the patient demonstrates a readiness to learn.

11. Mrs. Renton is hospitalized in the final stage of metastatic carcinoma. She tells her physician that she will accept her prognosis if he can keep her alive until her grandchild is born in 3 months. Mrs. Renton is in that stage of dying identified by Kubler-Ross as:

    a. isolation.

    b. anger.

    c. bargaining.

    d. depression.

SHORT ANSWER

Read each statement carefully. Write your response in the space provided.

1. It is estimated that approximately _____ percent of consumers in the United States follow holistic health practices.

2. Write the most commonly accepted definition of a mental disorder:

   _____

3. List the five major family functions described by Wright and Leahy (2000) that significantly influence an individual's response to illness.

   _____

   _____

   _____

   _____

   _____

4. Record seven traits identified by Burr and associates (1994) that enhance coping of family members under stress.

   _____

   _____

   _____

_____

_____

_____

_____

5. Identify five common emotional responses to posttraumatic stress disorder (PTSD).

_____

_____

_____

_____

_____

6. Three physiologic responses to PTSD are increased _____,
   _____, and _____.

7. List seven life events that are known to trigger symptoms of PTSD:

_____

_____

_____

_____

_____

_____

_____

8. List two criteria that distinguish clinical depression from everyday sadness:

_____

_____

9. The seven leading somatic complaints of individuals struggling with depression are:

_____

_____

_____

_____

_____

_____

_____

10. List two common substance abuse problems:

_____

_____

MATCHING

Match the classification of a complementary and alternative therapy listed in column II with a specific type of holistic care listed in column I.

Column I

1. _____ Hypnosis
2. _____ Reiki
3. _____ Acupuncture
4. _____ Chiropractic
5. _____ Dietary plans
6. _____ Ayurveda
7. _____ Therapeutic Touch
8. _____ Homeopathic medicine
9. _____ Dance and music
10. _____ Qi gong

Column II

a. Alternative medical systems
b. Biologically based systems
c. Energy therapies
d. Manipulative methods
e. Mind-body interventions

II. Critical Thinking Questions and Exercises

DISCUSSION AND ANALYSIS

Discuss the following topics with your classmates.

1. Compare and contrast the characteristics associated with mental health (Chart 7-3) to those characteristics associated with mental disorders (Chart 7- 4).

RECOGNIZING CONTRADICTIONS

Rewrite each statement correctly. Underline the key concepts.

1. Since 1980, there has been a gradual decline in the number of individuals who seek holistic health care treatment.

_____

2. The philosophical framework supporting holistic health care is emphasis on the spiritual domain of healing.

_____

3. Clinical depression is a common response to health problems, especially for the young and the elderly.

_____

4. The majority of people who commit suicide are depressed, isolated from friends, and have not sought personal or professional help.

_____

5. A diagnosis of clinical depression requires repeated episodes of sadness over a 4-week period.

_____

CLINICAL SITUATIONS

Read the following case studies. Circle the correct answer.

CASE STUDY: Hodgkin's Disease

Joan, a 29-year-old mother of two, works 20 hours a week as a secretary. She was diagnosed with Hodgkin's disease the week of her 29th birthday.

1. Joan's reaction to the diagnosis was to increase her working time to 40 hours per week and to increase her social activities. Joan's response is characteristic of the:
   a. first stage of illness.
   b. second stage of illness.
   c. third stage of illness.
   d. fourth stage of illness.

2. The most prominent emotion the nurse would expect Joan to experience at the time of her diagnosis is:
   a. acceptance.
   b. denial.
   c. depression.
   d. guilt.

3. Nursing intervention at the time of the diagnosis would *not* include:
   a. answering questions.
   b. listening to the patient ventilate.
   c. reinforcing reality.
   d. supporting denial.

CASE STUDY: Radical Mastectomy

Kathy, a 45-year-old, single executive with a major oil company, lives alone in a high-rise city apartment. She is recovering from a right radical mastectomy performed 3 days ago.

1. Kathy is firm about not bathing in the morning, because her normal home routine involves a nightly relaxing tub bath. The nurse should:
   a. document in the plan of care that bathing is to take place near bedtime.
   b. explain the clinical routine to Kathy to help her understand the necessity for each patient to comply so that all patients will receive optimum care.
   c. gently remind Kathy that she is not in control in a hospital; the nurses decide when baths will be taken.
   d. give Kathy a choice of morning bath care or evening shower care, because staffing on the evening shift is not sufficient to meet her needs.

2. Kathy refuses to acknowledge that her breast was removed. She believes that her breast is intact under the dressings. The nurse should:
   a. call the physician to change the dressings so that Kathy can see the incision.
   b. recognize that Kathy is experiencing denial, a normal stage of the grieving process.
   c. reinforce Kathy's belief for several days, until her body can adjust to the stress of surgery.
   d. remind Kathy that she needs to accept her diagnosis so that she can begin rehabilitation exercises.

3. Kathy screams at her nurse because the nurse is 10 minutes late administering Kathy's pain medication. The nurse is aware that anger:

   a. is a maladaptive response to a stressful situation.

   b. is an anticipated reaction to a change in body appearance.

   c. should be reinforced to help reality orientation.

   d. should be repressed so that Kathy can gain control of her surroundings.

4. To help Kathy adjust to her altered body image, the nurse should:

   a. offer acceptance.

   b. reinforce Kathy's concept of self-worth.

   c. understand Kathy's emotional responses to her illness and her surgery.

   d. all of the above.

CHAPTER 8

Perspectives in Transcultural Nursing

I. Interpretation, Completion, and Comparison

MULTIPLE CHOICE

Read each question carefully. Circle your answer.

1. Choose the minority group in the United States that is *not* federally recognized as a minority.
   a. Asian/Pacific Islanders
   b. Hispanic Americans
   c. Native Americans
   d. Islamic

2. The most common non-English language spoken in the United States is:
   a. German.
   b. French.
   c. Italian.
   d. Spanish.

3. Madeline Leininger's theory of transcultural nursing supports providing care that:
   a. allows for restructuring.
   b. can be accommodated.
   c. is congruent.
   d. reflects all of the above characteristics.

4. Personal space is a culturally defined phenomenon. In comparing cultures, individuals who require the *most* personal space between themselves and others would be from:
   a. Japan.
   b. Latin America.
   c. the Middle East.
   d. the United States.

5. Choose the culture that does *not* consider eye contact to be impolite when speaking with another person.
   a. American
   b. Arabian
   c. Indo-Chinese
   d. Native American

6. The cultural group in which staring at the floor during conversation is considered behavior conveying respect is the:
   a. Asian.
   b. Appalachian.
   c. Indo-Chinese.
   d. Native American.

7. The cultural group that maintains downcast eyes as a sign of appropriate deferential behavior toward others is the:
   a. Asian.
   b. Hispanic.
   c. Indo-Chinese.
   d. Native American.

8. The cultural group that has a wide frame of reference for attitudes about time is the:
   a. Hispanic.
   b. Arabian.
   c. Native American.
   d. Asian.

9. The nurse would expect that a woman from which of the following cultures would want only a female physician to examine her?
   a. Arabian
   b. Asian
   c. Japanese
   d. Latin American

10. For many in this cultural group, it is impolite to touch a person's head.
    a. Asian American
    b. Arabian
    c. Hispanic
    d. Japanese

11. Choose the religious group that shuns the use of caffeine-containing beverages.
    a. Hindu
    b. Jewish
    c. Mormon
    d. Seventh Day Adventist

12. It is estimated that approximately what percentage of adults in the United States use alternative medicine?
    a. 15%
    b. 25%
    c. 35%
    d. 60%

13. The yin-yang theory of harmony and illness is rooted in which paradigm of health and illness?
    a. Biomedical
    b. Holistic
    c. Religious
    d. Scientific

SHORT ANSWER

Read each statement carefully. Write your response in the space provided.

1. The founder of transcultural nursing is _____.

2. Name the four basic characteristics of culture.

   _____

   _____

   _____

   _____

3. Three elements frequently used to identify diversity are: _____,

   _____, and _____.

4. List four examples of American subcultures based on ethnicity:

   _____

   _____

   _____

   _____

5. Give at least five examples of other groupings that can be used to identity subcultures.

   _____

   _____

   _____

   _____

   _____

6. The two underlying goals of transcultural nursing are to provide _____ and
   _____ care.

7. Explain the concept of culturally competent and congruent nursing care: _____
   _____

8. List four strategies that individuals tend to use when communication has broken down.

   _____

   _____

   _____

   _____

9. Name four religious groups that routinely incorporate fasting into the religious practice.

   _____

   _____

   _____

   _____

10. Explain the concept of yin-yang: _____
    _____

II. Critical Thinking Questions and Exercises

DISCUSSION AND ANALYSIS

Discuss the following topics with your classmates.

1. Explain the goal of Madeleine Leininger's comprehensive research-based theory called "Culture Care Diversity and Universality."
2. Explain the concepts of culture care accommodation and culture care restructuring, according to Leininger's theory.
3. Distinguish between the terms *acculturation* and *cultural imposition*.
4. Explain the meaning of the term *general polymorphism*.
5. Distinguish between the five major categories of alternative medical interventions: alternative medical systems, mind-body interventions, biologically based therapies, manipulative and body-based methods, and energy therapies.

CHAPTER 9

Genetics Perspectives in Nursing

I. Interpretation, Completion, and Comparison

MULTIPLE CHOICE

Read each question carefully. Circle your answer.

1. The study of gene mapping and function is known as:
   a. genetics.
   b. genomics.
   c. meiosis.
   d. mitosis.

2. Chromosomes are located within the nucleus of a cell. The human body has how many chromosomes?
   a. 23
   b. 46
   c. 69
   d. 92

3. Gene mutations have significant implications for health and illness. A mutation in protein structure that alters the configuration of hemoglobin is known as:
   a. fragile X syndrome.
   b. Huntington's disease.
   c. muscular dystrophy.
   d. sickle cell anemia.

4. Trisomy refers to a condition in which cellular division results in an extra chromosome. An example of trisomy is:
   a. Down syndrome.
   b. sickle cell anemia.
   c. Tay-Sachs disease.
   d. Turner's syndrome.

5. Stephanie has learned that her ovarian cancer syndrome is an autosomal dominant inherited condition. Stephanie knows that her daughter has what chance of inheriting the gene mutation for this disease?
   a. 10% to 15%
   b. 25%
   c. 50%
   d. 60% to 80%

6. An example of an autosomal recessive inherited condition is:
   a. cystic fibrosis.
   b. hereditary breast cancer.
   c. Huntington's disease.
   d. familial hypercholesterolemia.

7. In autosomal recessive inheritance, each parent is a carrier and children have a 25% chance of inheriting the gene. All of the following are examples of autosomal recessive inheritance *except*:
   a. cystic fibrosis.
   b. Marfan's syndrome.
   c. phenylketonuria.
   d. sickle cell anemia.

8. An example of an X-linked, recessive inherited condition, in which a mother (carrier) has a 50% chance of passing the gene on to her son, is:

   a. cystic fibrosis.

   b. hemophilia.

   c. phenylketonuria.

   d. Tay-Sachs disease.

9. Katie has just been told that she has the *BRCA1* hereditary breast cancer gene mutation. At age 32, she knows that her risk of developing cancer by the age of 65 years is as high as:

   a. 25%.

   b. 50%.

   c. 80%.

   d. 100%.

10. Kurt and Kathy are carriers for thalassemia. They are thinking about starting a family. A nurse tells them that their risk of having a child who will inherit the gene is:

    a. 25%.

    b. 50%.

    c. 75%.

    d. 100%.

11. A multifactorial genetic condition that tends to cluster in families is:

    a. galactosemia.

    b. Duchenne muscular dystrophy.

    c. neurofibromatosis.

    d. neural tube defects.

12. When assessing patient information as part of genetic counseling, the nurse knows that Tay-Sachs disease is most common among:

    a. Ashkenazi Jews.

    b. Italian Americans.

    c. American Indians.

    d. African Americans.

SHORT ANSWER

Read each statement carefully. Write your response in the space provided.

1. The term *genomic medicine* refers to: _____

   _____

2. The nurse uses a framework for integrating genetics into nursing practice when he or she:

   _____, _____,

   _____, and _____.

3. A person's individual genetic makeup (composed of 30,000 to 40,000 genes) is called a _____ ; the person's set of characteristics of physical appearance and other traits is called a _____.

4. Genes are working subunits of DNA. Genes are arranged in linear order within _____. Twenty-two pairs of chromosomes, also called _____, are the same in males and females. The 23rd pair, the _____, is composed of two _____ for the female and _____ for the male. At conception, the sex of a child is determined because each parent gives _____.

5. Cite several examples of multifactorial inherited conditions:

   _____

   _____

   _____

   _____

6. The common chromosomal condition that occurs with greater frequency in pregnancies of women who are 35 years of age or older is _____.

7. The frequency of chromosomal abnormalities in newborns is _____, and chromosomal abnormalities account for _____ percent of all spontaneous first-trimester pregnancy losses.

8. Define the term *pharmacogenetics*: _____

_____

9. The most common adult-onset genetic condition in the Caucasian population is:

_____.

10. List five nursing activities in genetics-related nursing practice:

_____

_____

_____

_____

_____

MATCHING

Match the genetic term listed in column II with its specific definition listed in column I.

Column I

1. _____ The number of chromosomes normally present in humans ($N = 46$)

2. _____ The presence of one extra chromosome (e.g., Down syndrome)

3. _____ The genes and variations that a person inherits from his or her parents

4. _____ A single chromosome from any of the 22 pairs not involved in sex determination (i.e., not XX or XY)

5. _____ A person's entire physiologic and biologic makeup as determined by genotype and environment

6. _____ Primary genetic material (DNA)

7. _____ A heterozygous person who carries two different alleles of a gene pair

8. _____ The microscopic cell nucleus that contains genetic information

Column II

a. Autosome

b. Carrier

c. Chromosome

d. Deoxyribonucleic acid

e. Diploid

f. Genotype

g. Phenotype

h. Trisomy

Match the age of adult onset in column II with the specific disorder listed in column I.

Column I

1. _____ Spinocerebellar ataxia, type 2

2. _____ Huntington's disease

3. _____ Early-onset familial Alzheimer's disease

4. _____ Hereditary hemochromatosis

5. _____ Spinocerebellar ataxia, type 3

6. _____ Polycystic kidney disease

7. _____ Familial hypercholesterolemia

8. _____ Amyotrophic lateral sclerosis (ALS)

Column II

a. Mean age of 30 years

b. 30 to 40 years

c. 35 to 44 years

d. 35 to 50 years

e. less then 60 to 65 years

f. 50 to 70 years

II. Critical Thinking Questions and Exercises

DISCUSSION AND ANALYSIS

Discuss the following topics with your classmates.

1. Developing self-awareness about attitudes, experiences, and assumptions regarding genetics can help the nurse apply a genetic framework to patient care. To understand your own attitudes, experiences, and assumptions, consider the following topics for discussion: (a) level of genetic knowledge; (b) past and current experiences with birth defects, chronic illnesses, and genetic conditions; (c) understanding of DNA; (d) beliefs about genetic testing; and (e) approach to those with disabilities.

2. Nursing assessment includes a family history to establish the presence of genetic conditions that are inherited (mendelian conditions). Compare and contrast the following types of mendelian conditions: autosomal dominant, autosomal recessive, and X-linked. Discuss specific nursing roles in genetic counseling.

CHAPTER 10

Chronic Illness and Disability

I. Interpretation, Completion, and Comparison

MULTIPLE CHOICE

Read each question carefully. Circle your answer.

1. A medical condition is considered chronic when long-term management is required for a minimum of:
   a. 8 weeks.
   b. 3 months.
   c. 16 weeks.
   d. 6 months.

2. It is estimated that the number of people afflicted with chronic conditions in 2006 do what by the year 2030?
   a. decrease by 25%
   b. double
   c. increase by 50%
   d. triple

3. It is projected that the direct medical costs for those with chronic illness will do what from 2006 to 2010?
   a. decrease by 5%
   b. grow about 2% per year
   c. increase by 20%
   d. remain the same

4. It is projected that the percentage of health care costs associated with chronic illness over the next 5 years will be approximately:
   a. 30%.
   b. 40%.
   c. 50%.
   d. 75%.

5. The most disabling chronic condition in the United States is projected to be:
   a. extremity paralysis.
   b. mental retardation.
   c. multiple sclerosis.
   d. respiratory cancers.

6. Identify the chronic illness that is increasing rapidly and is directly related to an unhealthy lifestyle.
   a. diabetes mellitus
   b. breast cancer
   c. emphysema
   d. colorectal cancer

7. A major health-promoting behavior that can significantly improve the quality of life for those with a chronic condition is:
   a. diet.
   b. exercise.
   c. hydration.
   d. rest.

8. A person who is at risk for developing a chronic condition because of genetic factors is said to be in which phase of the Trajectory Model?
   a. pretrajectory
   b. trajectory
   c. unstable
   d. acute

9. Chronic illness can be monitored using the Trajectory Model. The phase in which a nursing diagnosis can help in care planning is known as:
   a. pretrajectory.
   c. crisis.
   b. trajectory.
   d. downward course.

10. Remission after an exacerbation represents the Trajectory Model phase known as:
    a. acute.
    c. comeback.
    b. crisis.
    d. downward course.

11. According to the most recent U.S. Census (2000), approximately what percentage of people have a disability?
    a. 10%
    c. 30%
    b. 20%
    d. 40%

12. An example of a developmental disability is:
    a. cerebral palsy.
    c. stroke.
    b. spinal cord injury.
    d. osteoarthritis.

13. Select the disability model that is most appropriate for nurses to use as a guide for planning care.
    a. Biopsychosocial Model
    c. Medical Model
    b. Interface Model
    d. Social Model

SHORT ANSWER

Read each statement carefully. Write your response in the space provided.

1. The three most frequently occurring chronic diseases that result from four preventable causes are:
   _____, _____, and _____.

2. List factors believed to significantly increase the occurrence of chronic conditions in the United States.
   _____
   _____
   _____
   _____

3. Three characteristics common to all forms of chronic illness are: _____,
   _____, and _____.

4. The two most frequent interferences with activities of daily living (ADL) related to chronic illness are:
   _____ and _____.

5. List six common management problems related to chronic conditions.
   _____
   _____
   _____
   _____
   _____
   _____

6. Define the concept of the Trajectory Model as it relates to chronic illness: _____

_____

II. Critical Thinking Questions and Exercises

DISCUSSION AND ANALYSIS

Discuss the following topics with your classmates.

1. Explain the differences between the terms *disability* and *handicap*.
2. Discuss the psychological and emotional reactions to chronic illness and those factors (e.g., lifestyle changes, financial resources) that affect adjustment.
3. Discuss some of the daily challenges of living with a chronic illness that can be helped by nursing intervention. Use as a reference *A Portrait of the Chronically Ill in America, 2001* (report from the Robert Wood Johnson Foundation).
4. Explain the differences between the Rehabilitation Act of 1973 and the Disabilities Act of 1990 and how they have helped protect disabled people from discrimination.

EXAMINING ASSOCIATIONS

Listed below are some characteristics of chronic illness. For each statement, write an explanation of how nursing care can improve the patient's and family's response to management and adaptation.

1. Managing chronic illness involves more than managing medical problems.

_____

_____

2. Chronic conditions are associated with different phases over a course of time.

_____

_____

3. Managing chronic conditions requires persistent adherence to a therapeutic regimen.

_____

_____

4. Chronic illness affects the whole family.

_____

_____

CLINICAL APPLICATIONS

Read the case study below and follow the steps.

CASE STUDY: Applying the Nursing Process to the Trajectory Model of Chronic Illness

The focus of care for patients with chronic illness is determined by their phase of illness (refer to Chart 10-2 in the text). Each of the nine phases can be correlated to a step in the nursing process. For each step below, discuss the role of nursing intervention. Use the example of a 32-year-old mother of one who works full-time as a teacher and has just been diagnosed with rheumatoid arthritis. She is in the Trajectory onset/stable phase of chronic illness.

Step 1: Identify the specific problems and the Trajectory Phase

_____

_____

Step 2: Establish and prioritize goals

_____

_____

Step 3: Define a plan of action to achieve desired outcomes

_____

_____

Step 4: Implement interventions

_____

_____

Step 5: Follow-up and evaluate outcomes

_____

_____

CHAPTER 11

Principles and Practices of Rehabilitation

I. Interpretation, Completion, and Comparison

MULTIPLE CHOICE

Read each question carefully. Circle your answer.

1. Rehabilitation, an integral part of nursing, should begin:
   a. after the patient feels comfortable in the clinical setting.
   b. after the physician has prescribed rehabilitative goals.
   c. when an exercise program has been initiated.
   d. with initial patient contact.

2. In the United States, approximately what percentage of Americans have some form of disability, and what percentage have a severe disability?
   a. 10% and 10%
   b. 20% and 10%
   c. 40% and 20%
   d. 60% and 30%

3. The normal first emotional reactions to a disability are:
   a. anger and hostility.
   b. confusion and denial.
   c. depression and regression.
   d. grief and mourning.

4. The most important member of the rehabilitation team is the:
   a. nurse.
   b. patient.
   c. physical therapist.
   d. physician.

5. The occurrence of spinal cord and traumatic brain injuries is directly associated with substance abuse, alcohol, and the use of illegal drugs. The percentage of patients who are under the influence at the time of injury is as high as:
   a. 50%.
   b. 75%.
   c. 80%.
   d. 95%.

6. The PULSES profile uses six components to evaluate self-care independence. The assessment of bladder control would be documented under:
   a. bowel/bladder function.
   b. lower extremity functions.
   c. physical condition.
   d. sensory functions.

7. The least common position used in positioning a patient in bed to prevent musculoskeletal complications is:
   a. prone.
   b. semi-Fowler's.
   c. side-lying.
   d. supine.

8. A nurse who wants to help a patient assume the side-lying position would:
   a. align the lower extremities in a neutral position.
   b. extend the legs with a firm support under the popliteal area.
   c. place the uppermost hip slightly forward in a position of slight abduction.
   d. position the trunk so that hip flexion is minimized.

9. A quick method used to measure for crutches is to use the patient's height and:
   a. add 6 inches.
   b. add 12 inches.
   c. subtract 8 inches.
   d. subtract 16 inches.

10. A pressure ulcer is associated with the presence of:
    a. dehydration and skin dryness.
    b. excessive skin moisture.
    c. inflammation and infection.
    d. small nutrient vessel compression.

11. Initial skin redness in a patient susceptible to pressure sores should be documented as tissue:
    a. anoxia.
    b. eschar.
    c. hyperemia.
    d. ischemia.

12. A patient at potential risk for a pressure ulcer is assessed by the nurse. A laboratory study the nurse should examine is:
    a. serum albumin.
    b. serum glucose.
    c. prothrombin time.
    d. sedimentation rate.

13. A diet recommended for hypoproteinemia that *spares* protein is one high in:
    a. carbohydrates.
    b. fats.
    c. minerals.
    d. vitamins.

14. Wound healing depends on collagen formation, which depends on:
    a. vitamin A.
    b. vitamin C.
    c. vitamin D.
    d. vitamin K.

15. A rehabilitation program for an elderly patient with a hip fracture must focus on the:
    a. impact of multiple system pathology on recovery.
    b. influence of mental status changes on health improvement.
    c. periodic physiologic evaluation of bone repair.
    d. value of all of the above factors.

16. Insufficient cerebral circulation can result from the use of the tilt table and can be identified by:
    a. diaphoresis.
    b. nausea.
    c. tachycardia.
    d. all of the above.

17. Weight bearing on long bones is essential for preventing:
    a. calcium loss.
    b. potassium loss.
    c. protein loss.
    d. sodium loss.

18. To initiate a schedule of bladder training, the nurse should:
    a. encourage the patient to wait 30 minutes after drinking a measured amount of fluid before attempting to void.
    b. give up to 2500 mL of fluid daily.
    c. teach bladder massage to increase intra-abdominal pressure.
    d. do all of the above.

19. Successful bowel training depends on:
    a. a daily defecation time that is within 15 minutes of the same time every day.
    b. an adequate intake of fiber-containing foods.
    c. fluid intake between 2 and 4 L/day.
    d. all of the above.

20. Sexual problems faced by the disabled include:
    a. impaired self-image.
    b. lack of opportunities to form friendships.
    c. limited access to information about sexuality.
    d. all of the above.

SHORT ANSWER

Read each statement carefully. Write your response in the space provided.

1. The goal of rehabilitation is to _____ or _____ and _____.

2. List five major goals for rehabilitation that are associated with the nursing diagnosis of Self-care deficit: bathing/hygiene, dressing/grooming, feeding, and toileting.

   _____

   _____

   _____

   _____

   _____

3. Four nursing diagnoses for patients with impaired physical mobility are _____, _____, _____, and _____, and four major rehabilitative goals are _____, _____, _____, and _____.

4. The Americans with Disabilities Act went into effect in July 1992. This act requires employers to provide access to facilitate employment of a person with a disability. The two phrases that mandate compliance are _____ and _____.

5. Define the term *contracture* as it relates to impaired physical mobility: _____ _____

6. List three complications commonly associated with prolonged or impaired physical immobility.

   _____

   _____

   _____

7. Two common musculoskeletal complications for patients who are in bed for prolonged periods are: _____ and _____.

8. Four factors that contribute to footdrop are _____, _____, _____, and _____.

9. A joint should be moved through its range of motion _____ times, at least once a day.

10. For crutch-walking, the sequence for the four-point gait begins with the _____ crutch and ends with the _____ foot.

11. Examples of orthotic devices include: _____

_____

12. List five of a possible twelve areas susceptible to pressure ulcers.

_____

_____

_____

_____

_____

13. Life-threatening complications of pressure sores include: _____

_____

14. Eschar covering an ulcer should be removed surgically because eschar: _____

_____

MATCHING

Match the explanations of range-of-motion techniques in column II with their associated terms listed in column I.

Column I

1. _____ Adduction

2. _____ Dorsiflexion

3. _____ Extension

4. _____ Inversion

5. _____ Pronation

6. _____ Abduction

Column II

a. Bending of the foot toward the leg

b. Increasing the angle of a joint

c. Movement away from the midline of the body

d. Movement that turns the sole of the foot inward

e. Movement toward the midline of the body

f. Rotating the forearm so that the palm is down

II. Critical Thinking Questions, Exercises, and Issues

DISCUSSION AND ANALYSIS

Discuss the following topics with your classmates.

1. Discuss the concerns of older adults facing disability; include personal, religious, and psychosocial concerns.
2. Compare and contrast the three assessment tools that are used to assess a patient's level of independence: the PULSES profile, the Barthel Index, and the Patient Evaluation Conference System (PECS).
3. Discuss at least four expected patient outcomes for a nursing plan of rehabilitation care based on the nursing diagnosis of self-care deficit.
4. Explain the physiologic basis for the development of a pressure ulcer.

5. Compare and contrast the physiologic differences in pressure ulcers in stages I through IV.

6. A 65-year-old woman is recovering from surgery to repair a compound fracture of the femur. She will be discharged to home in 24 hours. One nursing diagnosis is Self-care deficit, bathing and dressing. After assessing her limitations in performing activities of daily living (ADL), the nurse designs a plan of care. Refer to Chart 11-3 in the text to outline specific nursing activities related to teaching ADL.

7. A patient has been diagnosed with impaired physical mobility due to a lower leg deformity. After assessment, the nurse selects a nursing diagnosis that can be used to design a plan of care. List several possible nursing diagnoses.

CLINICAL SITUATIONS

View Figures 11-4 and 11-5 in the text, and answer the following clinically focused questions regarding impaired skin integrity.

1. Define the term *pressure ulcer:* _____

_____

2. The initial sign of pressure is _____ caused by _____.

3. The two most susceptible surfaces for pressure ulcer formation are the _____ and the _____.

4. The least favorable position to use to shift body weight is:

   a. prone.
   b. recumbent.

   c. semi-Fowler's.
   d. side-lying.

5. The patient should be repositioned:

   a. every 30 minutes.
   b. hourly.

   c. every 3 to 4 hours.
   d. once per shift.

6. Based on the _____ law, explain why a gel-type flotation pad and an air-fluidized bed reduce pressure: _____

_____

7. Explain why the shearing force is increased when the head of a bed is raised, even if only by a few centimeters: _____

_____

Read the following case studies. Circle the correct answers.

CASE STUDY: Traumatic Amputation Psychosocial Perspective

Oliver, a 42-year-old mechanical engineer, works at a major paper mill. While he was doing routine maintenance work, his foot slipped, and he fell against an industrial paper cutter. He suffered a traumatic amputation of his left hand.

1. The nurse expects Oliver's initial emotional reaction on admission to the emergency department to be one of:

   a. adjustment and acceptance.

   b. anger and regression.

   c. denial and confusion.

   d. grief and depression.

2. If Oliver begins to mourn for his missing body part, the nurse should:

   a. emphasize all the abilities he has with his remaining hand.

   b. encourage him to cheer up.

   c. listen as he talks about his loss.

   d. remind him of his limited abilities, to reinforce reality.

3. The nurse notices that Oliver blames his loss on his family, because he has rationalized that he had to work in a dangerous area to generate sufficient income to support his seven children and his dependent parents. A nursing care plan for Oliver should include:

   a. advising him about budgeting his income to minimize the stress associated with financial worries.

   b. allowing him to project his emotions.

   c. demonstrating self-assistive devices that will help him meet his activities of daily living.

   d. encouraging him to have a positive attitude toward his disability to facilitate his recovery.

4. After several weeks, Oliver seems to be adjusting to his disability. Behaviors consistent with this period include:

   a. acceptance of his limitations.

   b. interest in obtaining information about his disability.

   c. redirecting his energies toward coping.

   d. all of the above.

CASE STUDY: Buck's Extension Traction

Patricia is 67 years old and has limited mobility as a result of a right hip fracture. She is in Buck's extension traction awaiting surgery.

1. During morning care, the nurse suggests that Patricia attempt isometric exercises of her legs. This suggestion is based on the nurse's goal of:

   a. encouraging normal muscle function.

   b. maintaining muscle strength while immobilizing the joints.

   c. providing resistance to increase muscle strength.

   d. retaining as much joint range of motion as possible.

2. The nursing goals associated with therapeutic isometric exercises include all of the following *except*:

   a. enhanced joint mobility.

   b. improved patient well-being.

   c. increased strength of the musculature that controls the joints.

   d. prevention of venous stasis.

3. To assist Patricia with isometric exercises of her lower extremities, the nurse should teach her to:

   a. contract or tighten her thigh and calf muscles without moving her knees and hip joints, hold for several seconds, and then "let go."

   b. slowly move her legs through limited range of motion while the nurse stabilizes the proximal joint and supports the distal part.

   c. move her legs through their full range of motion while the nurse supports each distal part.

   d. put each leg through full range of motion while the nurse offers slight resistance to the movement.

CASE STUDY: Assisted Ambulation: Crutches

Rita, a 17-year-old college student, is in a full leg cast because of a compound fracture of the left femur. Rita is to be discharged from the hospital in several days. She lives with her parents in a split-level house.

1. The exercises that the nurse would recommend to strengthen Rita's upper extremity muscles are:
   a. isometric exercises of the biceps.
   b. push-ups performed in a sitting position.
   c. gluteal setting.
   d. quadriceps setting.

2. Rita is 5 feet 5 inches tall. Her crutches should measure:
   a. 45 inches.
   b. 49 inches.
   c. 54 inches.
   d. 59 inches.

3. Before teaching a crutch gait, the nurse directs Rita to assume the tripod position. In this basic crutch stance, the crutches are placed in front and to the side of Rita's toes, at an approximate distance of:
   a. 4 to 6 inches.
   b. 6 to 8 inches.
   c. 8 to 10 inches.
   d. 10 to 12 inches.

4. Because Rita is not allowed to bear weight on her casted leg, she should be taught the:
   a. two-point gait.
   b. three-point gait.
   c. four-point gait.
   d. swing-through gait.

CHAPTER 12

Health Care of the Older Adult

I. Interpretation, Completion, and Comparison

MULTIPLE CHOICE

Read each question carefully. Circle your answer.

1. The study of old age is referred to as:
   a. ageism.
   b. geriatrics.
   c. gerontonics.
   d. gerontology.

2. Psychological adjustment to aging is believed to be related to the successful completion of:
   a. aging.
   b. developmental tasks.
   c. physical adjustment.
   d. societal position.

3. Nursing interventions to help older people deal with psychological aging include:
   a. attentive listening.
   b. discussing their personal plans for the future.
   c. focusing their attention on the present.
   d. all of the above.

4. All of the following statements are true concerning Erikson's task of ego integrity *except:*
   a. one accepts one's lifestyle as it is.
   b. one feels dissatisfied with life.
   c. one is still in control of one's life.
   d. one has made the best choices for particular situations.

5. Choose the sociologic theory that suggests that adjustment to old age depends on the person's ability to continue life patterns throughout his or her lifetime.
   a. Activity
   b. Continuity
   c. Disengagement
   d. Adaptation

6. The process most sensitive to deterioration with aging seems to be:
   a. creativity.
   b. judgment.
   c. intelligence.
   d. short-term memory.

7. The leading cause of death in the aged is a disorder or dysfunction of which system?
   a. cardiovascular
   b. genitourinary
   c. integumentary
   d. reproductive

8. The primary cause of hospitalization among the elderly is:
   a. congestive heart failure.
   b. emphysema.
   c. chronic renal failure.
   d. cancer of the lung.

9. The cardiac condition most frequently seen among the aged is:
   a. aortic stenosis.
   b. coronary artery disease.
   c. mitral valve prolapse.
   d. ventricular tachycardia.

10. Respiratory changes associated with aging include all of the following *except*:
    a. decreased residual volume.
    b. changes in the anteroposterior diameter of the chest.
    c. loss of elastic tissue surrounding the alveoli.
    d. reduced vital capacity.

11. All of the following statements concerning genitourinary system changes in the older adult are true *except*:
    a. The renal filtration rate decreases.
    b. The acid-base balance is restored more slowly.
    c. Bladder capacity increases with advanced age.
    d. Urinary frequency, urgency, and incontinence are common problems.

12. Dietary intake should emphasize fruits, vegetables, and fish. The daily intake of carbohydrates should be about what percentage of total calories?
    a. 20% to 25%.
    b. 40% to 45%.
    c. 55% to 60%.
    d. 70% to 75%.

13. Bone changes associated with aging frequently result from a loss of:
    a. calcium.
    b. magnesium.
    c. vitamin A.
    d. vitamin C.

14. Nervous system changes associated with aging include all of the following *except*:
    a. a decrease in brain weight subsequent to the destruction of brain cells.
    b. an increase in blood flow to the brain to compensate for the gradual loss of brain cells.
    c. atrophy of the convolutions of the brain surface.
    d. widening and deepening of the spaces between the convolutions of the brain.

15. Nursing measures to deal with sensory changes in the aged include:
    a. increasing room lighting without increasing glare.
    b. speaking louder than normal.
    c. suggesting appetite stimulants before meals.
    d. all of the above actions.

16. The most common affective or mood disorder of old age is:
    a. Alzheimer's disease.
    b. delirium.
    c. depression.
    d. multi-infarct dementia.

17. The leading cause of injury and preventable source of mortality and morbidity in older adults is:
    a. dehydration.
    b. emphysema.
    c. falls.
    d. melanoma.

18. Drug dosages must be reduced in the elderly because:
    a. cardiac output is significantly reduced.
    b. the number of mucosal cells in the gastrointestinal tract is reduced.
    c. drug biotransformation takes longer in older persons.
    d. all of the above are true.

19. The medications that remain in the body longer in the elderly because of increased body fat are:
    a. anticoagulants.
    c. digitalis glycosides.
    b. barbiturates.
    d. diuretics.

20. The seventh leading cause of death in older persons is:
    a. accidents and injuries.
    c. elder abuse.
    b. drug toxicity.
    d. malnutrition.

21. The major source of public funding that provides nursing home care for the poor elderly is:
    a. Medicaid.
    b. Medicare.

SHORT ANSWER

Read each statement carefully. Write your response in the space provided.

1. In approximately _____ years, there will be a higher percentage (_____%) of people older than 65 years of age than of those younger than 18 years of age (_____%).

2. A 75-year old woman today can expect to live to be about _____ years of age.

3. The major cause of disability in those older than 65 years of age is _____.

4. The leading cause of death in those older than 65 years of age is _____, followed by _____ and _____.

5. According to Erickson and Havighurst, older adults experience six developmental tasks:
   _____, _____,
   _____, _____,
   _____, and _____.

6. The primary cause of age-related vision loss in the elderly is _____.

7. The ability to acquire new information and learn new skills significantly decreases after the age of _____ years.

8. The dementias in older adults are characterized by a decrease in the following intellectual skills:
   _____, _____,
   _____, and _____.

9. The least common affective or mood disorder of old age is _____.

10. List the five most common infections in the elderly.

_____

_____

_____

_____

_____

II. Critical Thinking Questions and Exercises

INTERPRETING DATA

Refer to Figure 12-1 in the text to answer the following questions.

1. In the decade between the years 2000 and 2010, the percentage of people older than 65 years of age will increase by the following amount: _____%.

2. In the decade between 2010 and 2020, the increase in the percentage of people older than 65 years of age will be _____%, more than _____ times the increase of the prior 10 years (2000–2010).

3. The percentage of people older than 65 years of age will continue to increase from 2020 to 2030 at a rate that is _____ (slower than, equal to, greater than) the rate in 2000–2010.[AQ4] The increase for this decade is projected to be _____%.

4. The number of persons older than 65 years of age increased at the same rate (_____%) over the two time spans of _____ and _____.

5. By the year 2030, approximately _____ million individuals will be older than 65 years of age.

RECOGNIZING CONTRADICTIONS

Rewrite each statement correctly. Underline the key concepts.

1. Bones are composed of postmiotic cells that diminish and cause bone density.

_____

2. Osteoporosis, accelerated by the loss of estrogen, can be reversed with a high-calcium diet.

_____

3. If the symptoms of delirium go untreated, they will eventually decrease, and the person will regain his or her previous level of consciousness.

_____

4. Older persons should "take it easy" and avoid vigorous activity.

_____

5. Baseline body temperature is usually 1°F higher than normal in an older person because dehydration is common.

_____

DISCUSSION AND ANALYSIS

Discuss the following topics with your classmates.

1. Compare and contrast the two sociologic theories of aging: the activity theory and the continuity theory.
2. Distinguish between the two major programs in the United States that finance health care: Medicare and Medicaid.
3. Explain the purpose and limitations of a living will and a durable power of attorney.
4. Explain the Patient Self-Determination Act (PSDA).

CLINICAL SITUATIONS

Read the following case studies. Circle the correct answer or fill in the blanks below.

CASE STUDY: Loneliness

Suzanne is an 80-year-old retired schoolteacher. She was recently widowed and lives alone. She is financially secure but socially isolated, because she has outlived most of her friends. Her children are self-sufficient and are very busy with their own lives.

1. Psychological threats that Suzanne may experience include:
   a. a deterioration of self-concept.
   b. a loss of self-esteem.
   c. extensive grief over frequently occurring losses.
   d. all of the above.

2. Suzanne is concerned about the dryness of her skin. Suggestions for skin care include:
   a. applying ointment to the skin several times a day.
   b. avoiding overexposure to the sun.
   c. patting the skin dry instead of rubbing it with a towel.
   d. all of the above measures.

3. Suzanne notices that food does not taste the same as before. She needs to be aware that this sensory change is most probably related to:
   a. a decrease in the number of taste buds.
   b. a loss of appetite associated with a decreased sense of smell.
   c. altered enzyme secretions.
   d. diminished gastric secretions.

4. An analysis of Suzanne's diet shows that it does not contain adequate protein. Her daily protein intake, for a body weight of 134 lb, should be about:
   a. 30 g.
   b. 40 g.
   c. 50 g.
   d. 60 g.

5. Most accidents among older people involve falls within the home. Preventive nursing measures include advising Suzanne to:
   a. avoid climbing and bending.
   b. keep personal items stored at a level between her hips and her eyes.
   c. make certain that all her shoes fit securely.
   d. do all of the above.

CASE STUDY: Alzheimer's Disease

Thomas, a 75-year-old retired bricklayer, lives at home with Anne, his 65-year-old wife, who is healthy and active. Lately Anne has noticed that Thomas is negative, hostile, and suspicious of her. He gets lost in his own home, and his conversations have been accompanied by forgetfulness. Recently, Thomas' physician has indicated a probable diagnosis of Alzheimer's disease.

1. Choose the statement that is *false* concerning Alzheimer's disease.
   a. It is found only in old persons.
   b. The disease process is irreversible.
   c. The probable cause is neuropathologic and biochemical.
   d. The cells that are affected by the disease are the ones that use acetylcholine.

2. Physiologically, an enzyme that produces the neurotransmitter _____ is decreased, and neural damage occurs primarily in the _____, causing decreased _____.

3. The nurse should suggest that Anne deal with Thomas' behavior by:

   a. reasoning with him.

   b. providing reality orientation.

   c. providing a calm and predictable environment.

   d. not structuring activities for him.

4. An important point to communicate to Anne is that:

   a. there are no realistic goals appropriate for Thomas.

   b. lists and written instructions will only tend to confuse Thomas.

   c. Thomas should be restrained when agitated.

   d. maintaining personal dignity and autonomy is still an important part of Thomas' life.

5. Caregivers of patients with Alzheimer's disease should be aware that:

   a. Alzheimer's support groups exist.

   b. Alzheimer's disease does not eliminate the need for intimacy.

   c. socializing with old friends may be comforting.

   d. all of the above are appropriate.

6. The physician explains that there is no cure for the disease and no way to slow its progression, which intensifies symptoms. Eventually, death occurs as a result of complications such as _____, _____, and _____.

CASE STUDY: Dehydration

Vera, an 89-year-old widow, was transferred from a nursing home to a hospital with a diagnosis of dehydration. Vera needs to be in bed because of her generalized weakness. She is occasionally confused and disoriented.

1. From knowledge of temperature regulation in the elderly, the nurse should:

   a. make sure that the environmental temperature is adequate.

   b. palpate Vera's skin periodically to assess for warmth.

   c. place extra blankets at Vera's bedside in case she becomes cold, especially in the evening.

   d. do all of the above.

2. The nurse initiates a 2-hour turning schedule for Vera, based on the knowledge that the underlying cause of all decubiti is:

   a. altered skin turgor.

   b. nutritional deficiency.

   c. pressure.

   d. vasoconstriction.

3. Vera has been incontinent of urine since admission. Nursing interventions include all of the following _except:_

   a. initiating a bladder training program.

   b. offering fluids frequently to maintain a minimum daily intake of 2 to 3 L.

   c. providing means for limited daily exercises and ambulation.

   d. securing a physician's order for urethral catheterization.

4. The nurse suggests that Vera sit in a rocking chair for 20 minutes, four times a day. This suggestion is based on the knowledge that rocking:

   a. discourages hypostatic pulmonary congestion.

   b. increases pulmonary ventilation.

   c. improves venous return through contraction of the calf muscles.

   d. does all of the above.

CHAPTER 13

Pain Management

I. Interpretation, Completion, and Comparison

MULTIPLE CHOICE

Read each question carefully. Circle your answer.

1. Although the criterion is arbitrary, pain can be classified as chronic when it has persisted for:
   a. 1 to 2 months.
   b. 3 months.
   c. 3 to 5 months.
   d. longer than 6 months.

2. Acute pain may be described as having the following characteristic.
   a. It does not usually respond well to treatment.
   b. It is associated with a specific injury.
   c. It serves no useful purpose.
   d. It responds well to placebos.

3. A physiologic response *not* usually associated with acute pain is:
   a. decreased cardiac output.
   b. altered insulin response.
   c. increased metabolic rate.
   d. decreased production of cortisol.

4. Chronic pain may be described as:
   a. attributable to a specific cause.
   b. prolonged in duration.
   c. rapidly occurring and subsiding with treatment.
   d. separate from any central or peripheral pathology.

5. An example of chronic benign pain is:
   a. a migraine headache.
   b. an exacerbation of rheumatoid arthritis.
   c. low back pain.
   d. sickle cell crisis.

6. A chemical substance thought to inhibit the transmission of pain is:
   a. acetylcholine.
   b. bradykinin.
   c. enkephalin.
   d. histamine.

7. All of the following statements about endorphins are true *except*:
   a. Their release inhibits the transmission of painful impulses.
   b. They represent the same mechanism of pain relief as non-narcotic analgesics.
   c. They are endogenous neurotransmitters structurally similar to opioids.
   d. They are found in heavy concentrations in the central nervous system.

8. The nurse assessing for pain should:
   a. believe a patient when he or she states that pain is present.
   b. doubt that pain exists when no physical origin can be identified.
   c. realize that patients frequently imagine and state that they have pain without actually feeling painful sensations.
   d. do all of the above.

9. When a nurse asks a patient to describe the quality of his or her pain, the nurse expects the patient to use a descriptive term such as:
   a. burning.
   b. chronic.
   c. intermittent.
   d. severe.

10. A physiologic indicator of acute pain is:
    a. diaphoresis.
    b. bradycardia.
    c. hypotension.
    d. lowered respiratory rate.

11. A nursing measure to manage anxiety during the anticipation of pain should include:
    a. focusing the patient's attention on another problem.
    b. teaching about the nature of the impending pain and associated relief measures.
    c. using an anxiety-reducing technique, such as desensitization.
    d. any or all of the above.

12. A nursing plan of care for pain management should include:
    a. altering factors that influence the pain sensation.
    b. determining responses to the patient's behavior toward pain.
    c. selecting goals for nursing intervention.
    d. all of the above.

13. The nurse's major area of assessment for a patient receiving patient-controlled analgesia (PCA) is assessment of which system?
    a. cardiovascular
    b. integumentary
    c. neurologic
    d. respiratory

14. Pain in the elderly requires careful assessment, because older people:
    a. are expected to experience chronic pain.
    b. have a decreased pain threshold.
    c. experience reduced sensory perception.
    d. have increased sensory perception.

15. Administration of analgesics to the elderly requires careful patient assessment, because older people:
    a. metabolize drugs more rapidly.
    b. have increased hepatic, renal, and gastrointestinal function.
    c. are more sensitive to drugs.
    d. have lower ratios of body fat and muscle mass.

16. A preventive approach to pain relief with nonsteroidal anti-inflammatory drugs (NSAIDs) means that the medication is given:
    a. before the pain becomes severe.
    b. before the pain is experienced.
    c. when pain is at its peak.
    d. when the level of pain tolerance has been exceeded.

17. The advantage of using intraspinal infusion to deliver analgesics is:
    a. reduced side effects of systemic analgesia.
    b. reduced effects on pulse, respirations, and blood pressure.
    c. reduced need for frequent injections.
    d. all of the above.

18. The drug of choice for epidural administration of analgesia is:
   a. codeine.
   b. Demerol.
   c. Dilaudid.
   d. morphine.

19. The most worrisome adverse effect of epidural opioids is:
   a. asystole.
   b. hypertension.
   c. bradypnea.
   d. tachycardia.

20. Cutaneous stimulation is helpful in reducing painful sensations, because it:
   a. provides distraction from the pain source and decreases awareness.
   b. releases endorphins.
   c. stimulates large-diameter nerve fibers and reduces the intensity of pain.
   d. accomplishes all of the above.

SHORT ANSWER

Read each statement carefully. Write your response in the space provided.

1. The definition of pain is: _____

_____

2. Name three categories used to describe pain.

_____

_____

_____

3. One pathophysiologic response to chronic pain is _____.

4. List five algogenic substances that are released into the tissues and affect the sensitivity of nociceptors.

_____

_____

_____

_____

5. List the six factors that directly influence an individual's response to pain.

_____

_____

_____

_____

_____

6. Define the term *placebo effect*: _____

_____

7. Identify the seven factors that a nurse needs to consider for complete pain assessment.

_____

_____

_____

_____

_____

_____

_____

8. List eight common physiologic responses to pain.

_____

_____

_____

_____

_____

_____

_____

_____

9. Define the term *balanced analgesia*: _____

_____

10. Name the three general categories of analgesic agents that are used in some combination form to achieve balanced anesthesia.

_____

_____

_____

11. The two most common types of electrical stimulation are _____ and

_____.

CROSSWORD PUZZLE: PAIN TRANSMISSION AND MANAGEMENT

Complete the following crossword puzzle using terminology associated with pain transmission and management.

DOWN
1. Pain receptors sensitive to noxious and damaging stimuli.
2. Nonsteroidal agents that decrease inflammation and increase the effects of analgesics.
3. A type of analgesia that is controlled by the patient using a special pump.
4. A drug is prescribed on an "as needed" basis for pain management (pro re nata).
5. The only commercially available transdermal opioid medication.
6. Significantly increases a person's response to pain.

ACROSS

1. Chemicals known to inhibit the transmission or perception of pain.
2. This substance, released in response to painful stimuli, causes vasodilation.
3. An inactive substance given in place of pain medication.
4. Medication administration directly into the subarachnoid space and cerebrospinal fluid.
5. A type of cutaneous stimulation that decreases pain transmission through the descending pain pathway.
6. Transcutaneous stimulation of nonpain receptors in the same area of an injury.
7. Term used to describe a pain's rhythm.

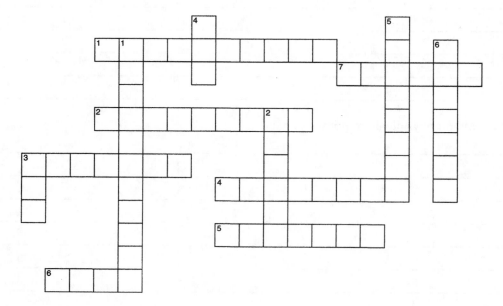

II. Critical Thinking Questions and Exercises

DISCUSSION AND ANALYSIS

Discuss the following topics with your classmates.

1. Explain the seven rights that patients have according to the Pain Care Bill of Rights officially enacted by the state of California.
2. Distinguish among acute, chronic (persistent, nonmalignant), and cancer-related pain and cite an example of each.
3. Describe the transmission and awareness of pain (nociception system) by explaining the role of the central nervous system and the ascending and descending sensory pathways.
4. Describe the classic Gate Control Theory of pain as described by Melzack and Well in 1965.
5. Discuss the possible side effects of opioid analgesic agents and nursing interventions to prevent or minimize potential side effects.
6. Explain the action and purpose of cyclo-oxygenase inhibitors (COX-1 and COX-2) and provide some examples of each.
7. Explain how the technique of distraction works to relieve acute and chronic pain.

CLINICAL SITUATIONS

Read the following case study. Circle the correct answer.

CASE STUDY: Pain Experience

Courtney is a young, healthy adult who slipped off the stairs going down to the basement and struck her forehead on the cement flooring. Courtney did not lose consciousness but did sustain a mild concussion and a hematoma that was 5 cm in width and protruded outward about 6 cm. She experienced immediate acute pain at the site of injury plus a pounding headache.

1. An immediate assessment of the localized pain, based on the patient's description, is that it should be:
   a. brief in duration.
   b. mild in intensity.
   c. persistent after healing has occurred.
   d. recurrent for 3 to 4 months.

2. During the assessment process, the nurse attempts to determine Courtney's physiologic and behavioral responses to her pain experience. The nurse is aware that a patient can be in pain yet appear to be "pain free." A behavioral response indicative of acute pain is:
   a. an expressionless face.
   b. clear verbalization of details.
   c. muscle tension.
   d. physical inactivity.

3. The nurse uses distraction to help Courtney cope with her pain experience. A suggested activity is:
   a. promoting relaxation.
   b. playing music or using a videotape.
   c. using cutaneous stimulation.
   d. any or all of the above.

4. After treatment, Courtney is discharged to home while still in pain. The nurse should:
   a. clarify that Courtney knows what type of pain signals a problem.
   b. remind Courtney that acute pain may persist for several days.
   c. review methods of pain management.
   d. do all of the above.

CHAPTER 14

Fluid and Electrolytes: Balance and Disturbances

I. Interpretation, Completion, and Comparison

MULTIPLE CHOICE

Read each question carefully. Circle your answer.

1. The average daily urinary output in an adult is:
   a. 0.5 L.
   b. 3.0 L.
   c. 1.5 L.
   d. 2.5 L.

2. A febrile patient's fluid output is in excess of normal because of diaphoresis. The nurse should plan fluid replacement based on the knowledge that insensible losses in an afebrile person are normally not greater than:
   a. 300 mL/24 h.
   b. 600 mL/24 h.
   c. 900 mL/24 h.
   d. 1200 mL/24 h.

3. A patient's serum sodium concentration is within the normal range. The nurse estimates that the serum osmolality should be:
   a. less than 136 mOsm/kg.
   b. 275 to 300 mOsm/kg.
   c. greater than 408 mOsm/kg.
   d. 350 to 544 mOsm/kg.

4. The nurse expects that a decrease in serum osmolality would occur with:
   a. diabetes insipidus.
   b. hyperglycemia.
   c. renal failure.
   d. uremia.

5. If the patient's serum sodium level is 140 mEq/L, a nurse can estimate that the serum osmolality is:
   a. 70 mOsm/kg.
   b. 140 mOsm/kg.
   c. 210 mOsm/kg.
   d. 280 mOsm/kg.

6. The nurse notes that a patient's urine osmolality is 980 mOsm/kg. The nurse knows to assess for the possible cause of:
   a. acidosis.
   b. fluid volume excess.
   c. diabetes insipidus.
   d. hyponatremia.

7. One of the best indicators of renal function is:
   a. blood urea nitrogen (BUN).
   b. serum creatinine.
   c. specific gravity.
   d. urine osmolality.

8. A patient is hemorrhaging from multiple trauma sites. The nurse expects that compensatory mechanisms associated with hypovolemia would cause all of the following symptoms *except*:
   a. hypertension.
   b. oliguria.
   c. tachycardia.
   d. tachypnea.

9. A clinical manifestation *not* found in hypovolemia is:
   a. muscle weakness.
   b. oliguria.
   c. postural hypotension.
   d. bradycardia.

10. Laboratory findings consistent with hypovolemia in a female would include all of the following *except*:
    a. hematocrit greater than 47%.
    b. BUN–serum creatinine ratio greater than 12:1.
    c. urine specific gravity of 1.027.
    d. urine osmolality greater than 450 mOsm/kg.

11. The nurse should expect that a patient with mild fluid volume excess would be prescribed a diuretic that blocks sodium reabsorption in the distal tubule, such as:
    a. Bumex.
    b. Demadex.
    c. HydroDIURIL.
    d. Lasix.

12. When assessing the weight of a patient who is on a sodium-restricted diet, the nurse knows that a weight gain of approximately two pounds (2.2 lb = 1 kg) is equivalent to a gain of how much fluid?
    a. 0.5 L.
    b. 1.0 L.
    c. 1.5 L.
    d. 2.0 L.

13. Nursing intervention for a patient with a diagnosis of hyponatremia includes all of the following *except*:
    a. assessing for symptoms of nausea and malaise.
    b. encouraging the intake of low-sodium liquids, such as coffee or tea.
    c. monitoring neurologic status.
    d. restricting tap water intake.

14. A patient with abnormal sodium losses is receiving a house diet. To provide 1600 mg of sodium daily, the nurse could supplement the patient's diet with:
    a. one beef cube and 8 oz of tomato juice.
    b. four beef cubes and 8 oz of tomato juice.
    c. one beef cube and 16 oz of tomato juice.
    d. one beef cube and 12 oz of tomato juice.

15. One of the dangers of treating hypernatremia is:
    a. red blood cell crenation.
    b. red blood cell hydrolysis.
    c. cerebral edema.
    d. renal shutdown.

16. A nurse is directed to administer a hypotonic intravenous solution. Looking at the following labeled solutions, she should choose:
    a. 0.45% sodium chloride.
    b. 0.90% sodium chloride.
    c. 5% dextrose in water.
    d. 5% dextrose in normal saline solution.

17. An isotonic solution that contains electrolytes similar to the concentration of electrolytes used in plasma is:
    a. 5% dextrose in water.
    b. lactated Ringer's solution.
    c. 3% NaCl solution.
    d. 5% NaCl solution.

18. A patient is admitted who has had severe vomiting for 24 hours. She states that she is exhausted and weak. The results of an admitting electrocardiogram (ECG) show flat T waves and ST-segment depression. Choose the most likely potassium (K^+) value for this patient.
    a. 4.0 mEq/L
    b. 8.0 mEq/L
    c. 2.0 mEq/L
    d. 2.6 mEq/L

19. The ECG change that is specific to hypokalemia is:

    a. a depressed ST segment.

    b. a flat T wave.

    c. an elevated U wave.

    d. an inverted T wave.

20. To supplement a diet with foods high in potassium, the nurse should recommend the addition of:

    a. fruits such as bananas and apricots.

    b. green leafy vegetables.

    c. milk and yogurt.

    d. nuts and legumes.

21. If a patient has severe hyperkalemia, it is possible to administer calcium gluconate intravenously to:

    a. immediately lower the potassium (K^+) level by active transport.

    b. antagonize the action of K^+ on the heart.

    c. prevent transient renal failure (TRF).

    d. accomplish all of the above.

22. Cardiac effects of hyperkalemia are usually present when the serum potassium level reaches:

    a. 5 mEq/L.

    b. 6 mEq/L.

    c. 7 mEq/L.

    d. 8 mEq/L.

23. The most characteristic manifestation of hypocalcemia and hypomagnesemia is:

    a. anorexia and nausea.

    b. constipation.

    c. lack of coordination.

    d. tetany.

24. A patient complains of tingling in his fingers. He has positive Trousseau's and Chvostek's signs. He says that he feels depressed. Choose the most likely serum calcium (Ca^{++}) value for this patient.

    a. 11 mg/dL.

    b. 9 mg/dL.

    c. 7 mg/dL.

    d. 5 mg/dL.

25. Management of hypocalcemia includes all of the following actions *except* administration of:

    a. fluid to dilute the calcium levels.

    b. the diuretic furosemide (Lasix), without saline, to increase calcium excretion through the kidneys.

    c. inorganic phosphate salts.

    d. intravenous phosphate therapy.

26. Cardiac arrest will probably occur with a serum calcium level of:

    a. 9 mg/dL.

    b. 12 mg/dL.

    c. 15 mg/dL.

    d. 18 mg/dL.

27. A patient is admitted with a diagnosis of renal failure. He also mentions that he has had stomach distress and has ingested numerous antacid tablets over the past 2 days. His blood pressure is 110/70 mm Hg, his face is flushed, and he is experiencing generalized weakness. Choose the most likely magnesium (Mg^{++}) value for this patient.

    a. 11 mEq/L.

    b. 5 mEq/L.

    c. 2 mEq/L.

    d. 1 mEq/L.

28. For the patient described in the previous question, management should include:

    a. a regular diet with extra fruits and green vegetables.

    b. potassium-sparing diuretics.

    c. discontinuance of any oral magnesium salts.

    d. all of the above measures.

29. A clinical indication of hypophosphatemia is:
    a. bone pain.
    b. paresthesia.
    c. seizures.
    d. tetany.

30. The most common buffer system in the body is the:
    a. plasma protein buffer system.
    b. hemoglobin buffer system.
    c. phosphate buffer system.
    d. bicarbonate–carbonic acid buffer system.

31. The kidneys regulate acid–base balance by all of the following mechanisms *except:*
    a. excreting hydrogen ions (H^+).
    b. reabsorbing or excreting HCO_3- into the blood.
    c. reabsorbing carbon dioxide into the blood.
    d. retaining hydrogen ions (H^+).

32. The lungs regulate acid–base balance by all of the following mechanisms *except:*
    a. excreting HCO_3- into the blood.
    b. slowing ventilation.
    c. controlling carbon dioxide levels.
    d. increasing ventilation.

33. Choose the condition that exhibits blood values with a low pH and a low plasma bicarbonate concentration.
    a. respiratory acidosis
    b. respiratory alkalosis
    c. metabolic acidosis
    d. metabolic alkalosis

34. The nursing assessment for a patient with metabolic alkalosis includes evaluation of laboratory data for all of the following *except:*
    a. hypocalcemia.
    b. hypoglycemia.
    c. hypokalemia.
    d. hypoxemia.

35. Choose the condition that exhibits blood values with a low pH and a high PCO_2.
    a. respiratory acidosis
    b. respiratory alkalosis
    c. metabolic acidosis
    d. metabolic alkalosis

36. A normal oxygen saturation value for arterial blood is:
    a. 90%.
    b. 92%.
    c. 93%.
    d. 95%.

SHORT ANSWER

Read each statement carefully. Write your response in the space provided.

1. About _____ percent of total body fluid is in the intracellular space; the major positively charged ion in intracellular fluid is _____. The extracellular space is divided into three compartments: _____, _____, and _____; the major positively charged ion in extracellular fluid is _____. About _____ percent of the _____ liters of total blood volume is _____.

2. Define *colloidal osmotic pressure:* _____
   _____

3. Distinguish between the terms *urine specific gravity*, *BUN*, and *creatinine*: _____

_____

_____

4. Distinguish between the terms *baroreceptors* and *osmoreceptors*: _____

_____

5. The primary concentration of phosphorous (85%) is located in the _____, and about 14% is located in _____.

6. Calcium levels are primarily regulated by _____.

7. The primary complication of hyperphosphatemia is _____, which occurs when the calcium–magnesium product exceeds 70 mg/dL.

8. The normal blood pH is _____.

9. The upper and lower blood pH levels that are incompatible with life are _____ and _____.

10. Indicate which of the following factors contribute to *hyponatremia* by writing "LOW" in the space provided, and indicate which contribute to *hypernatremia* by writing "HIGH" in the space provided.

    a. _____ vomiting

    b. _____ diarrhea

    c. _____ watery diarrhea

    d. _____ inability to quench thirst

    e. _____ burns over a large surface area

    f. _____ diuretics

    g. _____ heat stroke

    h. _____ adrenal insufficiency

    i. _____ syndrome of inappropriate antidiuretic hormone

    j. _____ status post therapeutic abortion

    k. _____ diabetes insipidus with water restriction

    l. _____ excessive parenteral administration of dextrose and water solution

11. Indicate which of the following factors contribute to *hypokalemia* by writing "LOW' in the space provided, and indicate which contribute to *hyperkalemia* by writing "HIGH" in the space provided.

    a. _____ alkalosis

    b. _____ too tight a tourniquet when collecting a blood sample

    c. _____ vomiting

    d. _____ gastric suction

    e. _____ leukocytosis

    f. _____ anorexia nervosa

    g. _____ hyperaldosteronism

    h. _____ furosemide (Lasix) administration

    i. _____ steroid administration

    j. _____ renal failure

    k. _____ penicillin administration

    l. _____ adrenal steroid deficiency

12. Indicate which of the following factors contribute to *hypocalcemia* by writing "LOW" in the space provided, and indicate which contribute to *hypercalcemia* by writing "HIGH" in the space provided.

    a. _____ hyperparathyroidism

    b. _____ massive administration of citrated blood

    c. _____ malignant tumors

    d. _____ immobilization because of multiple fractures

    e. _____ pancreatitis

    f. _____ thiazide diuretics

    g. _____ renal failure

    h. _____ aminoglycoside administration

13. Indicate which of the following factors contribute to *hypomagnesemia* by writing "LOW" in the space provided, and indicate which contribute to *hypermagnesemia* by writing "HIGH" in the space provided.

    a. _____ alcohol abuse

    b. _____ renal failure

    c. _____ diarrhea

    d. _____ gentamicin administration

    e. _____ untreated ketoacidosis

14. Indicate which of the following factors contribute to *hypophosphatemia* by writing "LOW" in the space provided, and indicate which contribute to *hyperphosphatemia* by writing "HIGH" in the space provided.

    a. _____ hyperparathyroidism

    b. _____ renal failure

    c. _____ major thermal burns

    d. _____ alcohol withdrawal

    e. _____ neoplastic disease chemotherapy

15. For each of the following factors, indicate the probable cause by writing "M-ACID" for metabolic acidosis, "M-ALKA" for metabolic alkalosis, "R-ACID" for respiratory acidosis, or "R-ALKA" for respiratory alkalosis.

    a. _____ sedative overdose

    b. _____ lactic acidosis

    c. _____ ketoacidosis

    d. _____ severe pneumonia

    e. _____ hypoxemia

    f. _____ acute pulmonary edema

    g. _____ diarrhea

    h. _____ vomiting

    i. _____ hypokalemia

    j. _____ gram-negative bacterial infection

16. Explain why the administration of a 3% to 5% sodium chloride solution requires intense monitoring:

    _____

    _____

17. List several symptoms associated with air embolism, a complication of intravenous therapy:

_____

18. The major complication of intravenous therapy is _____.

II. Critical Thinking Questions and Exercises

DISCUSSION AND ANALYSIS

Discuss the following topics with your classmates.

1. Explain why decreased urine output, despite adequate fluid intake, is an early indicator of a third space fluid shift.
2. Explain the important role of two opposing forces, hydrostatic pressure and osmotic pressure, in maintaining fluid movement through blood vessels.
3. Determine the normal daily urine output of an adult. Calculate the usual output per hour for adults with the following weights: 110 lb, 132 lb, and 176 lb.
4. Define the terms *osmolality* and *osmolarity,* and explain how each is measured.
5. Distinguish between hypervolemia and hypovolemia (pathophysiology, clinical manifestations, assessment, diagnostic findings, medical and nursing management).
6. Distinguish between the purposes of using isotonic, hypotonic, or hypertonic intravenous solutions.
7. Discuss the nursing care management for a patient receiving intravenous therapy.
8. Discuss the nurses' role in managing the common complications of intravenous therapy: infiltration, phlebitis, thrombophlebitis, hematoma, clotting, and obstruction.

APPLYING CONCEPTS

Examine Figure 14-1 in the text and answer the following questions.

1. Define the term *osmosis,* and explain how a fluid concentration gradient influences the movement between fluid compartments: _____

_____

_____

2. Explain how the osmolality of a solution is determined: _____

_____

_____

3. Explain the concept of tonicity and how it affects cell size: _____

_____

_____

4. Distinguish between osmotic pressure, oncotic pressure, and osmotic diuresis: _____

_____

_____

5. Clarify the differences between diffusion and filtration: _____

_____

_____

6. Give some examples of osmosis, diffusion, and filtration.

Osmosis: _____

Diffusion: _____

Filtration: _____

EXAMINING ASSOCIATIONS

Examine each of the following relationships and answer each question.

1. Describe the interaction of sodium and potassium that is involved in the sodium–potassium pump:

_____

_____

_____

2. Explain the interdependence of renin, angiotensin, and the aldosterone system on the fluid regulation cycle:

_____

_____

_____

MATCHING

Correlate the associations among body fluid compartments. First, match each statement about body fluid in column III with the appropriate body fluid space listed in column II; write the Roman numeral in the space provided. Then, match the fluid space in column II with an associated fact listed in column I; write the small letter in the space provided.

Column I

1. _____ Third space fluid shift

2. _____ The smallest compartment of the extracellular fluid space

3. _____ Space where plasma is contained

4. _____ Comprises the intravascular, interstitial, and transcellular fluid

5. _____ Comprises about 60% of body fluid

6. _____ Comprises fluid surrounding the cell

Column II

a. _____ Intracellular space

b. _____ Extracellular fluid compartment

c. _____ Intravascular space

d. _____ Transcellular space

e. _____ Interstitial space

f. _____ Intravascular fluid volume deficit

Column III

I. Comprises the cerebrospinal and pericardial fluids

II. Is equal to about 8 L in an adult

III. Signs include hypotension, edema, and tachycardia

IV. Found mostly in skeletal muscle mass

V. Comprises about one third of body fluid

VI. Comprises 50% of blood volume

EXTRACTING INFERENCES

Review Figure 14-4 in the text and answer the following questions.

1. Sodium, the most abundant electrolyte in extracellular fluid, is primarily responsible for maintaining fluid _____, whose purpose can be defined as _____.^{AQ3}

2. Sodium is regulated by _____, _____, and the _____ system.

3. Sodium establishes the electrochemical state necessary for _____ and the _____.

4. Signs of lethargy, increasing intracranial pressure, and seizures may occur when the serum sodium level reaches:

   a. 115 mEq/L.
   b. 130 mEq/L.

   c. 145 mEq/L.
   d. 160 mEq/L.

5. In a patient with excess fluid volume, hyponatremia is treated by restricting fluids to how many milliliters in 24 hours?

   a. 400
   b. 600

   c. 800
   d. 1200

6. To return a patient with hyponatremia to normal sodium levels, it is safer to restrict fluid intake than to administer sodium:

   a. in patients who are unconscious.
   b. to prevent fluid overload.

   c. to prevent dehydration.
   d. in patients who show neurologic symptoms.

7. Hypernatremia is associated with a:

   a. serum osmolality of 245 mOsm/kg.
   b. serum sodium concentration of 150 mEq/L.

   c. urine specific gravity lower than 1.003.
   d. combination of all of the above.

8. A semiconscious patient presents with restlessness and weakness. He has a dry, swollen tongue. His body temperature is 99.3°F, and his urine specific gravity is 1.020. Choose the most likely serum sodium (Na^+) value for this patient.

   a. 110 mEq/L
   b. 140 mEq/L

   c. 155 mEq/L
   d. 165 mEq/L

CLINICAL SITUATIONS

Read the following case studies. Circle the correct answer.

CASE STUDY: Extracellular Fluid Volume Deficit

Harriet, 30 years old, has been admitted to the burn treatment center with full-thickness burns over 30% of her upper body. Her diagnosis is consistent with extracellular fluid volume deficit (FVD).

1. The major indicator of extracellular FVD can be identified by assessing for:
   a. a full and bounding pulse.
   b. a drop in postural blood pressure.
   c. an elevated temperature.
   d. pitting edema of the lower extremities.

2. Manifestations of extracellular FVD include all of the following *except:*
   a. collapsed neck veins.
   b. decreased serum albumin.
   c. elevated hematocrit.
   d. weight loss.

3. A nursing plan of care for Harriet should include assessing blood pressure with the patient in the supine and upright positions. A diagnostic reading that should be recorded and reported is:
   a. supine, 140/90; sitting, 120/80; standing, 110/70 mm Hg.
   b. supine, 140/90; sitting, 130/90; standing, 130/90 mm Hg.
   c. supine, 140/90; sitting, 140/85; standing, 135/85 mm Hg.
   d. supine, 140/90; sitting, 140/90; standing, 130/90 mm Hg.

4. Nursing intervention for Harriet includes all of the following *except:*
   a. monitoring urinary output to assess kidney perfusion.
   b. placing the patient in the Trendelenburg position to maximize cerebral blood flow.
   c. positioning the patient flat in bed with legs elevated to maintain adequate circulating volume.
   d. teaching leg exercises to promote venous return and prevent postural hypotension when the patient stands.

CASE STUDY: Congestive Heart Failure

George, 88 years old, has congestive heart failure. He was admitted to the hospital with a diagnosis of extracellular fluid volume excess. He was frightened, slightly confused, and dyspneic on exertion.

1. During the assessment process, the nurse expects to identify all of the following *except:*
   a. a full pulse.
   b. decreased central venous pressure.
   c. edema.
   d. neck vein distention.

2. A manifestation of extracellular volume excess is:
   a. altered serum osmolality.
   b. hyponatremia.
   c. increased hematocrit when volume excess develops quickly.
   d. rapid weight gain.

3. A nursing plan of care for George should include:
   a. auscultating for abnormal breath sounds.
   b. inspecting for leg edema.
   c. weighing the patient daily.
   d. all of the above.

4. Nursing intervention for George should include all of the following *except:*

   a. administering diuretics, as prescribed, to help remove excess fluid.

   b. assisting the patient to a recumbent position to minimize his breathing effort.

   c. inspecting for sacral edema to note the degree of fluid retention.

   d. teaching dietary restriction of sodium to help decrease water retention.

CASE STUDY: Diabetes Mellitus

Isaac, 63 years old, was admitted to the hospital with a diagnosis of diabetes mellitus. On his admission, the nurse observed rapid respirations, confusion, and signs of dehydration.

1. Isaac's arterial blood gas values are as follows: pH, 7.27; HCO_3, 20 mEq/L; PaO_2, 33 mm Hg. These values are consistent with a diagnosis of compensated:

   a. metabolic acidosis.

   b. metabolic alkalosis.

   c. respiratory acidosis.

   d. respiratory alkalosis.

2. A manifestation *not* associated with altered acid–base balance is:

   a. bradycardia.

   b. hypertension.

   c. lethargy.

   d. hypokalemia.

3. In terms of cellular buffering response, the nurse should expect the major electrolyte disturbance to be:

   a. hyperkalemia.

   b. hypernatremia.

   c. hypocalcemia.

   d. hypokalemia.

4. The nurse should anticipate that the physician will attempt to reverse this acid–base imbalance by prescribing intravenous administration of:

   a. potassium chloride.

   b. potassium iodide.

   c. sodium bicarbonate.

   d. sodium chloride.

CHAPTER 15

Shock and Multisystem Failure

I. Interpretation, Completion, and Comparison

MULTIPLE CHOICE

Read each question carefully. Circle your answer.

1. Physiologic responses to all types of shock include all of the following *except*:
   a. activation of the inflammatory response.
   b. hypermetabolism.
   c. hypoperfusion of tissues.
   d. increased intravascular volume.

2. A patient's blood pressure is 110/70 mm Hg. What is his mean arterial pressure (MAP)?
   a. 65
   b. 73
   c. 83
   d. 91

3. Baroreceptors are a primary mechanism of blood pressure regulation which results from the initial stimulation of what type of receptors?
   a. chemical
   b. hormonal
   c. neural
   d. pressure

4. The initial stage of shock characterized by a normal blood pressure is the:
   a. initial stage.
   b. compensatory stage.
   c. progressive stage.
   d. irreversible stage.

5. The nurse knows to report an early indicator of compensatory shock such as a pulse pressure of:
   a. 25 mm Hg.
   b. 40 mm Hg.
   c. 55 mm Hg.
   d. 70 mm Hg.

6. In progressive stage shock, clinical hypotension is present if the systematic blood pressure is:
   a. 85 mm Hg.
   b. 90 mm Hg.
   c. 95 mm Hg.
   d. 100 mm Hg.

7. The nurse assesses a patient in compensatory shock whose lungs have decompensated. The nurse would *not* expect to find which of the following symptoms?
   a. a heart rate greater than 100 bpm
   b. crackles
   c. lethargy and mental confusion
   d. respirations fewer than 15 breaths/min

8. Oliguria occurs in the progressive stage of shock because the kidneys decompensate. To assess for this condition, the nurse should look for which of the following signs or symptoms?
   a. congestive heart failure
   b. decreased capillary permeability and localized edema
   c. increased blood urea nitrogen and serum creatinine
   d. systolic blood pressure greater than 120 mm Hg

9. Hematologic system changes in progressive shock would *not* be characterized by:
   a. generalized hypoxemia.
   b. hypertension.
   c. metabolic acidosis.
   d. sluggish blood flow.

10. The nurse would expect acute renal failure to develop when the mean arterial pressure (MAP) reaches:
    a. 65 mm Hg.
    b. 75 mm Hg.
    c. 80 mm Hg.
    d. 90 mm Hg.

11. Depleted adenosine triphosphate (ATP) stores and multiple organ failure are characteristic of which stage of shock?
    a. initial stage
    b. compensatory stage
    c. progressive stage
    d. irreversible stage

12. Patients receiving fluid replacement should frequently be monitored for:
    a. adequate urinary output.
    b. changes in mental status.
    c. vital sign stability.
    d. all of the above.

13. The most commonly used colloidal solution to treat hypovolemic shock is:
    a. blood products.
    b. 5% albumin.
    c. 6% dextran.
    d. 6% hetastarch.

14. Vasoactive agents are effective in treating shock because of their ability to:
    a. decrease blood pressure.
    b. decrease stroke volume.
    c. increase cardiac output.
    d. increase cardiac preload.

15. A common vasoactive agent used to improve cardiac contractility is:
    a. dopamine.
    b. epinephrine.
    c. nitroprusside.
    d. phenylephrine.

16. Hypovolemic shock occurs when intravascular volume decreases by:
    a. 5% to 10%.
    b. 15% to 25%.
    c. 30% to 50%.
    d. more than 60%.

17. Coronary cardiogenic shock is seen primarily in patients with:
    a. cardiomyopathies.
    b. dysrhythmias.
    c. myocardial infarction.
    d. valvular damage.

18. In cardiogenic shock, decreased cardiac contractility leads to all of the following compensatory responses *except:*
    a. decreased stroke volume.
    b. decreased tissue perfusion.
    c. increased stroke volume.
    d. pulmonary congestion.

19. The primary goal in treating cardiogenic shock is to:
    a. improve the heart's pumping mechanism.
    b. limit further myocardial damage.
    c. preserve the healthy myocardium.
    d. treat the oxygenation needs of the heart muscle.

20. The drug of choice for cardiac pain relief is intravenous:
    a. codeine.
    b. Demerol.
    c. Dilaudid.
    d. morphine.

21. Sympathomimetic drugs increase cardiac output by all of the following measures *except:*
    a. decreasing preload and afterload.
    b. increasing myocardial contractility.
    c. tachycardia.
    d. vasoconstriction.

22. The nurse assesses for the negative effect of intravenous nitroglycerin (Tridil) for shock management, which is:
    a. reduced preload.
    b. reduced afterload.
    c. increased cardiac output.
    d. increased blood pressure.

23. The vasoactive effects of dopamine are diminished when high doses are given, because vasoconstriction increases cardiac workload. Doses are titrated for therapeutic range. A *nontherapeutic* drug dose for a 154-lb (70-kg) man would be:
    a. 210 mg/min.
    b. 350 mg/min.
    c. 490 mg/min.
    d. 630 mg/min.

24. Intra-aortic balloon counterpulsation (IABC) is a mechanical, assistive device used as a temporary means of improving the heart's pumping ability. IABC is primarily meant to:
    a. decrease cardiac work.
    b. decrease stroke volume.
    c. increase preload.
    d. maintain current coronary circulation.

25. The primary cause of distributive shock is:
    a. arterial and venous dilatation.
    b. compromised cardiac contractility.
    c. decreased blood volume.
    d. obstructed blood flow.

26. A clinical sign of septic shock would *not* be:
    a. bradypnea.
    b. $PaCo_2$ less than 32 mm Hg.
    c. tachycardia.
    d. WBC count greater than 12,000 cells/mm^3

27. The sequence of organ failure in multiple-organ dysfunction syndrome (MODS) usually begins in the:
    a. heart.
    b. kidneys.
    c. liver.
    d. lungs.

SHORT ANSWER

Read each statement carefully. Write your response in the space provided.

1. The basic, underlying characteristic of shock is _____, which results in

   _____, _____, _____,

   _____, and _____.

2. Two other terms that are used to describe circulatory shock are _____ shock and

   _____ shock.

3. Energy metabolism occurs in the cells, where _____ is primarily responsible for

   cellular energy in the form of _____.

4. Define the term *mean arterial pressure (MAP):* _____

   _____

5. Baroreceptors are located in the _____ and _____, whereas

   chemoreceptors are located in the _____ and _____.

6. Shock progresses along a continuum of three stages: _____ (stage 1),

   _____ (stage 2), and _____ (stage 3).

7. A new cardiac marker, _____, which increases when the ventricle is overdistended,

   is being used to assess the cardiovascular effects of shock.

8. Two common intravenous fluids used for hypovolemic shock are _____ and

   _____.

9. The primary causes of circulatory shock are _____ and

   _____.

10. Neurogenic shock can be caused by _____, _____, or

    _____.

SCRAMBLEGRAM: SHOCK AND MULTISYSTEM FAILURE.

Read the definitions of the terms related to shock and multisystem failure. Find each term in the scramblegram and circle it. Terms may be written in any direction.

DEFINITIONS OF TERMS

1. A syndrome of inadequate blood flow to body tissues
2. Nutrients, chemically broken down within the cell, are stored in this form
3. Substance responsible for the conversion of angiotensin I
4. Hormone, secreted by the pituitary gland, that causes the kidneys to retain fluid
5. Insufficient oxygenation of the blood
6. The degree of stretch of cardiac muscle before its contraction
7. Urinary output of less than 30 mL/h
8. A colloid that rapidly expands plasma volume
9. A popular vasoactive agent that improves cardiac contractility
10. The most common type of distributive shock
11. A central line used to monitor venous pressure
12. The most common side effect of fluid replacement in shock
13. These solutions are used to expand intravascular volume in shock
14. Multiple organ failure usually begins in this organ
15. A vasodilator used to reduce the heart's demand for oxygen in conditions of shock

D	A	O	L	E	R	P	B	D	F	H	R
B	L	C	F	I	L	U	M	P	R	E	T
C	B	A	J	A	R	L	D	G	N	H	G
Y	U	D	K	S	E	M	J	I	L	F	K
L	M	G	W	F	B	O	N	E	D	N	O
M	I	S	P	T	G	N	S	G	N	U	L
A	N	D	T	C	R	A	R	M	I	H	I
I	V	I	A	D	H	Y	I	R	P	D	G
M	L	O	R	O	C	Y	P	J	R	K	U
E	A	L	T	P	X	E	L	S	I	O	R
X	C	L	B	A	I	D	M	N	D	M	I
O	S	O	K	M	W	E	S	O	E	P	A
P	V	C	O	I	L	M	A	H	K	I	F
Y	R	A	Q	N	F	A	N	T	O	C	P
H	T	R	C	E	S	E	P	T	I	C	J
C	K	G	P	N	W	T	U	C	M	B	K
F	H	J	M	E	S	B	M	E	D	I	A
H	A	D	G	K	O	R	H	L	O	B	F

MATCHING

Match the type of shock in column II with its associated cause listed in column I. An answer may be used more than once.

Column I

1. _____ Valvular damage
2. _____ Peritonitis
3. _____ Burns
4. _____ Bee sting allergy
5. _____ Immunosuppression
6. _____ Spinal cord injury
7. _____ Dysrhythmias
8. _____ Vomiting
9. _____ Pulmonary embolism
10. _____ Penicillin sensitivity

Column II

a. Hypovolemic, owing to an internal fluid shift
b. Hypovolemic, owing to an external fluid loss
c. Cardiogenic
d. Circulatory of a neurogenic nature
e. Circulatory of an anaphylactic nature
f. Circulatory of a septic nature
g. Noncoronary cardiogenic shock

II. Critical Thinking Questions and Exercises

IDENTIFYING PATTERNS

Chart the physiologic sequence of events.

Flow Chart: Blood Pressure Regulation Shock

A drop in blood pressure (baroreceptor response)

↓

release of _____ and _____ from _____

↓

_____ and _____ = _____.

↓

A drop in blood pressure (response by kidneys)

↓

release of the enzyme _____

↓

converts _____ to _____

↓

_____

↓

_____ from the adrenal cortex promotes retention of

↓

_____ and _____.

↓

Stimulates the release of _____ by the pituitary gland

↓

causes the kidneys to raise _____ and _____.

Flow Chart: Hypovolemic Shock

↓ _____ from hemorrhage or severe dehydration

results in

↓ _____ and ↓ _____

which causes

↓ _____ and ↓ _____

which leads to

↓ _____ and _____

CLINICAL SITUATIONS

Read the following case studies. Fill in the blanks or circle the correct answer.

CASE STUDY: Hypovolemic Shock

Mr. Mazda is a 57-year-old, 154-lb (70-kg) patient, who was received on the nursing unit from the recovery room after having a hemicolectomy for colon cancer. On initial assessment, Mr. Mazda was alert, yet anxious; his skin was cool, pale, and moist; and his abdominal dressings were saturated with bright red blood. Urinary output was 100 mL over 4 hours. The patient was receiving 1000 mL of lactated Ringer's solution. Vital signs were as follows: blood pressure, 80/60 mm Hg; heart rate, 126 bpm; and respirations 40 breaths/min. (Baseline vital signs were 130/70, 84, and 22, respectively.). The nurse assessed that the patient was experiencing hypovolemic shock.

1. The nurse understands that hypovolemic shock will occur with an intravascular volume reduction of 15% to 25%. Therefore, the nurse determines that Mr. Mazda, who weighs 70 kg, has probably lost:

   a. 200 mL of blood.   c. 500 mL of blood.

   b. 300 mL of blood.   d. 750 mL of blood.

2. The nurse knows to monitor vital signs every 5 to 15 minutes and to be concerned about the patient's pulse pressure of _____.

3. The nurse knows that the progressive pattern of changes in vital signs is more important than the exact readings. A _____ in pulse rate, followed by a _____ in blood pressure, is indicative of shock.

4. The nurse understands that a systolic reading of 80 mm Hg is serious, because a systolic reading lower than _____ mm Hg in a normotensive person indicates well-advanced shock.

5. Urinary output will be measured hourly. An output of less than _____ mL/h is indicative of decreased glomerular filtration.

6. Nursing interventions include notifying the physician, reinforcing the abdominal dressings, and treating the patient for shock by administering fluids ordered, such as:

   a. _____

   b. _____

   c. _____

CASE STUDY: Septic Shock

Mr. Dressler, a 43-year-old Caucasian, was admitted to the medical-surgical unit on the third postoperative day after a vertical bonded gastroplasty for morbid obesity. He had initially transferred to the intensive care unit from the recovery room. Mr. Dressler had a normal postoperative recovery period until his first afternoon on the unit. The RN went into his room to assess 4 PM vital signs and noted that his temperature was 102°F, he was shaking with chills, his skin was warm and dry, yet his extremities were cool to the touch. The nurse, assessing that Mr. Dressler was probably experiencing septicemia, immediately notified the physician.

Answer the following questions based on your knowledge of septicemia and shock.

1. Septic shock is most commonly caused by gram-negative organisms. Give an example of a common gram-negative bacteria: _____.

2. The nurse knows that the mortality rate associated with septic shock is between _____% and _____%.

3. The nurse expects that the physician will request body fluid specimens for culture and sensitivity tests. The nurse prepares to collect specimens of: _____, _____, _____, and _____.

4. Four modalities of treatment are essential to manage the septic shock: _____, _____, _____, and _____.

5. The two most common and serious side effects of fluid replacement are: _____ and _____.

6. A central venous pressure line (CVP) helps monitor fluid replacement. A normal CVP value is: _____.

CHAPTER 16

Oncology: Nursing Management in Cancer Care

I. Interpretation, Completion, and Comparison

MULTIPLE CHOICE

Read each question carefully. Circle your answer.

1. As a cause of death in the United States, cancer ranks:
   a. first.
   b. second.
   c. third.
   d. fourth.

2. Cancer mortality in the United States is highest among:
   a. African Americans.
   b. American Indians.
   c. Caucasians.
   d. Hispanics.

3. The etiology of cancer can be associated with specific agents or factors such as:
   a. dietary and genetic factors.
   b. hormonal and chemical agents.
   c. viruses.
   d. all of the above.

4. David, age 67 years, is admitted for diagnostic studies to rule out cancer. He is white, has been employed as a landscaper for 40 years, and has a 36-year history of smoking one pack of cigarettes a day. David has three risk factors associated with the development of cancer. Choose the *least* significant risk factor among the following:
   a. age
   b. sex
   c. occupation
   d. race

5. Cancer cells can affect the immune system by:
   a. stimulating the release of T lymphocytes into the circulation.
   b. suppressing the patient's natural defenses.
   c. mobilizing macrophages.
   d. all of the above.

6. To reduce nitrate intake because of possible carcinogenic action, the nurse suggests that a patient decrease his or her intake of:
   a. eggs and milk.
   b. fish and poultry.
   c. ham and bacon.
   d. green, leafy vegetables.

7. An endoscopic procedure can be used to remove an entire piece of suspicious tissue growth. The diagnostic biopsy method used for this procedure is known as:
   a. excisional biopsy.
   b. incisional biopsy.
   c. needle biopsy.
   d. staging.

8. A patient is admitted for an excisional biopsy of a breast lesion. The nurse should do all of the following *except:*

   a. clarify information provided by the physician.

   b. provide aseptic care to the incision postoperatively.

   c. provide time for the patient to discuss her concerns.

   d. counsel the patient about the possibility of losing her breast.

9. Surgery done to remove lesions that are likely to develop into cancer is known as:

   a. diagnostic.

   b. palliative.

   c. prophylactic.

   d. reconstructive.

10. An example of palliative surgery is a:

    a. colectomy.

    b. cordotomy.

    c. mastectomy.

    d. nephrectomy.

11. The *incorrect* rationale for the effectiveness of radiation therapy is its ability to:

    a. cause cell death.

    b. break the strands of the DNA helix.

    c. disrupt mitosis by slowing dividing cells.

    d. interrupt cellular growth when a nonsurgical approach is needed.

12. Radiation therapy for the treatment of cancer is administered over several weeks to:

    a. allow time for the patient to cope with the treatment.

    b. allow time for the repair of healthy tissue.

    c. decrease the incidence of leukopenia and thrombocytopenia.

    d. accomplish all of the above.

13. A patient with uterine cancer is being treated with internal radiation therapy. A primary nursing responsibility is to:

    a. explain to the patient that she will continue to emit radiation for approximately 1 week after the implant is removed.

    b. maintain as much distance as possible from the patient while in the room.

    c. alert family members that they should restrict their visiting to 5 minutes at any one time.

    d. wear a lead apron when providing direct patient care.

14. A major disadvantage of chemotherapy is that it:

    a. attacks cancer cells during their vulnerable phase.

    b. functions against disseminated disease.

    c. is systemic.

    d. targets normal body cells as well as cancer cells.

15. When a patient takes vincristine, a plant alkaloid, the nurse should assess for symptoms of toxicity affecting the:

    a. gastrointestinal system.

    b. nervous system.

    c. pulmonary system.

    d. urinary system.

16. Initial nursing action for extravasation of a chemotherapeutic agent includes all of the following *except:*

    a. applying warm compresses to the phlebitic area.

    b. immediately discontinuing the infusion.

    c. injecting an antidote, if required.

    d. placing ice over the site of infiltration.

17. Realizing that chemotherapy can result in renal damage, the nurse should:
    a. encourage fluid intake to dilute the urine.
    b. take measures to acidify the urine and thus prevent uric acid crystallization.
    c. withhold medication when the blood urea nitrogen level exceeds 20 mg/dL.
    d. limit fluids to 1000 mL daily to prevent accumulation of the drugs' end products after cell lysis.

18. Allopurinol may be prescribed for a patient who is receiving chemotherapy to:
    a. stimulate the immune system against the tumor cells.
    b. treat drug-related anemia.
    c. prevent alopecia.
    d. lower serum and urine uric acid levels.

19. The use of hyperthermia as a treatment modality for cancer may cause:
    a. fatigue, nausea, and vomiting.
    b. hypotension, skin burn, and tissue damage.
    c. thrombophlebitis, diarrhea, and peripheral neuropathies.
    d. all of the above side effects.

20. Bacille Calmette-Guerin (BCG) is a nonspecific biologic response modifier that is a standard form of treatment for cancer of the:
    a. bladder.
    b. breast.
    c. lungs.
    d. skin.

21. The nurse should assess a cancer patient's nutritional status by:
    a. weighing the patient daily.
    b. monitoring daily calorie intake.
    c. observing for proper wound healing.
    d. doing all of the above.

22. The most frequently occurring gram-positive cause of infection in cancer patients is:
    a. *Candida albicans.*
    b. *Escherichia coli.*
    c. *Pseudomonas aeruginosa.*
    d. *Staphylococcus.*

23. The most common cause of bleeding in cancer patients is:
    a. anemia.
    b. coagulation disorders.
    c. hypoxemia.
    d. thrombocytopenia.

DEFINE

Write the definition for each of the following words.

1. anaplasia _____

2. alopecia _____

3. carcinogenesis _____

4. cytokines _____

5. metastasis _____

6. nadir _____

7. vesicant _____

8. xerostomia _____

SHORT ANSWER

Read each statement carefully. Write your response in the space provided.

1. List in order of frequency the three leading causes of cancer deaths in the United States.

Men

   a. _____

   b. _____

   c. _____

Women

   a. _____

   b. _____

   c. _____

2. Define, in very simple language, the cause of cancer: _____

   _____

   _____

3. List two significant tumor-specific antigens present in cancer cells that help with diagnosis and treatment:

   _____

   _____

4. About _____% of all cancers are thought to be related to the environment around us.

5. The single most lethal chemical carcinogen is _____.

6. List four cancers that are associated with familial inheritance.

   _____

   _____

   _____

   _____

7. Three cruciferous vegetables that appear to reduce cancer risk are _____,
   _____, and _____, whereas three dietary substances that
   tend to increase the risk of cancer are _____, _____,
   _____, and _____.

8. Identify five substances produced by the immune system in response to cancer cells:

   _____

   _____

   _____

   _____

   _____

9. Toxicity occurs with radiation therapy. For each of the following, list three common side effects of radiation therapy.

  a. Skin: _____, _____, and _____.

  b. Oral mucosal membrane: _____, _____, and

   _____.

  c. Stomach or colon: _____, _____, and

   _____.

  d. Bone marrow-producing sites: _____, _____, and

   _____.

10. List five signs that indicate that an extravasation of an infusion of a cancer chemotherapeutic agent has occurred.

   _____

   _____

   _____

   _____

   _____

11. The two most common side effects of chemotherapy are: _____ and

   _____.

MATCHING

Match the type of neoplasm in column II with its associated description listed in column I.

Column I

1. _____ Cells bear little resemblance to the normal cells of the tissue from which they arose.

2. _____ Rate of growth is usually slow.

3. _____ Tumor tissue is encapsulated.

4. _____ Tumor spreads by way of blood and lymph channels to other areas of the body.

5. _____ Growth tends to recur when removed.

Column II

a. Benign

b. Malignant

Match the drug category in column II with an associated antineoplastic agent listed in column I; write the letter in the space provided. Then, for each drug, list a common side effect. An answer may be used more than once. Refer to Table 16-6 in the text.

Column I

1. _____ vincristine (VCR) _____

2. _____ 5-fluorouracil (5-FU) _____

3. _____ cisplatin _____

4. _____ estrogens _____

5. _____ thiotepa _____

6. _____ lomustine (CCNU) _____

7. _____ doxorubicin _____

8. _____ ifosfamide _____

9. _____ methotrexate _____

10. _____ asparaginase _____

Column II

a. alkylating agent

b. nitrosourea

c. antimetabolite

d. antitumor antibiotic

e. plant alkaloid/natural product

f. hormonal agent

g. miscellaneous agent

II. Critical Thinking Questions and Exercises

DISCUSSION AND ANALYSIS

Discuss the following topics with your classmates.

1. Distinguish between the terms *invasion* and *metastasis* as they relate to the spread of cancerous cells.
2. Distinguish between primary and secondary prevention of cancer, and provide an example of how nurses can participate in both types of prevention.
3. Distinguish between three diagnostic tests used to detect cancer: magnetic resonance imaging (MRI), computed tomography (CT), and positron emission tomography (PET).
4. Explain the modes of action for the following two classifications of chemotherapeutic agents: cell cycle–specific and cell cycle–nonspecific.
5. Describe the role of interferons in the treatment of cancer.
6. Discuss the nurse's role in managing the side effects of chemotherapy.
7. Select at least three nursing diagnoses and collaborative problems for patients with cancer and discuss nursing interventions for treatment.

EXAMINING ASSOCIATIONS

Read each analogy. Write the best response in the space provided.

1. Primary cancer prevention : preventing or reducing the risk of cancer :: Secondary prevention :

   _____.

2. Staging of tumor cells : tumor size and existence of metastasis :: Grading :

   _____.

3. Excisional biopsy : malignant melanoma :: _____ biopsy : prostate cancer.

4. Oophorectomy : prophylactic surgery :: Abdominal shunt placement : _____ surgery.

5. Allogenic bone marrow transplant : an unrelated donor :: Syngenic bone marrow transplant : _____.

6. Cytokines : interferons :: lymphokines : _____.

7. Stomatitis : oral tissue inflammation :: Alopecia : _____.

8. Anorexia : loss of appetite :: Cachexia : _____.

9. Streptococcus : gram positive :: _____ : gram negative.

10. Avastin : metastatic colorectal cancer :: Mylotarg : _____.

CLINICAL SITUATIONS

Read the following case studies. Fill in the space or circle the correct answer.

CASE STUDY: Cancer of the Breast

Kim is a 45-year-old mother of four who, after a needle aspiration biopsy, is diagnosed as having a malignant breast tumor, stage III. She was scheduled for a modified radical mastectomy. On assessment, her breast tissue had a dimpling or "orange-peel" appearance. Nursing diagnoses included (a) Fear and ineffective coping related to the diagnosis and (b) Disturbance in self-concept related to the nature of the surgery.

1. Realizing that Kim's mother died of breast cancer, the nurse correlates the cause of Kim's diagnosis to:
   a. environmental factors.
   b. genetics.
   c. dietary factors.
   d. chemical agents.

2. To assist Kim in adapting to the loss of her breast, the nurse should assess Kim's:
   a. attitude toward her body image.
   b. feelings of self-esteem.
   c. social and sexual values.
   d. attitudes and values regarding all of the above.

3. Kim's husband refuses to participate in any discussion about his wife's diagnosis. The nurse realizes that he is using the defense mechanism of:
   a. denial.
   b. depression.
   c. rationalization.
   d. repression.

4. Postoperatively, Kim experiences severe incisional pain. The nurse realizes that Kim's perception of pain is possibly influenced by:
   a. tissue manipulation during surgery.
   b. apprehension regarding the prognosis of her condition.
   c. anger stemming from her change in body image.
   d. all of the above.

5. Kim is scheduled to begin radiation therapy, followed by chemotherapy with 5-fluorouracil. Realizing the side effects of radiation therapy, the nurse should prepare Kim for all of the following *except*:
   a. her lungs may possibly produce more mucus.
   b. the skin at the treatment area may become red and inflamed.
   c. she may tire more easily and require additional rest periods.
   d. alopecia will occur as a result of the quickly growing hair follicles.

6. The nurse should teach Kim what she can do to protect her skin between radiation treatments. Measures include all of the following *except*:

a. handle the area gently.

b. avoid irritation with soap and water.

c. use a heat lamp once a day directed to the radiation site to promote tissue repair.

d. wear loose-fitting clothing.

7. After radiation therapy, Kim begins a regimen of chemotherapy with 5-fluorouracil. Three weeks after treatment begins, Kim develops a fever, sore throat, and cold symptoms. The nurse knows that Kim's symptoms could be due to all of the following *except*:

a. hypercalcemia.

b. bone marrow depression.

c. altered nutrition.

d. leukopenia.

8. Nursing assessment during Kim's chemotherapy includes observing for:

a. evidence of stomatitis.

b. renal and hepatic abnormalities.

c. symptoms of infection owing to granulocytopenia.

d. all of the above.

9. Kim is diagnosed as having thrombocytopenia. The nurse should assess for all of the following *except*:

a. hematuria.

b. fever.

c. hematemesis.

d. ecchymosis.

CASE STUDY: Cancer of the Lung

Mr. Donato is a 48-year-old accountant who has been a one-pack-a-day smoker for 23 years. He has had a persistent cough for 1 year that is hacking and nonproductive and has had repeated unresolved upper respiratory tract infections. He went to see his physician because he was fatigued, had been anorexic, and had lost 12 pounds over the last 3 months. Diagnostic evaluation led to the diagnosis of a localized tumor with no evidence of metastatic spread. Mr. Donato is scheduled for a lobectomy in 3 days.

1. Because infection is the leading cause of mortality in the oncology population, the nurse preoperatively notes the significance of:

a. a basophil count of 1.3%.

b. an eosinophil count of 4.5%.

c. a lymphocyte count of 23%.

d. a neutrophil count of 20%.

2. The nurse is concerned that the patient's nutritional status is compromised based on his recent weight loss. Impaired nutritional status contributes to _____, _____, _____, and _____.

3. List five factors that the nurse would assess to determine the patient's experience with pain, in order to develop a plan of care for pain management.

_____

_____

_____

_____

_____

4. The nurse knows that a diagnosis of cancer is accompanied by grieving. Usually the first reaction in the grieving process is:

   a. bargaining.

   b. acceptance.

   c. denial.

   d. depression.

5. List four activities the nurse can do to support the patient and family during the grieving process.

   _____

   _____

   _____

   _____

6. The nurse knows that postoperative care needs to be directed toward the prevention of _____, the leading cause of death in cancer patients.

7. Two major gram-negative bacilli that cause infection in an immunosuppressed patient are _____ and _____.

8. The nurse will also assess for the postoperative complication of septic shock, which is associated with all of the following *except:*

   a. dysrhythmias.

   b. hypertension.

   c. metabolic acidosis.

   d. oliguria.

CHAPTER **17**

End-of-Life Care

I. Interpretation, Completion, and Comparison

MULTIPLE CHOICE

Read each question carefully. Circle your answer.

1. The major causes of death in this century are diseases of what type?
   a. communicable
   b. degenerative
   c. genetic
   d. infectious

2. A common, initial patient response to the seriousness of a terminal illness is:
   a. acceptance.
   b. anger.
   c. denial.
   d. bargaining.

3. The only state in the United States that has legalized assisted suicide (1994) is:
   a. California.
   b. Colorado.
   c. Oregon.
   d. Vermont.

4. Patients enrolled in hospice care are terminally ill with a life expectancy of about:
   a. 3 months.
   b. 6 months.
   c. 6 to 9 months.
   d. 1 year.

5. Hospice care is utilized by about what percentage of eligible patients?
   a. 15%
   b. 30%
   c. 50%
   d. 75%

6. When a person authorizes another to make medical decisions on his or her behalf, the person has written:
   a. an advance directive.
   b. a living will.
   c. a standard addendum to a will.
   d. a proxy directive.

7. A dying patient wants to talk to the nurse about his fears. The patient states, "I know I'm dying, aren't I?" An appropriate nursing response would be:
   a. "This must be very difficult for you."
   b. "Tell me more about what's on your mind."
   c. "I'm so sorry. I know just how you feel."
   d. "You know you're dying?"

8. One of the most common and feared responses to terminal illness is:
   a. anorexia.
   b. cachexia.
   c. dyspnea.
   d. pain.

9. The anorexia-cachexia syndrome that is common toward the end of life is characterized by:

a. anemia.

b. alterations in carbohydrate metabolism.

c. endocrine dysfunction.

d. all of the above, plus altered fat and altered protein metabolism.

SHORT ANSWER

Read each statement carefully. Write your response in the space provided.

1. Dr. _____, who spearheaded a movement to increase awareness of the dying process among health care practitioners, published a landmark book, _____, in 1969.

2. Distinguish between the terms *assisted suicide* and *physician-assisted suicide:* _____
   _____

3. Define the terms *palliative care* and *hospice care:* _____
   _____

4. The concept of hospice care was originally implemented in the country of _____ by Dr. _____, who founded the world-renowned _____.

5. The first hospice program in the United States began in the state of _____ in the year _____.

6. The Medicare Hospice Benefit was implemented to cover hospice care for Medicare beneficiaries. Its benefits were recently expanded in the year _____.

7. Two types of medications that are routinely used to treat the underlying obstructive pathology associated with dyspnea are _____ and _____.

8. List four medications that are commonly used to stimulate appetite in anorexic patients.

   _____

   _____

   _____

   _____

II. Critical Thinking Questions and Exercises

DISCUSSION AND ANALYSIS

Discuss the following topics with your classmates.

1. Discuss the following major ethical question: "Because medical professionals can prolong life through a particular intervention, does it necessarily follow that they must do so?"
2. Explain how Dr. Kubler-Ross's work helped the medical and nursing community view the dying process in a more personalized way.
3. Explain the position of the American Nurses Association on the role of nursing and assisted suicide.

4. Distinguish between the terms *living will* and *durable power of attorney*.

5. How a person and his or her family cope with the dying process is influenced by many cultural, psychological, and socioeconomic factors. Analyze the role of the nurse in assessing values, preferences, and practices for a patient influenced by the Western culture of autonomy over care decisions and for a patient influenced by an Eastern culture of interdependence with care decisions.

6. Consider a recent clinical experience involving a dying patient. Draft an outline of nursing interventions that were or could have been used to support the patient's ability to maintain "hope" within the context of realism for the patient.

7. Review Dr. Kubler-Ross's five stages of dying and discuss nursing implications for each stage. Use some recent clinical examples if possible.

CHAPTER 18

Preoperative Nursing Management

I. Interpretation, Comparison, and Completion

MULTIPLE CHOICE

Read each question carefully. Circle your answer.

1. An example of a surgical procedure classified as urgent is:
   a. an appendectomy.
   b. an exploratory laparotomy.
   c. a repair of multiple stab wounds.
   d. a face lift.

2. A mammoplasty would be classified as surgery that is:
   a. urgent.
   b. optional.
   c. required.
   d. reconstructive.

3. An informed consent is required for:
   a. closed reduction of a fracture.
   b. insertion of an intravenous catheter.
   c. irrigation of the external ear canal.
   d. urethral catheterization.

4. Protein replacement for nutritional balance can be accomplished with a diet that:
   a. is high in carbohydrates.
   b. is high in protein.
   c. is low in fats.
   d. includes all of the above.

5. A significant mortality rate exists for those alcoholics who experience "delirium tremens" postoperatively. When caring for the alcoholic, the nurse should assess for symptoms of alcoholic withdrawal:
   a. within the first 12 hours.
   b. about 24 hours postoperatively.
   c. on the second or third day.
   d. 4 days after surgery.

6. It is recommended that those who smoke cigarettes should stop smoking how long before surgery?
   a. at least 2 months
   b. at least 3 months
   c. at least 2 weeks
   d. at least 3 weeks

7. Because liver disease is associated with a high surgical mortality rate, the nurse knows to alert the physician for:
   a. a blood ammonia concentration of 180 mg/dL.
   b. a lactate dehydrogenase concentration of 300 U/L.
   c. a serum albumin concentration of 5.0 g/dL.
   d. a serum globulin concentration of 2.8 g/dL.

8. Surgery would be contraindicated for a renal patient with:
   a. a blood urea nitrogen level of 42 mg/dL.
   b. a creatine kinase level of 120 U/L.
   c. a serum creatinine level of 0.9 mg/dL.
   d. a urine creatinine level of 1.2 mg/dL.

9. The chief life-threatening hazard for surgical patients with uncontrolled diabetes is:
   a. dehydration.
   b. hypertension.
   c. hypoglycemia.
   d. glucosuria.

10. The goal for the diabetic patient undergoing surgery is to maintain a blood glucose level of:
    a. 140 to 200 mg/dL.
    b. 200 to 240 mg/dL.
    c. 250 to 300 mg/dL.
    d. 300 to 350 mg/dL.

11. A nursing history of prior drug therapy is based on the particular concern that:
    a. phenothiazines may increase the hypotensive action of anesthetics.
    b. thiazide diuretics may cause excessive respiratory depression during anesthesia.
    c. tranquilizers may cause anxiety and even seizures if withdrawn suddenly.
    d. all of the above potential complications could occur.

12. The potential effects of medication therapy must be evaluated before surgery. A drug classification that can cause electrolyte imbalance is:
    a. corticosteroids.
    * b. diuretics.
    c. phenothiazines.
    d. insulin.

13. Assessment of a gerontologic patient reveals bilateral dimmed vision. This information alerts the nurse to plan for:
    a. a safe environment.
    b. restrictions of the patient's unassisted mobility activities.
    c. probable cataract extractions.
    d. referral to an ophthalmologist.

14. Hazards of surgery for the geriatric patient are directly related to the:
    a. number of coexisting health problems.
    b. type of surgical procedure.
    c. severity of the surgery.
    d. all of the above.

15. Obesity is positively correlated with surgical complications of:
    a. the cardiovascular system.
    b. the gastrointestinal system.
    c. the pulmonary system.
    d. all of the systems listed.

16. The purpose of the nursing goal of encouraging postoperative body movement is:
    a. to contribute to optimal respiratory function.
    b. to improve circulation.
    c. to prevent venous stasis.
    d. all of the above.

17. Food and water are usually withheld beginning at midnight of the surgical day. However, if necessary, water may be given up to:
    a. 8 hours before surgery.
    b. 6 hours before surgery.
    c. 4 hours before surgery.
    d. 2 hours before surgery.

18. The primary goal in withholding food before surgery is to prevent:
    a. aspiration.
    b. distention.
    c. infection.
    d. obstruction.

19. Expected patient outcomes for relief of anxiety related to a surgical procedure include all of the following *except:*

   * a. understands the nature of the surgery and voluntarily signs an informed consent.
   b. verbalizes an understanding of the preanesthetic medication.
   c. requests a visit with a member of the clergy.
   d. questions the anesthesiologist about anesthesia-related concerns.

20. Choose a statement that indicates that a patient is knowledgeable about his or her impending surgery. The patient:

   * a. participates willingly in the preoperative preparation.
   b. discusses stress factors that are making him or her depressed.
   c. expresses concern about postoperative pain.
   d. verbalizes his or her fears to family.

21. Hidden fears may be indicated when a patient:

   a. avoids communication.
   b. repeatedly asks questions that have previously been answered.
   c. talks incessantly.
   d. does all of the above.

22. Choose the appropriate response to the statement, "I'm so nervous about my surgery."

   a. "Relax. Your recovery period will be shorter if you're less nervous."
   b. "Stop worrying. It only makes you more nervous."
   c. "You needn't worry. Your doctor has done this surgery many times before."
   * d. "You seem nervous about your surgery."

23. The purpose of preoperative skin preparation is:

   a. to reduce the number of microorganisms.
   b. to remove all resident bacteria.
   c. to render the skin sterile.
   d. all of the above.

24. The *least* desirable method of hair removal is use of:

   a. electric clippers.
   b. a depilatory cream in nonsensitive patients.
   c. a razor with an extruded blade.
   d. scissors for long hair (more than 3 mm).

25. Purposes of preanesthetic medication include all of the following *except:*

   a. facilitation of anesthesia induction.
   b. lowering of the dose of the anesthetic agent used.
   c. potentiation of the effects of anesthesia.
   d. reduction of preoperative pain.

SHORT ANSWER

Read each statement carefully. Write your response in the space provided.

1. The preoperative phase begins _____ and ends when the patient _____.

2. The intraoperative phase begins when the patient _____ and ends when _____.

3. Informed consent for a surgical procedure is necessary when a procedure meets the following four

   conditions: _____, _____, _____, and

   _____.

4. Diabetics undergoing surgery are at risk for four complications: _____,

   _____, _____, and _____.

5. Aspirin is withheld _____ days before surgery, if possible, because it acts by

   _____.

6. List three significant nutritional concerns for the elderly surgical patient.

   _____

   _____

   _____

7. Name three primary goals necessary to promote postoperative mobility.

   _____

   _____

   _____

8. List the seven primary National Patient Safety Goals as issued by JCAH (2005).

   a. _____

   b. _____

   c. _____

   d. _____

   e. _____

   f. _____

   g. _____

MATCHING

Match the nutrient in column II with its associated rationale for use listed in column I.

Column I

1. _____ Essential for normal blood clotting
2. _____ Allows collagen deposition to occur
3. _____ Necessary for DNA synthesis
4. _____ Increases inflammatory response in wounds
5. _____ Vital for capillary formation

Column II

a. Protein
b. Vitamin C
c. Vitamin A
d. Vitamin K
e. Zinc

II. Critical Thinking Questions and Exercises

EXAMINING ASSOCIATIONS

Medication Administration

For each drug classification, list the potential effects of interaction with anesthetics.

1. Anticoagulants _____
2. Antiseizure agents _____
3. Corticosteroids _____
4. Diuretics _____
5. Insulin _____
6. Phenothiazines _____
7. Tranquilizers _____
8. Monoamine oxidase inhibitors (MAO) _____

Preoperative Nursing

For each essential preoperative nursing activity, write an appropriate nursing goal. An example is provided.

1. (Example) Restriction of nutrition and fluids   Prevent aspiration
2. Intestinal preparation _____
3. Preoperative skin preparation (cleansing) _____
4. Urinary catheterization _____
5. Administration of preoperative medications _____
6. Transportation of patient to presurgical suite _____

CLINICAL APPLICATIONS

Please refer to Chart 18-4 in the text. List five preoperative teaching points the nurse would cover to instruct a patient (1) how to cough correctly and (2) how to perform leg exercises to prevent postoperative complication.

Splinting When Coughing

a. _____

b. _____

c. _____

d. _____

e. _____

Leg Exercises

a. _____

b. _____

c. _____

d. _____

e. _____

CHAPTER 19

Intraoperative Nursing Management

I. Interpretation, Completion, and Comparison

MULTIPLE CHOICE

Read each question carefully. Circle your answer.

1. The circulating nurse's responsibilities, in contrast to the scrub nurse's responsibilities, include:
   a. assisting the surgeon.
   b. monitoring the surgical team.
   c. setting up the sterile tables.
   d. all of the above functions.

2. Preoperatively, an anesthesiologist is responsible for:
   a. assessing pulmonary status.
   b. inquiring about preexisting pulmonary infections.
   c. knowing the patient's history of smoking.
   d. all of the above.

3. The anesthesiologist classifies a person's physical status for anesthesia before surgery. There are six classifications a nurse knows that a preoperative classification of II refers to patients with:
   a. mild systemic disease.
   b. no systemic abnormality.
   c. severe systemic disease.
   d. an incapacitating systemic disease.

4. A nurse knows that perioperative risks increase with age because:
   a. ciliary action decreases, reducing the cough reflex.
   b. fatty tissue increases, prolonging the effects of anesthesia.
   c. liver size decreases, reducing the metabolism of anesthetics.
   d. all of the above biologic changes exist.

5. The most commonly used inhalation gas anesthetic agent is:
   a. Ethrane.
   b. Florane.
   c. nitrous oxide.
   d. Ultrane.

6. The nurse should know that, postoperatively, a general anesthetic is primarily eliminated by:
   a. the kidneys.
   b. the lungs.
   c. the skin.
   d. all of these routes.

7. An example of a stable and safe nondepolarizing muscle relaxant is:
   a. Anectine (succinylcholine chloride).
   b. Norcuron (vecuronium bromide).
   c. Pavulon (pancuronium bromide).
   d. Syncurine (decamethonium).

8. An intravenous anesthetic that has a powerful respiratory depressant effect sufficient to cause apnea is:
   a. Amidate.
   b. Ketalar.
   c. Pentothal.
   d. Versed.

9. Postoperative nursing assessment for a patient who has received a depolarizing neuromuscular blocking agent includes careful monitoring of the:

a. cardiovascular system.

b. endocrine system.

c. gastrointestinal system.

d. genitourinary system.

10. A factor involved in post–spinal anesthesia headaches is the:

a. degree of patient hydration.

b. leakage of spinal fluid from the subarachnoid space.

c. size of the spinal needle used.

d. combination of the above mechanisms.

11. Epinephrine is often used in combination with a local infiltration anesthetic, because it:

a. causes vasoconstriction.

b. prevents rapid absorption of the anesthetic drug.

c. prolongs the local action of the anesthetic agent.

d. does all of the above.

12. A local infiltration anesthetic can last for up to:

a. 1 hour.

b. 3 hours.

c. 5 hours.

d. 7 hours.

13. Recent research has indicated that inadvertent hypothermia in gerontologic patients can be effectively and inexpensively prevented by:

a. placing the patient on a hyperthermia blanket.

b. maintaining environmental temperature at 37°C.

✳ c. covering the top of the patient's head with an ordinary plastic shower cap during anesthesia.

d. frequent massage of the extremities with warmed skin lotion.

14. The nurse caring for a patient who is at risk for malignant hyperthermia subsequent to general anesthesia would assess for the most frequent early sign of:

a. hypertension.

b. muscle rigidity ("tetany-like" movements).

c. oliguria.

✳ d. tachycardia.

15. If an operating room nurse is to assist a patient to the Trendelenburg position, she would place him:

a. flat on his back with his arms next to his sides.

b. on his back with his head lowered so that the plane of his body meets the horizontal on an angle.

c. on his back with his legs and thighs flexed at right angles.

d. on his side with his uppermost leg adducted and flexed at the knee.

SHORT ANSWER

Read each statement carefully. Write your response in the space provided.

1. Anesthesia dosage is reduced with age, because _____.

2. List four responsibilities of a Registered Nurse First Assistant (RNFA).

_____

_____

_____

_____

3. Five health hazards associated with the surgical environment are _____,
_____, _____, _____, and
_____.

4. The type of anesthesia most likely to be used for a patient undergoing a colonoscopy is
_____, and the most frequently used agents are _____ and
_____.

5. The anesthetic most commonly used for general anesthesia by intravenous injection is
_____, which can cause _____ as a serious, toxic side effect.

6. Spinal anesthesia is a conduction nerve block that occurs when a local anesthetic is injected into
_____.

7. The conduction block anesthesia commonly used in labor is the _____.

8. What nursing assessment indicates that a patient has recovered from the effects of spinal anesthesia?
_____

9. List six potential intraoperative complications:

_____

_____

_____

_____

_____

_____

10. With malignant hypothermia, the core body temperature can increase 1° to 2° every 5 minutes, reaching
or exceeding a body temperature of _____ degrees in a short amount of time.

MATCHING

Match the inhalation anesthetic agent in column II with its associated nursing implication listed in column I.

Column I

1. _____ Monitor for chest pain and stroke

2. _____ Monitor blood pressure frequently

3. _____ Observe for respiratory depression

4. _____ Monitor respirations closely

5. _____ Monitor for malignant hypothermia

Column II

a. Ethrane

b. Fluothane

c. Forane

d. Nitrous oxide

e. Suprane

Match the commonly used intravenous medication in column II with its associated common usage listed in column I.

Column I

1. _____ Sedation with regional anesthesia

2. _____ Hypnotic and anxiolytic

3. _____ Epidural infusion for postoperative analgesia

4. _____ Intubation and relaxation

Column II

a. Fentanyl

b. Midazolam

c. Pancuronium

d. Propofol

e. Rocuronium

II. Critical Thinking Questions and Exercises

DISCUSSION AND ANALYSIS

Discuss the following topics with your classmates.

1. Describe 10 potential adverse effects of surgery and anesthesia and their associated causes.
2. Explain why the elderly are at a higher risk of complications from anesthesia because of biologic changes that occur in later life.
3. Briefly describe the basic guidelines for maintaining surgical asepsis.
4. Explain what is meant by "anesthesia awareness."
5. Identify and discuss several nursing diagnoses for a patient during surgery.

RECOGNIZING CONTRADICTIONS

Rewrite each statement correctly. Underline the key concepts.

1. Older patients need more anesthetic agent to produce anesthesia, because they eliminate anesthetic agents more quickly.

   _____

2. A scrub nurse controls the environment, coordinates the activities of other personnel, and monitors the patient.

   _____

3. If there is any doubt about the sterility of an area, it is considered sterile.

   _____

4. A draped table is considered sterile from the top to the edge of the drapes.

   _____

5. Only the circulating nurse can extend an arm over the sterile area to deliver sterile supplies.

   _____

CLINICAL SITUATIONS

Read the following case studies. Circle the correct answer.

CASE STUDY: General Anesthesia

Anne, age 34, is in excellent health and is scheduled for open reduction of a fractured femur. The general anesthetic drugs to be used include enflurane and nitrous oxide.

1. The nurse knows that the advantages of enflurane (Ethrane) include all of the following *except*:
   a. fast recovery.
   b. low incidence of respiratory depression.
   c. potent analgesia.
   d. rapid induction.

2. The major disadvantage of nitrous oxide is its ability to cause:
   a. hypertension.
   b. hypoxia.
   c. liver damage.
   d. nausea and vomiting.

3. The major postoperative nursing assessment after administration of Ethrane is observation for:
   a. anuria.
   b. laryngospasm.
   c. respiratory depression.
   d. tachycardia.

CASE STUDY: Intravenous Anesthesia

Brian is scheduled to have a wisdom tooth extracted. The anesthetic agent of choice is thiopental sodium (Pentothal).

1. The nurse anticipates that the route of administration will be:
   a. by inhalation.
   b. by mask.
   c. intramuscular.
   d. intravenous.

2. The nurse is aware that after anesthetic administration, Brian will be unconscious in:
   a. 30 seconds.
   b. 60 seconds.
   c. 2 minutes.
   d. 3 minutes.

3. The chief danger with thiopental sodium is its:
   a. beta-adrenergic blocking action.
   b. depressant action on the respiratory system.
   c. nephrotoxicity.
   d. rapid onset and prolonged duration.

CHAPTER 20

Postoperative Nursing Management

I. Interpretation, Completion, and Comparison

MULTIPLE CHOICE

Read each question carefully. Circle your answer.

1. The primary nursing goal in the immediate postoperative period is maintenance of pulmonary function and prevention of:
   a. laryngospasm.
   b. hyperventilation.
   * c. hypoxemia and hypercapnia.
   d. pulmonary edema and embolism.

2. Unless contraindicated, any unconscious patient should be positioned:
   a. flat on his or her back, without elevation of the head, to facilitate frequent turning and minimize pulmonary complications.
   b. in semi-Fowler's position, to promote respiratory function and reduce the incidence of orthostatic hypotension when the patient can eventually stand.
   c. in Fowler's position, which most closely simulates a sitting position, thus facilitating respiratory as well as gastrointestinal functioning.
   d. on his or her side with a pillow at the patient's back and his or her chin extended, to minimize the dangers of aspiration.

3. A major postoperative nursing responsibility is assessing for cardiovascular function by monitoring:
   a. arterial blood gases.
   b. central venous pressure.
   c. vital signs.
   d. all of the above.

4. In the immediate postoperative period, a nurse should immediately report:
   a. a systolic blood pressure lower than 90 mm Hg.
   b. a temperature reading between 97°F and 98°F.
   c. respirations between 20 and 25 breaths/min.
   d. all of the above assessments.

5. Patients remain in the recovery room or postanesthesia care unit (PACU) until they are fully recovered from anesthesia. This is evidenced by:
   a. a patent airway.
   b. a reasonable degree of consciousness.
   c. a stable blood pressure.
   * d. indication that all of the above have occurred.

6. When a PACU room scoring guide is used, a patient can be transferred out of the recovery room with a minimum score of:
   a. 5.
   b. 6.
   * c. 7.
   d. 8.

7. With the PACU room scoring guide, a nurse would give a patient an admission cardiovascular score of 2 if the patient's systolic arterial pressure is what percentage of his or her preanesthetic level?

   a. 80%
   b. 75% to 60%

   c. 60% to 50%
   d. less than 50%

8. When vomiting occurs postoperatively, the most important nursing intervention is to:

   a. measure the amount of vomitus to estimate fluid loss, in order to accurately monitor fluid balance.
   b. offer tepid water and juices to replace lost fluids and electrolytes.

   c. support the wound area so that unnecessary strain will not disrupt the integrity of the incision.
   d. turn the patient's head to prevent aspiration of vomitus into the lungs.

9. Postoperatively, the nurse monitors urinary function. An abnormal outcome that should be reported to the physician is a 2-hour output of:

   a. less than 30 mL.
   b. between 75 and 100 mL.

   c. between 100 and 200 mL.
   d. greater than 200 mL.

10. Most surgical patients are encouraged to be out of bed:

    a. within 6 to 8 hours after surgery.
    b. between 10 and 12 hours after surgery.

    c. as soon as it is indicated.
    d. on the second postoperative day.

11. The most common postoperative respiratory complication in elderly patients is:

    a. pleurisy.
    b. pneumonia.

    c. hypoxemia.
    d. pulmonary edema.

12. The proliferative stage of wound healing is characterized by:

    a. deposition of a fibrinoplatelet clot.
    b. histamine release and increased capillary permeability.

    c. fibroblast stimulation of collagen synthesis.
    d. scar formation.

13. A nurse wants to document the presence of granulation tissue in a healing wound. She describes the tissue as:

    a. necrotic and hard.
    b. pale yet able to blanch with digital pressure.

    c. pink to red and soft, noting that it bleeds easily.
    d. white with long, thin areas of scar tissue.

14. A physician's admitting note lists a wound as healing by second intention. The nurse expects to see:

    a. a deep, open wound that was previously sutured.
    b. a sutured incision with a little tissue reaction.

    c. a wound with a deep, wide scar that was previously resutured.
    d. a wound in which the edges were not approximated.

15. A wound that has hemorrhaged carries an increased risk of infection, because:

    a. reduced amounts of oxygen and nutrients are available.
    b. the tissue becomes less resilient.

    c. retrograde bacterial contamination may occur.
    d. dead space and dead cells provide a culture medium.

16. Postoperative abdominal distention seems to be directly related to:

    a. a temporary loss of peristalsis and gas accumulation in the intestines.
    b. beginning food intake in the immediate postoperative period.

    c. improper body positioning during the recovery period.
    d. the type of anesthetic administered.

17. A nursing measure for evisceration is to:

   a. apply an abdominal binder snugly so that the intestines can be slowly pushed back into the abdominal cavity.

   b. approximate the wound edges with adhesive tape so that the intestines can be gently pushed back into the abdomen.

   c. carefully push the exposed intestines back into the abdominal cavity.

   d. cover the protruding coils of intestines with sterile dressings moistened with sterile saline solution.

18. The characteristic sign of a paralytic ileus is:

   a. abdominal tightness.

   b. abdominal distention.

   c. absence of peristalsis.

   d. increased abdominal girth.

19. The most common postoperative nosocomial infections occur in the incisional area in what percentage of surgical patients?

   a. 5% to 15%

   b. 15% to 25%

   c. 25% to 50%

   d. approximately 67%

20. One of the major dangers associated with deep venous thrombosis is:

   a. pulmonary embolism.

   b. immobility because of calf pain.

   c. marked tenderness over the anteromedial surface of the thigh.

   d. swelling of the entire leg owing to edema.

21. Nursing measures to prevent thrombophlebitis include:

   a. assisting the patient with leg exercises.

   b. encouraging early ambulation.

   c. avoiding placement of pillows or blanket rolls under the patient's knees.

   d. all of the above.

22. One of the most effective nursing procedures for reducing nosocomial infections is:

   a. administration of prophylactic antibiotics.

   b. aseptic wound care.

   c. control of upper respiratory tract infections.

   d. proper hand-washing techniques.

23. The nurse recognizes that a clean-contaminated wound has a relative probability of infection of:

   a. 1% to 3%.

   b. 7% to 16%.

   c. 3% to 7%.

   d. more than 16%.

SHORT ANSWER

Read each statement carefully. Write your response in the space provided.

1. List five areas of concern for a recovery room PACU nurse who has just received a patient from the operating room.

   _____

   _____

   _____

   _____

   _____

2. The primary nursing priorities during immediate postoperative assessment are evaluation of
   _____.

3. Distinguish among the three classifications of hemorrhage (primary, intermediary, and secondary) and include the defining characteristics of each:

   Primary: _____

   Intermediary: _____

   Secondary: _____

4. The most serious and most frequent postoperative complications involve the _____ system.

5. List five potential postoperative complications.

   _____

   _____

   _____

   _____

   _____

6. Several psychological factors that can influence a patient's pain experience are: _____

   _____

   _____

   _____

7. Explain patient-controlled analgesia (PCA): _____

   _____

8. Explain why the postoperative complications of atelectasis and hypostatic pneumonia are reduced as a result of early ambulation: _____

   _____

9. Name three criteria that must be met before a postoperative patient can be given fluids.

   _____

   _____

   _____

10. The return of peristalsis in the postoperative period can be determined by the presence of
    _____ and _____, both of which are assessed by the nurse.

11. Distinguish between *wound dehiscence* and *evisceration*: _____

    _____

II. Critical Thinking Questions and Exercises

DISCUSSION AND ANALYSIS

Discuss the following topics with your classmates.

1. Discuss the system assessment that a nurse would need to perform in determining a patient's readiness for discharge from the PACU.
2. Explain how various factors (age, edema, nutritional deficits, oxygen deficit, medications, and systemic disorders) affect the progress of wound healing.
3. Review common nursing diagnoses and collaborative problems for the postoperative patient.
4. Describe three postoperative conditions that put a patient at risk for common respiratory complications.
5. Describe expected nursing interventions to treat hypopharyngeal obstruction.

IDENTIFYING PATTERNS

Read the case study. Fill in the spaces provided.

CASE STUDY: Postoperative Pain

Mr. Flynn's pain medication was frequently delayed because his staff nurses were busy with other patients. As a nursing supervisor, you emphasized the necessity of preventing or managing postoperative pain, knowing that there is a positive correlation between pain experience and the frequency of complications. Support your argument by filling in these blank spaces.

1. Pain stimulates _____, which increases _____ and _____.

2. Noxious impulses stimulate _____, which increases _____ and _____.

3. Hypothalamic stress responses increase _____ and _____, which can lead to _____ and _____.

CLINICAL SITUATIONS

Read the following case studies. Circle the correct answer.

CASE STUDY: Hypovolemic Shock

Mario is admitted to the emergency department with a diagnosis of hypovolemic shock secondary to a 30% blood volume loss resulting from a motorcycle accident.

1. A primary nursing objective is to:
   a. administer vasopressors.
   b. ensure a patent airway.
   c. minimize energy expenditure.
   d. provide external warmth.

2. With a diagnosis of hypovolemic shock, the nurse expects to assess all of the following *except*:
   a. a decreased and concentrated urinary output.
   b. an elevated central venous pressure reading.
   c. hypotension with a small pulse pressure.
   d. tachycardia and a thready pulse.

3. The nurse takes blood pressure readings every 5 minutes. She knows that shock is well advanced when the systolic pressure drops to less than:
   a. 90 mm Hg.
   b. 100 mm Hg.
   c. 110 mm Hg.
   d. 120 mm Hg.

4. A urinary catheter is inserted to measure hourly output. The nurse knows that inadequate volume replacement is reflected by an output of less than:
   a. 30 mL/h.
   b. 50 mL/h.
   c. 80 mL/h.
   d. 100 mL/h.

5. The physician prescribes crystalloid solution to be administered to restore blood volume. The nurse knows that a crystalloid solution is:
   a. a blood transfusion.
   b. lactated Ringer's solution.
   c. plasma or a plasma substitute.
   d. serum albumin.

CASE STUDY: Hypopharyngeal Obstruction

Daena is unconscious when she is transferred to the recovery room. She has experienced prolonged anesthesia, and all her muscles are relaxed.

1. During the initial assessment, the nurse diagnosed hypopharyngeal obstruction. This difficulty is signaled by:
   a. choking.
   b. cyanosis.
   c. irregular respirations.
   d. all of the above.

2. To treat hypopharyngeal obstruction, the nurse would:
   a. flex the neck and pull the lower jaw down toward the chest.
   b. hyperextend the neck and push forward on the angle of the lower jaw.
   c. raise the head and open the mouth as far as possible.
   d. rotate the head to either side and unclench the teeth.

3. The nurse knows that the most accurate way to determine whether Daena is breathing is to:
   a. auscultate for breath sounds.
   b. inspect for diaphragmatic movement.
   c. palpate for thoracic changes.
   d. place his or her palm over Daena's nose and mouth.

4. The anesthesiologist chose to leave a plastic airway in Daena's mouth. The nurse knows that an airway should not be removed:
   a. without a physician's order.
   b. until the patient's secretions have been aspirated.
   c. until signs indicate that reflexes are returning.
   d. until arterial blood gas measurements indicate adequate PO_2 levels.

CASE STUDY: Wound Healing

Elizabeth is returned from the recovery room to a patient care area after a routine cholecystectomy.

1. The nurse expects that the inflammatory phase of wound healing should last for about:
   a. 7 days.
   b. 3 days.
   c. 5 days.
   d. 6 days.

2. When both sides of the wound approximate within 24 to 48 hours, the healing is said to be by:
   a. first intention.
   b. second intention.
   c. third intention.
   d. spontaneous intention.

3. Those clinical manifestations associated with the inflammatory phase of wound healing that the nurse would expect to see postoperatively are:
   a. pain.
   b. redness.
   c. warmth.
   d. all of the above.

4. Nursing measures to promote adequate tissue oxygenation during the inflammatory phase of wound healing include:
   a. applying warm compresses to the incision every 4 hours for 2 to 3 days to stimulate vasodilation.
   b. encouraging coughing and deep breathing to enhance pulmonary and cardiovascular functions.
   c. helping Elizabeth stay in bed for 4 to 6 days to prevent unnecessary strain on the suture line.
   d. leaving soiled dressings in place to prevent airborne microorganisms from entering the wound and setting up a localized infection.

CHAPTER 21

Assessment of Respiratory Function

I. Interpretation, Completion, and Comparison

MULTIPLE CHOICE

Read each question carefully. Circle your answer.

1. The purpose of the cilia is to:
   a. produce mucus.
   b. phagocytize bacteria.
   c. contract smooth muscle.
   d. move the mucus back to the larynx.

2. A patient with sinus congestion points to the area on the inside of the eye as a point of pain. The nurse knows that the patient is referring to which sinus?
   a. frontal
   b. ethmoidal
   c. maxillary
   d. sphenoidal

3. The lungs are enclosed in a serous membrane called the:
   a. diaphragm.
   b. mediastinum.
   c. pleura.
   d. xiphoid process.

4. The left lung, in contrast to the right lung, has:
   a. one less lobe.
   b. one more lobe.
   c. the same number of lobes.
   d. two more lobes.

5. The divisions of the lung lobe proceed in the following order, beginning at the mainstem bronchi:
   a. lobar bronchi, bronchioles, segmented bronchi, subsequent bronchi.
   b. segmented bronchi, subsegmented bronchi, lobar bronchi, bronchioles.
   c. lobar bronchi, segmented bronchi, subsegmented bronchi, bronchioles.
   d. subsegmented bronchi, lobar bronchi, bronchioles, segmented bronchi.

6. Choose the initial part of the respiratory tract that is *not* considered part of the gas-exchange airways.
   a. bronchioles
   b. respiratory bronchioles
   c. alveolar duct
   d. alveolar sacs

7. Choose the alveolar cells that secrete surfactant.
   a. type I cells
   b. type II cells
   c. type III cells
   d. type I and type II cells

8. Gas exchange between the lungs and blood and between the blood and tissues is called:
   a. active transport.
   b. respiration.
   c. ventilation.
   d. cellular respiration.

9. The exchange of oxygen and carbon dioxide from the alveoli into the blood occurs by:
   a. active transport.
   b. diffusion.
   c. osmosis.
   d. pinocytosis.

10. Airflow into the lungs during inspiration depends on all of the following *except:*
    a. contraction of the muscles of respiration.
    b. enlargement of the thoracic cavity.
    c. lowered intrathoracic pressure.
    d. relaxation of the diaphragm.

11. The pulmonary circulation is considered a:
    a. high-pressure, high-resistance system.
    b. low-pressure, low-resistance system.
    c. high-pressure, low-resistance system.
    d. low-pressure, high-resistance system.

12. The symbol used to identify the partial pressure of oxygen is:
    a. PO_2
    b. PAO_2
    c. PaO_2
    d. $PV\text{-}O_2$

13. Gerontologic changes in the respiratory system include all of the following *except:*
    a. decreased alveolar duct diameter.
    b. decreased gag reflex.
    c. increased presence of collagen in alveolar walls.
    d. decreased presence of mucus.

14. The maximum volume of air that can be inhaled after a normal inhalation is known as:
    a. inspiratory reserve volume.
    b. expiratory reserve volume.
    c. tidal volume.
    d. residual volume.

15. Tidal volume, which may not significantly change with disease, has a normal value of approximately:
    a. 300 mL.
    b. 500 mL.
    c. 800 mL.
    d. 1000 mL.

16. Uneven perfusion of the lung is primarily due to:
    a. pulmonary artery pressure.
    b. gravity.
    c. alveolar pressure.
    d. all of the above.

17. A nurse caring for a patient with a pulmonary embolism understands that a high ventilation–perfusion ratio may exist. This means that:
    a. perfusion exceeds ventilation.
    b. there is an absence of perfusion and ventilation.
    c. ventilation exceeds perfusion.
    d. ventilation matches perfusion.

18. A nurse understands that a safe but low level of oxygen saturation provides for adequate tissue saturation but allows no reserve for situations that threaten ventilation. A safe but low oxygen saturation level is:
    a. 40 mm Hg.
    b. 75 mm Hg.
    c. 80 mm Hg.
    d. 95 mm Hg.

19. When taking a respiratory history, the nurse should assess:
    a. the previous history of lung disease in the patient or family.
    b. occupational and environmental influences.
    c. smoking and exposure to allergies.
    d. all of the above.

20. Bacterial pneumonia can be indicated by the presence of all of the following *except:*
    a. green, purulent sputum.
    b. thick, yellow sputum.
    c. thin, mucoid sputum.
    d. rusty sputum.

21. Nursing assessment for a patient with chest pain includes:
    a. determining whether there is a relationship between the pain and the patient's posture.
    b. evaluating the effect of the phases of respiration on the pain.
    c. looking for factors that precipitate the pain.
    d. all of the above.

22. Chest pain described as knifelike on inspiration would most likely be diagnostic of:
    a. bacterial pneumonia.
    b. bronchogenic carcinoma.
    c. lung infarction.
    d. pleurisy.

23. Hemoptysis, a symptom of cardiopulmonary disorders, is characterized by all of the following *except:*
    a. a coffeeground appearance.
    b. an alkaline pH.
    c. a sudden onset.
    d. bright red bleeding mixed with sputum.

24. A patient exhibits cyanosis when how much hemoglobin is unoxygenated?
    a. 0.77 g/dL
    b. 2.3 g/dL
    c. 15.0 g/dL
    d. 5.0 g/dL

25. The nurse inspects the thorax of a patient with advanced emphysema. The nurse expects chest configuration change consistent with a deformity known as:
    a. barrel chest.
    b. funnel chest.
    c. kyphoscoliosis.
    d. pigeon chest.

26. Breath sounds that originate in the smaller bronchi and bronchioles and are high-pitched, sibilant, and musical are called:
    a. wheezes.
    b. rhonchi.
    c. rales.
    d. crackles.

27. Crackles, noncontinuous breath sounds, would be assessed for a patient with:
    a. asthma.
    b. bronchospasm.
    c. collapsed alveoli.
    d. pulmonary fibrosis.

28. During a preadmission assessment the nurse would expect to find decreased tactile fremitus and hyperresonant percussion sounds with a diagnosis of:
    a. bronchitis.
    b. emphysema.
    c. atelectasis.
    d. pulmonary edema.

29. The arterial blood gas measurement that best reflects the adequacy of alveolar ventilation is the:
    a. PaO_2.
    b. $PaCO_2$.
    c. pH.
    d. SaO_2.

30. Nursing directions to a patient from whom a sputum specimen is to be obtained should include all of the following *except* directing the patient to:
    a. initially clear his or her nose and throat.
    b. spit surface mucus and saliva into a sterile specimen container.
    c. take a few deep breaths before coughing.
    d. use diaphragmatic contractions to aid in the expulsion of sputum.

31. A physician wants a study of diaphragmatic motion because of suspected pathology. The physician would most likely order a:

    a. barium swallow.

    b. bronchogram.

    c. fluoroscopy.

    d. tomogram.

32. Nursing instructions for a patient who is scheduled for a perfusion lung scan should include informing the patient that:

    a. a mask will be placed over his or her nose and mouth during the test.

    b. he or she will be expected to lie under the camera.

    c. the imaging time will amount to 20 to 40 minutes.

    d. all of the above will occur.

33. The nurse should advise the patient who is scheduled for bronchoscopy that he or she will:

    a. have his or her nose sprayed with a topical anesthetic.

    b. be required to fast before the procedure.

    c. receive preoperative medication.

    d. experience all of the above.

SHORT ANSWER

Read each statement carefully. Write your response in the space provided.

1. Distinguish between *ventilation* and *respiration*: _____

   _____

2. Describe the function of the epiglottis: _____

   _____

3. List four conditions that cause low compliance.

   _____

   _____

   _____

   _____

4. Define the term *partial pressure*: _____

   _____

5. Name two centers in the brain that are responsible for the neurologic control of ventilation.

   _____

   _____

6. The alveoli begin to lose elasticity at about age _____ years, resulting in decreased gas diffusion.

7. List five of the eight major signs and symptoms of respiratory disease.

   _____

   _____

   _____

   _____

   _____

6. Explain the breathing pattern characterized as Cheyne-Stokes respirations: _____

_____

II. Critical Thinking Questions and Exercises

DISCUSSION AND ANALYSIS

Discuss the following topics with your classmates.

1. Describe four common phenomena that can alter bronchial diameter.
2. Explain the difference between the terms *diffusion* and *pulmonary perfusion*.
3. Explain how oxygen is carried in the blood.

CLINICAL SITUATIONS

Read the following case studies. Circle the correct answer.

CASE STUDY: Bronchoscopy

Mr. Kecklin is scheduled for a bronchoscopy for the diagnostic purpose of locating a pathologic process.

1. Because a bronchoscopy was ordered, the nurse knows that the suspected lesion was *not* in the:
   a. bronchus.
   b. larynx.
   c. pharynx.
   d. trachea.

2. Nursing measures before the bronchoscopy include:
   a. obtaining an informed consent.
   b. supplying information about the procedure.
   c. withholding food and fluids for 6 hours before the test.
   d. all of the above.

3. The nurse is aware that possible complications of bronchoscopy include all of the following *except*:
   a. aspiration.
   b. gastric perforation.
   c. infection.
   d. pneumothorax.

4. After the bronchoscopy, Mr. Kecklin must be observed for:
   a. dyspnea.
   b. hemoptysis.
   c. tachycardia.
   d. all of the above.

5. After the bronchoscopy, Mr. Kecklin:
   a. may be given ice chips and fluids after he demonstrates that he can perform the gag reflex.
   b. should immediately be given a house diet to alleviate the hunger resulting from the required fast.
   c. should initially be given iced ginger ale to prevent vomiting and possible aspiration of stomach contents.
   d. will need to remain NPO for 6 hours to prevent pharyngeal irritation.

CASE STUDY: Thoracentesis

Mrs. Lomar is admitted to the clinical area for a thoracentesis. The physician wants to remove excess air from the pleural cavity.

1. Nursing responsibilities before the thoracentesis should include:
   a. informing Mrs. Lomar about pressure sensations that will be experienced during the procedure.
   b. making sure that chest roentgenograms ordered in advance have been completed.
   c. seeing that the consent form has been explained and signed.
   d. all of the above.

2. For the thoracentesis, the patient is assisted to any of the following positions *except:*
   a. lying on the unaffected side with the bed elevated 30 to 40 degrees.
   b. lying prone with the head of the bed lowered 15 to 30 degrees.
   c. sitting on the edge of the bed with her feet supported and her arms and head on a padded overbed table.
   d. straddling a chair with her arms and head resting on the back of the chair.

3. Nursing intervention includes exposing the entire chest even though the thoracentesis site is normally in the midclavicular line between the:
   a. first and second intercostal spaces.
   b. second and third intercostal spaces.
   c. third and fourth intercostal spaces.
   d. fourth and fifth intercostal spaces.

4. Nursing observations after the thoracentesis include assessment for:
   a. blood-tinged mucus.
   b. signs of hypoxemia.
   c. tachycardia.
   d. all of the above.

5. A chest x-ray film is usually ordered after the thoracentesis to rule out:
   a. pleurisy.
   b. pneumonia.
   c. pneumothorax.
   d. pulmonary edema.

INTERPRETING DATA

Review the accompanying figure and explain in your own words what the oxyhemoglobin dissociation curve depicts. Also explain expected changes with clinical conditions.

The oxyhemoglobin dissociation curve is marked to show three oxygen levels: (1) normal levels (PaO$_2$ greater than 70 mm Hg), (2) relatively safe levels (PaO$_2$ of 45 to 70 mm Hg), and (3) dangerous levels (PaO$_2$ lower than 40 mm Hg). The normal (middle) curve shows that 75% saturation occurs at a PaO$_2$ of 40 mm Hg. If the curve shifts to the right, the same saturation (75%) occurs at the higher PaO$_2$ of 57 mm Hg. If the curve shifts to the left, 75% saturation occurs at a PaO$_2$ of 25 mm Hg.

Explain the concepts supporting the basis for the oxyhemoglobin dissociation curve in your own words. Interpret the relevance of the data depicted in the oxyhemoglobin dissociation curve.

_____

_____

_____

_____

_____

CHAPTER 22

Management of Patients With Upper Respiratory Tract Disorders

I. Interpretation, Completion, and Comparison

MULTIPLE CHOICE

Read each question carefully. Circle your answer.

1. Nursing measures associated with the uncomplicated common cold include all of the following *except:*
   a. administering prescribed antibiotics to decrease the severity of the viral infection.
   b. informing the patient about the symptoms of secondary infection, the major complication of a cold.
   c. suggesting adequate fluid intake and rest.
   d. teaching people that the virus is contagious for 2 days before symptoms appear and during the first part of the symptomatic phase.

2. Health teaching for viral rhinitis (common cold) includes advising the patient to:
   a. blow his or her nose gently to prevent spread of the infection.
   b. blow through both nostrils to equalize the pressure.
   c. rest, to promote overall comfort.
   d. do all of the above.

3. The herpes virus, which remains latent in cells of the lips or nose, usually subsides spontaneously in:
   a. 5 days.
   b. 1 week.
   c. 10 to 14 days.
   d. 3 to 4 weeks.

4. Acyclovir, an antiviral agent, is recommended for:
   a. herpes simplex infection.
   b. rhinitis.
   c. sinusitis.
   d. bronchitis.

5. About 60% of cases of acute sinusitis are caused by bacterial organisms. A second-line antibiotic used is:
   a. Augmentin
   b. Amoxil.
   c. erythromycin.
   d. Septra.

6. Nursing suggestions for a patient with acute or chronic sinusitis include:
   a. adequate fluid intake.
   b. increased humidity.
   c. local heat applications to promote drainage.
   d. all of the above.

7. An antibiotic that decreases nasal secretions and polyp size in chronic sinusitis is:
   a. Augmentin.
   b. Biaxin.
   c. Cefzil.
   d. Vantin.

8. Acute pharyngitis of a bacterial nature is most commonly caused by:
   a. group A, beta-hemolytic streptococci.
   b. gram-negative *Klebsiella*.
   c. *Pseudomonas.*
   d. *Staphylococcus aureus.*

9. A complication of acute pharyngitis can be:
   a. mastoiditis.
   b. otitis media.
   c. peritonsillar abscess.
   d. all of the above.

10. Nursing management for a patient with acute pharyngitis includes:
   a. applying an ice collar for symptomatic relief of a severe sore throat.
   b. encouraging bed rest during the febrile stage of the illness.
   c. suggesting a liquid or soft diet during the acute stage of the disease.
   d. all of the above measures.

11. The most common organism associated with tonsillitis and adenoiditis is:
   a. group A, beta-hemolytic streptococcus.
   b. gram-negative *Klebsiella*.
   c. *Pseudomonas.*
   d. *Staphylococcus aureus.*

12. Potential complications of enlarged adenoids include all of the following *except*:
   a. bronchitis.
   b. nasal obstruction.
   c. allergies.
   d. acute otitis media.

13. To assess for an upper respiratory tract infection, the nurse should palpate:
   a. the frontal and maxillary sinuses.
   b. the trachea.
   c. the neck lymph nodes.
   d. all of the above areas.

14. To assess for an upper respiratory tract infection, the nurse should inspect:
   a. the nasal mucosa.
   b. the frontal sinuses.
   c. the tracheal mucosa.
   d. all of the above.

15. Airway clearance in a patient with an upper airway infection is facilitated by all of the following *except*:
   a. decreasing systemic hydration.
   b. humidifying inspired room air.
   c. positional drainage of the affected area.
   d. administering prescribed vasoconstrictive medications.

16. Nursing intervention for a patient with a fractured nose includes all of the following *except*:
   a. applying cold compresses to decrease swelling and control bleeding.
   b. assessing respirations to detect any interference with breathing.
   c. observing for any clear fluid drainage from either nostril.
   d. packing each nostril with a cotton pledget to minimize bleeding and help maintain the shape of the nose during fracture setting.

17. Surgical reduction of nasal fractures is usually performed how long after the fracture?
   a. within 24 hours
   b. 7 to 10 days
   c. 2 to 3 weeks
   d. 2 months

18. Angioedema as a risk factor that leads to laryngeal obstruction is usually caused by:
   a. heavy alcohol use.
   b. history of airway problems.
   c. presence of foreign body.
   d. use of angiotensin-converging enzyme (ACE) inhibitors.

19. To correctly perform the Heimlich maneuver, a person should forcefully apply pressure against the victim's:

   a. abdomen.

   b. diaphragm.

   c. lungs.

   d. trachea.

20. An early sign of cancer of the larynx in the glottic area (66% of cases) is:

   a. affected voice sounds.

   b. burning of the throat when hot liquids are ingested.

   c. enlarged cervical nodes.

   d. dysphagia.

21. A patient with a total laryngectomy would no longer have:

   a. natural vocalization.

   b. protection of the lower airway from foreign particles.

   c. a normal effective cough.

   d. all of the above mechanisms.

22. Patient education for a laryngectomy includes:

   a. advising that large amounts of mucus can be coughed up through the stoma.

   b. cautioning about preventing water from entering the stoma.

   c. telling the patient to expect a diminished sense of taste and smell.

   d. doing all of the above.

SHORT ANSWER

Read each statement carefully. Write your response in the space provided.

1. Explain how rhinitis can lead to sinusitis: _____

   _____

2. Name three bacterial organisms that account for more than 60% of all cases of acute sinusitis.

   _____

   _____

   _____

3. If untreated, acute sinusitis can lead to severe complications such as _____,

   _____, and _____.

4. The most serious complication of a tonsillectomy is: _____

   _____

5. The most common cause of laryngitis is _____, with symptoms including

   _____, _____, and _____.

6. List four possible nursing diagnoses and collaborative problems for a patient with an upper airway infection.

   _____

   _____

   _____

   _____

7. List five potential complications of an upper airway infection.

_____

_____

_____

_____

_____

8. List the clinical manifestations that are used to diagnose obstructive sleep apnea: _____

_____

9. List three types of alaryngeal communication.

_____

_____

_____

II. Critical Thinking Questions and Exercises

CLINICAL SITUATIONS

Read the following case studies. Fill in the blanks or circle the correct answer.

CASE STUDY: Tonsillectomy and Adenoidectomy

Isabel, a 14-year-old girl, has just undergone a tonsillectomy and adenoidectomy. The staff nurse assists her with transport from the recovery area to her room.

1. Based on knowledge about tonsillar disease, the nurse knows that Isabel must have experienced symptoms that required surgical intervention. Clinical manifestations may have included:
   a. hypertrophy of the tonsils.
   b. repeated attacks of otitis media.
   c. suspected hearing loss secondary to otitis media.
   d. all of the above.

2. The nurse assesses Isabel's postoperative vital signs and checks for the most significant postoperative complication, which is:
   a. epiglottis.
   b. eustachian tube perforation.
   c. hemorrhage.
   d. oropharyngeal edema.

3. The nurse maintains Isabel in the recommended postoperative position of:
   a. prone with her head on a pillow and turned to the side.
   b. reverse Trendelenburg with the neck extended.
   c. semi-Fowler's with the neck flexed.
   d. supine with her neck hyperextended and supported with a pillow.

4. Isabel is to be discharged the same day of her tonsillectomy. The nurse makes sure that her family knows to:
   a. encourage her to eat a house diet to build up her resistance to infection.
   b. offer her only clear liquids for 3 days, to prevent pharyngeal irritation.
   c. offer her soft foods for several days to minimize local discomfort and supply her with necessary nutrients.
   d. supplement her diet with orange and lemon juices because of the need for vitamin C to heal tissues.

CASE STUDY: Epistaxis

Gilberta, a 14-year-old high school student, is sent with her mother to the emergency department of a local hospital for uncontrolled epistaxis.

1. Describe what the school nurse should tell Gilberta to manage the bleeding site while being transported to the hospital: _____

   _____

2. Initial nursing measures in the emergency room that can be used to stop the nasal bleeding include:
   a. compressing the soft outer portion of the nose against the midline septum continuously for 5 to 10 minutes.
   b. keeping Gilberta in the upright position with her head tilted forward to prevent swallowing and aspiration of blood.
   c. telling Gilberta to breathe through her mouth and to refrain from talking.
   d. all of the above.

3. The nurse expects that emergency medical treatment may include insertion of a cotton pledget moistened with:
   a. an adrenergic blocking agent.
   b. aqueous epinephrine.
   c. protamine sulfate.
   d. vitamin K.

4. The nurse can advise the mother that nasal packing used to control bleeding can be left in place:
   a. no longer than 2 hours.
   b. an average of 12 hours.
   c. an average of 24 hours.
   d. anywhere from 2 to 6 days.

CASE STUDY: Cancer of the Larynx

Brenda, a 64-year-old woman with a long-term history of smoking, recently retired from the chemical laboratory department of a large company. After months of complaining of a persistent cough, sore throat, and pain and burning in the throat, Brenda was admitted to the hospital with a diagnosis of cancer of the larynx.

1. During her assessment, the nurse knows that a number of risk factors are associated with laryngeal cancer. List 10 of 20 possible factors.

   _____

   _____

   _____

   _____

   _____

   _____

   _____

   _____

   _____

   _____

2. The most common form of cancer of the larynx is _____.

3. Assessment of a patient admitted for laryngeal carcinoma includes:

   a. palpation of the frontal and maxillary sinuses to detect infection or inflammation.

   b. palpation of the neck for swelling.

   c. inspection of the nasal mucosa for polyps.

   d. all of the above techniques.

4. The nurse advises Brenda that the likelihood of lymph node involvement is less than _____%.

   Without lymph node metastasis, recovery is expected in _____% of patients.

5. The nurse knows that Brenda's stage I cancer will most likely be treated by

   _____.

6. The nurse advises Brenda to be vigilant about her follow-up care, because the highest risk for laryngeal

   cancer is in the first _____ to _____ years.

CASE STUDY: Laryngectomy

Jerome, a 52-year-old widower, is admitted for a laryngectomy owing to a malignant tumor.

1. Before developing a care plan, the nurse needs to know whether Jerome's voice will be preserved. The surgical procedure that would not damage the voice box is a:

   a. partial laryngectomy.

   b. supraglottic laryngectomy.

   c. thyrotomy.

   d. total laryngectomy.

2. Jerome is scheduled for a total laryngectomy. Preoperative education includes:

   a. informing him that there are ways he will be able to carry on a conversation without his voice.

   b. making sure that he knows he will require a permanent tracheal stoma.

   c. reminding him that he will not be able to sing, whistle, or laugh.

   d. all of the above.

3. Postoperative nutrition is usually maintained by way of a nasogastric catheter. The nurse needs to tell Jerome that oral feedings usually begin after:

   a. 24 hours.

   b. 2 to 3 days.

   c. 5 to 6 days.

   d. 1 week.

4. The nurse knows to assess for the most common postoperative complications of

   _____, _____, _____,

   _____, _____, and _____.

5. Postoperative nursing measures to promote respiratory effectiveness include:

   a. assisting with turning and early ambulation.

   b. positioning Jerome in semi-Fowler's to high Fowler's position.

   c. reminding Jerome to cough and take frequent deep breaths.

   d. all of the above.

6. List at least four signs of postoperative infection that the nurse should monitor.

_____

_____

_____

_____

7. Jerome needs to know that the laryngectomy tube will be removed when:

   a. esophageal speech has been perfected.

   b. he requests that it be removed.

   c. oral feedings are initiated.

   d. the stoma is well healed.

8. A lethal complication of wound breakdown is _____.

APPLYING CONCEPTS

Examine Chart 22-6 in the text and answer the following questions.

A woman is signaling that she is choking. The nurse is performing an abdominal thrust maneuver (the Heimlich maneuver). List the eight steps suggested by the AHA to dislodge the foreign object.

1. _____

2. _____

3. _____

4. _____

5. _____

6. _____

7. _____

8. _____

CHAPTER 23

Management of Patients With Chest and Lower Respiratory Tract Disorders

I. Interpretation, Comprehension, and Comparison

MULTIPLE CHOICE
Read each question carefully. Circle your answer.

1. Nursing management for a person diagnosed as having acute tracheobronchitis includes:
   a. increasing fluid intake to remove secretions.
   b. encouraging the patient to remain in bed.
   c. using cool-vapor therapy to relieve laryngeal and tracheal irritation.
   d. all of the above.

2. The nurse knows that a sputum culture is necessary to identify the causative organism for acute tracheobronchitis. If the culture identifies a fungal agent, the nurse knows it would most likely be:
   a. *Aspergillus.*
   b. *Haemophilus.*
   c. *Mycoplasma pneumoniae.*
   d. *Streptococcus pneumoniae.*

3. In the United States, the most common cause of death from infectious diseases is:
   a. atelectasis.
   b. pulmonary embolus.
   c. pneumonia.
   d. tracheobronchitis.

4. *Streptococcus pneumoniae* is the organism most commonly responsible for which of the following types of pneumonia?
   a. hospital-acquired
   b. immunocompromised
   c. aspiration-specific
   d. community-acquired

5. Characteristics of the *Mycobacterium tuberculosis* include all of the following *except:*
   a. it can be transmitted only by droplet nuclei.
   b. it is acid-fast.
   c. it is able to lie dormant within the body for years.
   d. it survives in anaerobic conditions.

6. It is estimated that *Mycobacterium tuberculosis* infects about what percentage of the world's population?
   a. 10%
   b. 25%
   c. 35%
   d. 50%

7. For the tubercle bacillus to multiply and initiate a tissue reaction in the lungs, it must be deposited in:
   a. the alveoli.
   b. the bronchi.
   c. the trachea.
   d. all of the above.

8. A Mantoux skin test is considered to be *not* significant if the size of the induration is:
   a. 3 to 4 mm.
   b. 5 to 6 mm.
   c. 7 to 8 mm.
   d. 9 mm.

9. Prophylactic INH drug treatment is necessary for about how many months?
   a. 3
   b. 3 to 5
   c. 6 to 12
   d. 13 to 18

10. Diagnostic confirmation of a lung abscess is made by:
    a. chest radiograph.
    b. bronchoscopy.
    c. sputum culture.
    d. evaluating all of the above studies.

11. The most diagnostic clinical symptom of pleurisy is:
    a. dullness or flatness on percussion over areas of collected fluid.
    b. dyspnea and coughing.
    c. fever and chills.
    d. stabbing pain during respiratory movement.

12. A pleural effusion results when fluid accumulation in the pleural space is greater than:
    a. 5 mL.
    b. 10 mL.
    c. 15 mL.
    d. 20 mL.

13. Auscultation can be used to diagnose the presence of pulmonary edema when the following adventitious breath sounds are present:
    a. crackles in the posterior bases.
    b. low-pitched rhonchi during expiration.
    c. pleural friction rub.
    d. sibilant wheezes.

14. Acute respiratory failure (ARF) occurs when the oxygen tension (PaO_2) falls to less than _____ mm Hg (hypoxemia) and carbon dioxide tension ($PaCO_2$) rises to greater than _____ mm Hg (hypercapnia).
    a. 50 and 50
    b. 60 and 60
    c. 75 and 75
    d. 80 and 80

15. The pathophysiology of ARF is directly related to:
    a. decreased respiratory drive.
    b. chest wall abnormalities.
    c. dysfunction of lung parenchyma.
    d. all of the above mechanisms.

16. Neuromuscular blockers are given to patients with ARF who are on ventilator assistance to accomplish all of the following *except:*
    a. maintain positive end-expiratory pressure (PEEP).
    b. maintain better ventilation.
    c. increase the respiratory rate.
    d. keep the patient from fighting the ventilator.

17. A key characteristic feature of adult respiratory distress syndrome (ARDS) is:
    a. arterial hypoxemia.
    b. diminished alveolar dilation.
    c. tachypnea.
    d. increased PaO_2.

18. A 154-lb, 60-year-old woman is being treated for ARDS. The nurse knows that the minimum daily caloric intake to meet normal requirements is:
    a. 1200 to 1800 cal.
    b. 1800 to 2200 cal.
    c. 2000 to 2400 cal.
    d. 2500 to 3000 cal.

19. A nurse knows to assess a patient with pulmonary arterial hypertension for the primary symptom of:
    a. ascites.
    b. dyspnea.
    c. hypertension.
    d. syncope.

20. Clinical manifestations directly related to cor pulmonale include all of the following *except*:
    a. dyspnea and cough.
    b. diminished peripheral pulses.
    c. distended neck veins.
    d. edema of the feet and legs.

21. The nurse assesses a patient for a possible pulmonary embolism. The nurse looks for the most frequent sign, which is:
    a. cough.
    b. hemoptysis.
    c. syncope.
    d. tachypnea.

22. Anticoagulation with heparin is administered in an attempt to maintain the partial thromboplastin time (PTT) at how many times the normal value?
    a. 0.5 to 1.0
    b. 1.5 to 2.5
    c. 2.5 to 3.0
    d. 3.0

23. Nursing measures to assist in the prevention of pulmonary embolism in a hospitalized patient include all of the following *except*:
    a. a liberal fluid intake.
    b. assisting the patient to do leg elevations above the level of the heart.
    c. encouraging the patient to dangle his or her legs over the side of the bed for 30 minutes, four times a day.
    d. the use of elastic stockings, especially when decreased mobility would promote venous stasis.

24. To assess for a positive Homans' sign, the nurse should:
    a. dorsiflex the foot while the leg is elevated to check for calf pain.
    b. elevate the patient's legs for 20 minutes and then lower them slowly while checking for areas of inadequate blood return.
    c. extend the leg, plantar flex the foot, and check for the patency of the dorsalis pedis pulse.
    d. lower the patient's legs and massage the calf muscles to note any areas of tenderness.

25. As a cause of death among men in the United States, lung cancer ranks:
    a. first.
    b. second.
    c. third.
    d. fourth.

26. More than 80% of all lung cancers are primarily caused by:
    a. cigarette smoking.
    b. fibrosis.
    c. inhalation of environmental carcinogens.
    d. tuberculosis.

27. The most prevalent lung carcinoma that is peripherally located and frequently metastasizes is:
    a. adenocarcinoma.
    b. bronchioalveolar.
    c. large cell.
    d. squamous cell.

28. The most frequent symptom of lung cancer is:
    a. copious sputum production.
    b. coughing.
    c. dyspnea.
    d. severe pain.

29. The nurse is aware that the most common surgical procedure for a small, apparently curable tumor of the lung is a:

    a. lobectomy.

    b. pneumonectomy.

    c. segmentectomy.

    d. wedge resection.

30. Paradoxical chest movement is associated with which chest disorder?

    a. pneumothorax

    b. flail chest

    c. ARDS

    d. tension pneumothorax

31. An initial characteristic symptom of a simple pneumothorax is:

    a. ARDS.

    b. severe respiratory distress.

    c. sudden onset of chest pain.

    d. tachypnea and hypoxemia.

SHORT ANSWER

Read each statement carefully. Write your response in the space provided.

1. Atelectasis, which refers to closure or collapse of alveoli, may be chronic or acute in nature. List 10 possible causes of atelectasis.

2. Name eight possible clinical manifestations of atelectasis.

3. Identify eight nursing measures that can be used to prevent atelectasis.

_____

_____

_____

_____

_____

_____

_____

_____

4. The diagnosis of hospital-acquired pneumonia is usually associated with the presence of one of three conditions: _____, _____, and

_____.

5. Name three common pathogens that cause aspiration pneumonia.

_____

_____

_____

6. Pneumonia tends to occur in patients with one or more of these five underlying disorders:

_____, _____, _____,

_____, and _____.

7. Three severe complications of pneumonia are: _____,

_____, and _____.

8. Explain the meaning of the term _superinfection:_ _____

_____

9. According to the World Health Organization (WHO), the leading cause of death among people who are infected with the human immunodeficiency virus (HIV) people is _____.

10. List four respiratory system mechanisms that can lead to acute respiratory failure (ARF).

_____

_____

_____

_____

11. The mortality rate with ARDS is as high as _____%. The cause of death is usually

_____.

12. A characteristic and diagnostic feature of ARDS is: _____.

13. Identify the cause of cor pulmonale: _____

_____

II. Critical Thinking Questions and Exercises

DISCUSSION AND ANALYSIS

Discuss the following topics with your classmates.

1. Explain the pathophysiology of atelectasis.
2. Discuss a variety of risk factors and associated preventive measures for pneumonia (eg, immunosuppression, age, smoking, sedation).
3. In simple terms, explain the pathophysiology of pulmonary edema.
4. Discuss at least six etiologic factors and nursing assessments for patients with ARDS.
5. Discuss the risk factors and nursing assessments for patients with a pulmonary embolism.
6. Distinguish between the pathophysiology and clinical manifestations of sarcoidosis, pneumoconiosis, silicosis, and asbestosis.

INTERPRETING PATTERNS

Fill out the following flow charts according to the directions.

1. Diagram the sequence of the pathophysiologic events that lead to pneumonia.

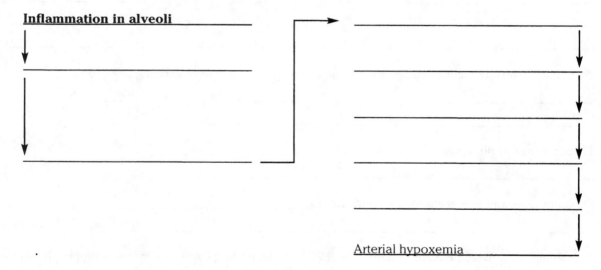

Inflammation in alveoli

Arterial hypoxemia

2. Diagram the sequence of the pathophysiologic events that lead to ARDS.

Inflammatory Event

Stiff lungs and severe hypoxemia

CLINICAL SITUATIONS

Read the following case studies. Circle the correct answer.

CASE STUDY: Community-Acquired Pneumonia

Theresa, a 20-year-old college student, lives in a small dormitory with 30 other students. Four weeks into the spring semester, she was diagnosed as having bacterial pneumonia and was admitted to the hospital.

1. The nurse is informed that Theresa has the strain of bacteria most frequently found in community-acquired pneumonia. The nurse suspects that the infecting agent is:
   a. *Haemophilus influenzae.*
   b. *Klebsiella.*
   c. *Pseudomonas aeruginosa.*
   d. *Streptococcus pneumoniae.*

2. All of the following are manifestations of bacterial pneumonia *except*:
   a. fever.
   b. bradycardia.
   c. stabbing or pleuritic chest pain.
   d. tachypnea.

3. The nurse expects that Theresa will be medicated with the usual antibiotic of choice, which is:
   a. cephalosporin.
   b. clindamycin.
   c. erythromycin.
   d. penicillin G.

4. The nurse is aware that Theresa may develop arterial hypoxemia, because:
   a. bronchospasm causes alveolar collapse, which decreases the surface area necessary for perfusion.
   b. mucosal edema occludes the alveoli, thereby producing a drop in alveolar oxygen.
   c. venous blood is shunted from the right to the left side of the heart.
   d. all of the above are true.

5. Theresa is expected to respond to antibiotic therapy:
   a. within 6 hours.
   b. between 1 and 2 days.
   c. by the fourth day.
   d. after 7 days.

6. Nursing management includes assessment for complications such as:
   a. atelectasis.
   b. hypotension and shock.
   c. pleural effusion.
   d. all of the above.

CASE STUDY: Tuberculosis

Mr. Carrera, a 67-year-old retired baker and pastry chef, is admitted to the clinical area for confirmation of suspected tuberculosis. He is anorexic and fatigued and suffers from "indigestion." His temperature is slightly elevated every afternoon.

1. Mr. Carrera's Mantoux tuberculin test yields an induration area of 10 mm. This result is interpreted as indicating that:
   a. active disease is present.
   b. he has been exposed to *M. tuberculosis* or has been vaccinated with BCG.
   c. preventive treatment should be initiated.
   d. the reaction is doubtful and should be repeated.

2. After Mr. Carrera has undergone a series of additional tests, the diagnosis is confirmed by:

   a. a chest radiograph.

   b. acid-fast bacilli in a sputum smear.

   c. a positive multiple-puncture skin test.

   d. repeated Mantoux tests that yield indurations of 10 mm or greater.

3. Mr. Carrera is started on a multiple-drug regimen. Nursing management includes observing for hepatotoxicity when which drug is used?

   a. ethambutol

   b. isoniazid

   c. rifampin

   d. pyrazinamide

4. Mr. Carrera needs to know that the initial intensive treatment is usually given daily for:

   a. 2 weeks.

   b. 2 to 4 weeks.

   c. 2 months.

   d. 4 to 6 months.

5. Mr. Carrera is informed that he will no longer be considered infectious after:

   a. repeat Mantoux tests are negative.

   b. serial chest radiographs show improvement.

   c. two consecutive sputum specimens are negative.

   d. all of the above parameters are met.

CASE STUDY: Acute Respiratory Distress Syndrome

Anne, 71 years of age and single, is admitted to the unit with a diagnosis of ARDS. She was receiving treatment at home for viral pneumonia and had appeared to be improving until yesterday.

1. During assessment, the nurse notes symptoms positively correlated with ARDS, including:

   a. dysrhythmias and hypotension.

   b. contraction of the accessory muscles of respiration.

   c. tachypnea and tachycardia.

   d. all of the above.

2. The nurse also observes symptoms of cerebral hypoxia, including:

   a. drowsiness.

   b. confusion.

   c. irritability.

   d. all of the above.

3. The nurse observes that Anne is receiving oxygen by way of a nasal cannula at 6 L/min. The nurse knows that Anne's FiO_2 is:

   a. 24%.

   b. 34%.

   c. 44%.

   d. 54%.

4. Indications for ventilator support for ARDS include all of the following *except*:

   a. O_2 saturation greater than 90%.

   b. PaO_2 greater than 60%.

   c. respiratory rate greater than 35 breaths/min.

   d. vital capacity equal to 60 mL/kg of body weight.

5. It is decided that Anne needs a ventilator to help her breathe. Her physician prescribes PEEP. When PEEP is used, all of the following occur *except*:

   a. improved arterial oxygenation.

   b. improved ventilation–perfusion.

   c. increased alveolar dilation.

   d. increased functional residual capacity.

CASE STUDY: Pulmonary Embolism

Sandy, a 37-year-old woman recovering from multiple fractures sustained in a car accident, was admitted to the intensive care unit for treatment of a pulmonary embolism. Before admission, she was short of breath after walking up a flight of stairs.

1. On the basis of Sandy's medical history, the nurse suspects that a predisposing condition may have been:
   a. hypercoagulability.
   b. postoperative immobility.
   c. venous stasis.
   d. all of the above factors.

2. As part of her assessment information, the nurse knows that the majority of pulmonary emboli originate in the:
   a. deep leg veins.
   b. lung tissue.
   c. pelvic area.
   d. right atrium of the heart.

3. The most common symptom of pulmonary embolism is:
   a. chest pain.
   b. dyspnea.
   c. fever.
   d. hemoptysis.

4. The nurse knows that treatment must be immediate, because death from a pulmonary embolism can occur:
   a. within 1 hour.
   b. within 24 hours.
   c. in the first 48 hours.
   d. in 3 to 5 days.

5. Based on Sandy's diagnosis, the nurse knows to look for a decrease in:
   a. alveolar dead space.
   b. cardiac output.
   c. pulmonary arterial pressure.
   d. right ventricular work load of the heart.

6. A primary nursing problem for Sandy would be:
   a. atelectasis.
   b. bradycardia.
   c. dyspnea.
   d. hypertension.

7. The nurse knows that Sandy's diagnosis was probably confirmed by:
   a. a bronchogram.
   b. a chest roentgenogram.
   c. an electrocardiogram.
   d. a lung scan.

APPLYING CONCEPTS

Examine Figure 23-2 in the text and answer the following two questions.

1. Look at the right lobes of the lung and explain how the figure illustrates lobar pneumonia:

   _____

2. Look at the left lobes and explain how the figure illustrates bronchopneumonia:

   _____

CHAPTER 24

Management of Patients With Chronic Obstructive Pulmonary Disease

I. Interpretation, Completion, and Comparison

MULTIPLE CHOICE

Read each question carefully. Circle your answer.

1. As a cause of death in the United States, chronic obstructive pulmonary disease (COPD) ranks:
   a. second.
   b. third.
   c. fourth.
   d. fifth.

2. The current new definition of COPD leaves only one disorder under its classification, and that disorder is:
   a. asthma.
   b. bronchiectasis.
   c. cystic fibrosis.
   d. emphysema.

3. The underlying pathophysiology of COPD is:
   a. inflamed airways that obstruct airflow.
   b. mucus secretions that block airways.
   c. overinflated alveoli that impair gas exchange.
   d. characterized by variations of all of the above.

4. The abnormal inflammatory response in the lungs occurs primarily in:
   a. the airways.
   b. the parenchyma.
   c. the pulmonary vasculature.
   d. all of the above.

5. Two diseases common to the etiology of COPD are:
   a. asthma and atelectasis.
   b. chronic bronchitis and emphysema.
   c. pneumonia and pleurisy.
   d. tuberculosis and pleural effusions.

6. For a patient with chronic bronchitis, the nurse expects to see the major clinical symptoms of:
   a. chest pain during respiration.
   b. sputum and a productive cough.
   c. fever, chills, and diaphoresis.
   d. tachypnea and tachycardia.

7. The major cause of emphysema is:
   a. air pollution.
   b. allergens.
   c. infectious agents.
   d. smoking.

8. The pathophysiology of emphysema is directly related to airway obstruction. The end result of deterioration is:
   a. diminished alveolar surface area.
   b. hypercapnia resulting from decreased carbon dioxide elimination.
   c. hypoxemia secondary to impaired oxygen diffusion.
   d. respiratory acidosis due to airway obstruction.

9. The primary presenting symptom of emphysema is:
   a. chronic cough.
   b. dyspnea.
   c. tachypnea.
   d. wheezing.

10. Bronchodilators are prescribed in emphysema primarily because they:
    a. improve gas exchange.
    b. interfere with mucosal edema.
    c. improve airflow.
    d. reverse bronchospasm.

11. A nurse notes that the FEV_1/FVC ratio is less than 70% for a patient with COPD. The nurse documents that the patient is in stage:
    a. 0.
    b. I.
    c. II.
    d. III.

12. Nursing assessment of a patient with bronchospasm associated with COPD would include assessment for:
    a. compromised gas exchange.
    b. decreased airflow.
    c. wheezes.
    d. all of the above.

13. A commonly prescribed methylxanthine used as a bronchodilator is:
    a. albuterol.
    b. levalbuterol.
    c. theophylline.
    d. terbutaline.

14. The physician orders a common bronchodilator that is only administered by inhaler. The nurse knows this would be:
    a. Alupent.
    b. Foradil.
    c. Maxair.
    d. Volmax.

15. The nurse should be alert for a complication of bronchiectasis that results from a combination of retained secretions and obstruction. This complication is known as:
    a. atelectasis.
    b. emphysema.
    c. pleurisy.
    d. pneumonia.

16. Histamine, a mediator that supports the inflammatory process in asthma, is secreted by:
    a. eosinophils.
    b. lymphocytes.
    c. mast cells.
    d. neutrophils.

17. Obstruction of the airway in the patient with asthma is caused by all of the following *except*:
    a. thick mucus.
    b. swelling of bronchial membranes.
    c. destruction of the alveolar wall.
    d. contraction of muscles surrounding the bronchi.

18. A commonly prescribed mast cell stabilizer used for asthma is:
    a. albuterol.
    b. budesonide.
    c. cromolyn sodium.
    d. theophylline.

19. The nurse understands that a patient with status asthmaticus will likely initially evidence symptoms of:
    a. metabolic acidosis.
    b. metabolic alkalosis.
    c. respiratory acidosis.
    d. respiratory alkalosis.

20. A definitive diagnosis of cystic fibrosis is based on the following diagnostic test:
    a. bronchoscopy.
    b. computed tomography scan of lungs.
    c. pulmonary function tests.
    d. sweat chloride test.

SHORT ANSWER.

Read each statement carefully. Write your response in the space provided.

1. Chronic airway inflammation in COPD results in: _____
    _____

2. Define the term *emphysema:* _____
    _____

3. The most important risk factor for COPD is: _____
    _____

4. A genetic risk factor for COPD is: _____
    _____

5. The three primary symptoms associated with COPD are _____,
    _____, and _____.

6. List at least five of the nine major factors that determine the clinical course and survival of patients with COPD.

    _____

    _____

    _____

    _____

    _____

7. The single most effective intervention to prevent COPD or slow its progression is
    _____.

8. Primary causes for an acute exacerbation of emphysema are _____ and
    _____.

9. List five nursing diagnoses for a patient with COPD.

    _____

    _____

    _____

    _____

    _____

10. The strongest predisposing factor for asthma is _____, and the three most
    common symptoms are _____, _____, and
    _____.

11. Complications of asthma may include _____, _____,
    _____, and _____.

II. Critical Thinking Questions and Exercises

DISCUSSION AND ANALYSIS

Discuss the following topics with your classmates.

1. Outline a health education teaching plan for a program at your local YMCA to present and explain the risk factors associated with COPD. You are aware that about 29% of high school students smoke.
2. Explain the Haldane effect of oxygen and carbon dioxide transport as it relates to the hypoxic drive theory of respiration.
3. Explain the pathophysiology of asthma.

IDENTIFYING PATTERNS

Fill out the following flow charts according to the directions.

1. Chart the sequence of events that illustrate the pathophysiology of chronic bronchitis.

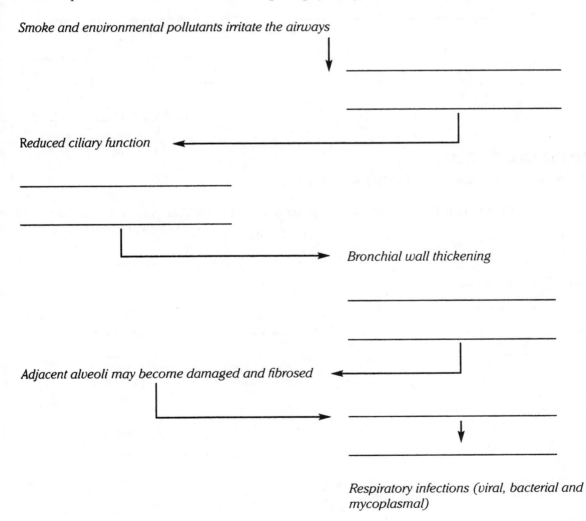

Smoke and environmental pollutants irritate the airways

_____

_____

Reduced ciliary function

_____

_____

Bronchial wall thickening

_____

_____

Adjacent alveoli may become damaged and fibrosed

_____

_____

Respiratory infections (viral, bacterial and mycoplasmal)

2. Chart the sequence of events that illustrate the pathophysiology of emphysema.

Alveolar walls are destroyed causing an increase in dead space ⟶ } _____

_____

In later stage emphysema, carbon dioxide elimination is impaired ⟶ } _____

_____

As the alveolar walls break down, the pulmonary capillary bed is reduced, causing increased pulmonary blood flow

⬇

_____ ⟶ } _____

_____

⬇

Cardiac failure _____

EXAMINING ASSOCIATIONS

Consider the following conditions and write your answers.

1. Compare the pathophysiologic changes and symptomatology for panlobular and centrilobular emphysema.

Panlobular   Centrilobular

_____   _____

_____   _____

_____   _____

_____   _____

_____   _____

CLINICAL SITUATIONS

Read the following case studies. Circle the correct answer.

CASE STUDY: Emphysema

Lois, who has had emphysema for 25 years, is admitted to the hospital with a diagnosis of bronchitis.

1. During assessment, the nurse notes the presence of a "barrel chest," which the nurse knows is caused by:
   a. a compensatory expansion of the bronchial airway.
   b. a decrease in intrapleural pressure.
   c. "air trapping" in the lungs.
   d. a progressive increase in vital capacity.

2. The nurse recognizes the need to be alert for the major presenting symptom of emphysema, which is:
   a. bradypnea.
   b. dyspnea.
   c. expiratory wheezing.
   d. fatigue.

3. Arterial blood gas measurements that are consistent with a diagnosis of emphysema are:
   a. pH, 7.32; PaO_2, 70 mm Hg; $PaCO_2$, 50 mm Hg.
   b. pH, 7.37; PaO_2, 90 mm Hg; $PaCO_2$, 42 mm Hg.
   c. pH, 7.39; PaO_2, 80 mm Hg; $PaCO_2$, 35 mm Hg.
   d. pH, 7.40; PaO_2, 85 mm Hg; $PaCO_2$, 42 mm Hg.

4. Lois is being medicated with a bronchodilator to reduce airway obstruction. Nursing actions include observing for the side effect of:
   a. dysrhythmias.
   b. central nervous system excitement.
   c. tachycardia.
   d. all of the above.

5. Diaphragmatic breathing is recommended for Lois because it does all of the following *except*:
   a. decrease respiratory rate.
   b. decrease tidal volume.
   c. increase alveolar ventilation.
   d. reduce functional residual capacity.

6. Oxygen is prescribed for Lois. The nurse knows that the most effective delivery system is:
   a. a rebreathing bag that delivers oxygen at a concentration greater than 60%.
   b. an oxygen mask set 8 L/min.
   c. a nasal cannula set at 6 L/min.
   d. a Venturi mask that delivers a predictable oxygen flow at about 24%.

CHAPTER 25

Respiratory Care Modalities

I. Interpretation, Completion, and Comparison

MULTIPLE CHOICE

Read each question carefully. Circle your answer.

1. The nurse knows that hypoxemia can be detected by noting a decrease in:
   a. PaO_2.
   b. PaO_2.
   c. pH.
   d. PCO_2.

2. A patient with bradycardia and hypotension would most likely exhibit:
   a. anemic hypoxia.
   b. circulatory hypoxia.
   c. histotoxic hypoxia.
   d. hypoxic hypoxia.

3. Carbon monoxide poisoning results in:
   a. anemic hypoxia.
   b. histotoxic hypoxia.
   c. hypoxic hypoxia.
   d. stagnant hypoxia.

4. Decreased gas exchange at the cellular level resulting from a toxic substance is classified as:
   a. circulatory
   b. histotoxic.
   c. hypoxemic.
   d. hypoxic.

5. Oxygen therapy administered to a pulmonary patient who retains carbon dioxide:
   a. can cause a dangerous rise in $PaCO_2$ levels.
   b. can suppress ventilation.
   c. should bring the patient's PO_2 level to 60 to 70 mm Hg.
   d. is able to accomplish all of the above.

6. When oxygen therapy is being used, "No Smoking" signs are posted, because oxygen:
   a. is combustible.
   b. is explosive.
   c. prevents the dispersion of smoke particles.
   d. supports combustion.

7. A patient has been receiving 100% oxygen therapy by way of a non-rebreather mask for several days. He complains of tingling in his fingers and shortness of breath. He is extremely restless and states that he has pain beneath his breastbone. The nurse should suspect:
   a. oxygen-induced hypoventilation.
   b. oxygen toxicity.
   c. oxygen-induced atelectasis.
   d. all of the above.

8. Oxygen concentrations of 70% can usually be delivered with the use of:
   a. a nasal cannula.
   b. an oropharyngeal catheter.
   c. a partial rebreathing mask.
   d. a Venturi mask.

9. The method of oxygen administration primarily used for patients with chronic obstructive pulmonary disease (COPD) is:

   a. a nasal cannula.

   b. an oropharyngeal catheter.

   c. a nonrebreathing mask.

   d. a Venturi mask.

10. Intermittent positive-pressure breathing differs from incentive spirometry in all of the following ways *except:*

    a. it is a mechanical aid to lung expansion.

    b. it is used to encourage hyperinflation.

    c. it produces a forced flow of air into the lungs during inhalation.

    d. it provides for the breathing of air or oxygen.

11. To help a patient use a mini-nebulizer, the nurse should encourage the patient to do all of the following *except:*

    a. hold his or her breath at the end of inspiration for a few seconds.

    b. cough frequently.

    c. take rapid, deep breaths.

    d. frequently evaluate his or her progress.

12. To assist a patient with the use of an incentive spirometer, the nurse should:

    a. make sure the patient is in a flat, supine position.

    b. tell the patient to try not to cough during and after each session, because doing so will cause pain.

    c. set an unrealistic goal so that the patient will try to maximize effort.

    d. encourage the patient to take approximately 10 breaths per hour between treatments, while awake.

13. Nursing actions associated with postural drainage include:

    a. encouraging the patient to cough after the procedure.

    b. auscultating the lungs before and after the procedure.

    c. encouraging the patient to exhale through pursed lips.

    d. all of the above.

14. When using percussion to aid in secretion removal, the nurse should avoid:

    a. the sternum and spine.

    b. the liver and kidneys.

    c. the spleen and female breast area.

    d. all of the above areas.

15. Percussion is accomplished by continuing the process for:

    a. 3 to 5 minutes while the patient uses diaphragmatic breathing.

    b. 10 to 15 minutes while the patient uses diaphragmatic breathing.

    c. 3 to 5 minutes while the patient breathes normally.

    d. 10 to 15 minutes while the patient breathes normally.

16. When vibrating the patient's chest, the nurse applies vibration:

    a. while the patient is inhaling.

    b. during both inhalation and exhalation.

    c. while the patient is exhaling.

    d. while the patient is holding the breath.

17. The purpose of pursed lips during exhalation is to:

    a. prolong exhalation.

    b. slow down the respiratory rate to allow for maximum lung expansion during inspiration.

    c. widen the airways.

    d. do all of the above.

18. Signs of an upper airway obstruction include:

    a. drawing in of the upper chest, sternum, and intercostal spaces.

    b. prolonged contraction of the abdominal muscles.

    c. tracheal tug.

    d. all of the above.

19. The suggested sequence of nursing actions for management of an upper airway obstruction is:

    a. clear airway, extend head, lift chin, use cross-finger technique, and perform a Heimlich maneuver.

    b. extend head, lift chin, clear airway, and perform a Heimlich maneuver.

    c. extend head, clear airway, lift chin, and insert airway.

    d. lift chin, clear airway, and perform a Heimlich maneuver.

20. Nursing management of a patient with an endotracheal tube includes:

    a. ensuring oxygen administration with high humidity.

    b. repositioning the patient every 2 hours.

    c. suctioning the oropharynx as needed.

    d. all of the above.

21. When suctioning secretions from a tracheostomy tube, it is helpful to first instill:

    a. less than 1 mL of sterile normal saline solution.

    b. 1 to 2 mL of sterile normal saline solution.

    c. 3 to 5 mL of sterile normal saline solution.

    d. 6 to 8 mL of sterile normal saline solution.

22. When suctioning a tracheostomy tube, the nurse needs to remember that each aspiration should not exceed:

    a. 15 seconds.

    b. 30 seconds.

    c. 45 seconds.

    d. 60 seconds.

23. Choose the blood gas sequence that indicates a need for mechanical ventilation.

    a. Decreasing PO_2, decreasing PCO_2, normal pH.

    b. Increasing PO_2, decreasing PCO_2, increasing pH.

    c. Decreasing PO_2, increasing PCO_2, decreasing pH.

    d. Increasing PO_2, decreasing PCO_2, decreasing pH.

24. The most commonly used positive-pressure ventilator currently is the:

    a. chest cuirass.

    b. time-cycled ventilator.

    c. pressure-cycled ventilator.

    d. volume-cycled ventilator.

25. With positive-pressure ventilation, positive intrathoracic pressure:

    a. increases venous return and decreases cardiac output.

    b. decreases venous return and increases cardiac output.

    c. decreases venous return and decreases cardiac output.

    d. increases venous return and increases cardiac output.

26. The sigh mechanism on an assist-control ventilator needs to be adjusted to provide _____ sigh(s) per hour at a volume that is _____ times the tidal volume.

    a. 1 and 1

    b. 1 to 2 and 2

    c. 1 to 3 and 1.5

    d. 3 to 6 and 3.5

27. The term used to describe thoracic surgery in which an entire lung is removed is:
    a. lobectomy.
    b. pneumonectomy.
    c. segmentectomy.
    d. wedge resection.

28. The patient who is scheduled for thoracic surgery needs to know that, postoperatively:
    a. chest tubes and drainage bottles may be necessary.
    b. he or she will be turned frequently and will be asked to cough and breathe deeply.
    c. oxygen will be administered to facilitate breathing if the need arises.
    d. all of the above treatments will be incorporated into a plan of care.

29. The water seal used in a disposable chest drainage system is effective if the water seal chamber is filled to the level of:
    a. 0.5 cm H_2O.
    b. 1.0 cm H_2O.
    c. 1.5 cm H_2O.
    d. 2.0 cm H_2O.

SHORT ANSWER

Read each statement carefully. Write your response in the space provided.

1. Oxygen transport to the tissues is dependent on four factors: _____, _____, _____, and _____.

2. Oxygen toxicity may occur if oxygen at greater than _____% concentration is administered for longer than _____.

3. List five signs and symptoms of oxygen toxicity.

   _____
   _____
   _____
   _____
   _____

4. For a patient with COPD, the stimulus for respiration is _____.

5. Four examples of low-flow oxygen delivery systems are _____, _____, _____, and _____.

6. The oxygen flow rate for a nasal cannula should not exceed _____ to _____ L/min.

7. List three goals of chest physiotherapy (CPT).

   _____
   _____
   _____

8. Cuff pressure for an endotracheal tube should be maintained at _____ mm Hg.

9. List three types of negative-pressure ventilators.

   _____

   _____

   _____

10. Positive-pressure ventilators work by: _____

    _____

11. Explain what is meant when the patient is said to be "bucking the ventilator": _____

    _____

12. For a patient to be safely weaned from a ventilator, the vital capacity should be

    _____, the minute ventilation should be _____, and the

    tidal volume should be _____.

13. List five complications that may occur after thoracic surgery.

    _____

    _____

    _____

    _____

    _____

COMPLETE THE CHART

Look at the accompanying figure of a disposable chest drainage system, and label the figure using the terms provided.

suction control
water seal
vent
drainage collection chambers
suction source
ventilation source

II. Critical Thinking Questions and Exercises

EXAMINING ASSOCIATIONS

Read each analogy. Write the best response in the space provided.

1. Hypoxia : decreased oxygen supply to the tissues :: Hypoxemia :

   _____.

2. Arterial oxygen pressure (PaO_2) : 60 to 95 mm Hg :: Oxygen saturation : _____ (%).

3. Partial rebreather mask : a flow rate of 8 to 11 L/min and 50% to 75% oxygen concentration ::

   Non-rebreather mask : a flow rate of _____ and _____

   % oxygen concentration.

4. Anemic hypoxia : decreased effective hemoglobin concentration :: Circulatory hypoxia :

   _____.

5. Ventilator tidal volume : 6 to 12 mL/kg (IBW) :: Ventilator rate : _____.

DISCUSSION AND ANALYSIS

Discuss the following topics with your classmates.

1. Distinguish between the clinical manifestations of hypoxia and hypoxemia.
2. Explain the pathophysiologic process involved with oxygen-induced hypoventilation for a patient with COPD.
3. Describe the proper hand position and technique used for chest percussion and vibration.
4. Explain the steps necessary to teach a patient diaphragmatic breathing and effective coughing techniques.
5. Describe the steps you would use to clear an obstructed airway.
6. Describe the techniques of tracheal tube suctioning.
7. Discuss in detail the guidelines for nursing interventions for weaning a patient from mechanical ventilation.
8. Explain the nursing interventions for managing a chest drainage system.

APPLYING CONCEPTS: CARE OF A PATIENT WITH AN ENDOTRACHEAL TUBE

Examine Figure 25-6 in the text. Immediately after intubation, the nurse completes a number of interventions. Consider each activity and explain the nursing role.

1. Check symmetry of chest expansion. To do this, the nurse would do four things,

   _____, _____,

   _____, and _____, to verify tube

   placement _____ every 8 hours _____.

2. To ensure high humidity, the nurse would _____.

3. Describe how the tube would be secured to prevent displacement: _____

   _____

4. To prevent the patient from biting the tube, the nurse would _____.

5. The patient would be repositioned every 2 hours for the purpose of _____.

6. Describe the suctioning technique: _____

   _____

7. List at least 5 of 10 interventions that a nurse would do to prevent complications.

   _____

   _____

   _____

   _____

   _____

   _____

CLINICAL SITUATIONS

Read the following case studies. Circle the correct answer.

CASE STUDY: Pneumonectomy: Preoperative Concerns

Mrs. Miley, a 66-year-old widow, is admitted to the clinical area as a preoperative patient scheduled for a pneumonectomy for lung cancer.

1. Nursing assessment during the admission history and physical examination includes obtaining data about the patient's:
   a. breathing patterns during exertion.
   b. cardiac status during exercise.
   c. smoking history.
   d. history relevant to all of the above.

2. The nurse knows that medical clearance for surgery is based primarily on evaluation of the:
   a. cardiopulmonary system.
   b. endocrine system.
   c. neurologic system.
   d. renal–urinary system.

3. A battery of preoperative tests are ordered. The nurse evaluates the serum creatinine level, because it reflects:
   a. cardiac status.
   b. endocrine status.
   c. pulmonary function.
   d. renal function.

4. The nurse knows that Mrs. Miley's functional lung capacity can be assessed by evaluating:
   a. arterial blood gases.
   b. blood urea nitrogen levels.
   c. chest radiographs.
   d. serum protein levels.

CASE STUDY: Pneumonectomy: Postoperative Concerns

Mrs. Miley is returned to the clinical area after being in the intensive care unit. She is recovering from a right pneumonectomy.

1. The major postoperative nursing objective is to:

    a. maintain a patent airway.

    b. provide for maximum remaining lung expansion.

    c. provide rehabilitative measures.

    d. recognize early indicators of complications.

2. Mrs. Miley has a central venous pressure line in place. Readings are to be taken to detect:

    a. hypothermia.

    b. hypovolemia.

    c. hypoxemia.

    d. hypoxia.

3. Pulmonary edema is a potential danger owing to the possible rapid infusion of intravenous fluids and a reduced vascular bed. Early symptoms of pulmonary edema include:

    a. dyspnea.

    b. frothy sputum.

    c. crackles (rales).

    d. all of the above.

4. The nurse should always be alert for signs of impending respiratory insufficiency, which would include all of the following *except:*

    a. bradycardia.

    b. dyspnea.

    c. hypertension.

    d. tachypnea.

CASE STUDY: Ventilator Patient

Mr. Brown, a 25-year-old man with a drug overdose, has been maintained on a volume-cycled ventilator for 3 weeks.

1. A major nursing assessment for Mr. Brown would be:

    a. breath sounds.

    b. nutritional needs.

    c. psychological status.

    d. spontaneous ventilatory efforts.

2. Positive-pressure ventilation can alter cardiac function. The nurse assesses for indicators of hypoxia and hypoxemia, which would include all of the following *except:*

    a. bradycardia and bradypnea.

    b. diaphoresis and oliguria.

    c. restlessness and confusion.

    d. transient hypertension.

3. A primary nursing intervention for Mr. Brown is maintaining optimal gas exchange. This can be accomplished by:

    a. conservative use of analgesics so that pain is relieved but the respiratory drive is not decreased.

    b. daily monitoring of fluid balance to prevent fluid overload.

    c. frequent repositioning to diminish the pulmonary effects of immobility.

    d. all of the above measures.

4. The nurse wants to determine early whether Mr. Brown is "bucking" his ventilator (breathing out during the ventilator's mechanical inspiratory phase) so that he or she can initiate preventive measures if necessary. The nurse should assess for signs and symptoms related to:

    a. hypercarbia.

    b. hypoxia.

    c. inadequate minute volume.

    d. all of the above.

CASE STUDY: Weaning From Ventilator

Mr. O'Day, a 71-year-old trauma victim, is to be weaned from his ventilator.

1. Before weaning, Mr. O'Day's ventilatory capacity should be such that he:
   a. can maintain an inspiratory force of at least 20 cm H_2O pressure.
   b. has a PaO_2 greater than 60% and an FiO_2 lower than 40%.
   c. is able to generate a minimum vital capacity of 10 to 15 mL/kg of body weight.
   d. is capable of all of the above.

2. Criteria to determine whether Mr. O'Day's endotracheal tube can be removed include:
   a. active pharyngeal and laryngeal gag reflexes.
   b. adequate spontaneous ventilation.
   c. voluntary cough mechanisms.
   d. all of the above.

3. Mr. O'Day will be weaned from oxygen when he can breathe room air and maintain a PaO_2 in the range of:
   a. 40 to 50 mm Hg.
   b. 50 to 60 mm Hg.
   c. 60 to 70 mm Hg.
   d. 70 to 100 mm Hg.

CHAPTER 26

Assessment of Cardiovascular Function

I. Interpretation, Completion, and Comparison

MULTIPLE CHOICE

Read each question carefully. Circle your answer.

1. The nurse who is caring for a patient with pericarditis understands that there is inflammation involving the:
   a. thin fibrous sac encasing the heart.
   b. inner lining of the heart and valves.
   c. heart's muscle fibers.
   d. exterior layer of the heart.

2. The coronary arteries arise from the:
   a. aorta near the origin of the left ventricle.
   b. pulmonary artery at the apex of the right ventricle.
   c. pulmonary vein near the left atrium.
   d. superior vena cava at the origin of the right atrium.

3. The pacemaker for the entire myocardium is the:
   a. atrioventricular junction.
   b. bundle of His.
   c. Purkinje fibers.
   d. sinoatrial node.

4. The intrinsic pacemaker rate of ventricular myocardial cells is:
   a. more than 80 bpm.
   b. 60 to 80 bpm.
   c. 40 to 60 bpm.
   d. fewer than 40 bpm.

5. An example of a beta-blocker that is administered to decrease automaticity is:
   a. Cardizem.
   b. Cordarone.
   c. Lopressor.
   d. Rythmol.

6. So that blood may flow from the right ventricle to the pulmonary artery, which of the following conditions is *not* required?
   a. the atrioventricular valves must be closed.
   b. the pulmonic valve must be open.
   c. right ventricular pressure must be less than pulmonary arterial pressure.
   d. right ventricular pressure must rise with systole.

7. Heart rate is stimulated by all of the following *except*:
   a. excess thyroid hormone.
   b. increased levels of circulating catecholamines.
   c. the sympathetic nervous system.
   d. the vagus nerve.

8. Stroke volume of the heart is determined by:
   a. the degree of cardiac muscle strength (precontraction).
   b. the intrinsic contractility of the cardiac muscle.
   c. the pressure gradient against which the muscle ejects blood during contraction.
   d. all of the above factors.

9. Changes in cardiac structure associated with aging include all of the following *except*:
   a. elongation of aorta.
   b. endocardial fibrosis.
   c. increased sensitivity to baroreceptors.
   d. increased size of left atrium.

10. A nonmodifiable risk factor for atherosclerosis is:
    a. stress.
    b. obesity.
    c. positive family history.
    d. hyperlipidemia.

11. The difference between the systolic and the diastolic pressure is called the:
    a. pulse pressure.
    b. auscultatory gap.
    c. pulse deficit.
    d. Korotkoff sound.

12. The nurse assessing a patient for postural hypotension recognizes the following positive sign:
    a. a heart rate of 5 to 20 bpm above the resting rate
    b. an unchanged systolic pressure
    c. a decrease of 10 mm Hg in the reading
    d. an increase of 5 mm Hg in diastolic pressure

13. If the sphygmomanometer cuff is too small for the patient, the blood pressure reading will probably be:
    a. falsely elevated.
    b. falsely decreased.
    c. an accurate reading.
    d. significantly different with each reading.

14. The first heart sound is generated by:
    a. closure of the aortic valve.
    b. closure of the atrioventricular valves.
    c. opening of the atrioventricular valves.
    d. opening of the pulmonic valve.

15. Exercise stress testing is a noninvasive procedure that can be used to assess certain aspects of cardiac function. After the test, the patient is instructed to:
    a. rest for a time.
    b. avoid stimulants.
    c. avoid extreme temperature changes.
    d. do all of the above.

16. Postcatheterization nursing measures for a patient who has had a cardiac catheterization include:
    a. assessing the peripheral pulses in the affected extremity.
    b. checking the insertion site for hematoma formation.
    c. evaluating temperature and color in the affected extremity.
    d. all of the above.

SHORT ANSWER

Read each statement carefully. Write your response in the space provided.

1. List the five categories of cardiovascular disease (CVD).

   _____

   _____

   _____

   _____

   _____

2. Distinguish between the functions of the atrioventricular and the semilunar valves:

_____

3. Briefly explain depolarization as it relates to cardiac physiology: _____

_____

4. Estimate the cardiac output (per beat) for an adult heart rate of 76 bpm with an average stroke volume of 70 mL: _____

_____

5. Describe Starling's law of the heart: _____

_____

6. List four physiologic effects on the cardiovascular system that are associated with the aging process.

_____

_____

_____

_____

7. List three major cardiovascular risk factors.

_____

_____

_____

8. If coronary artery disease (CAD) is present, the American Heart Association (AHA) recommends the following laboratory values: low-density lipoprotein (LDL), _____; blood pressure (BP), _____; serum glucose concentration, _____; and a body mass index (BMI) of _____.

9. To assess the apical pulse, the nurse would find the following location: _____

_____

10. Two most specific enzymes traditionally used to analyze an acute myocardial infarction (MI) are _____ and _____; two new biomarkers, _____ and _____, are early indicators of MI.

11. List several purposes of cardiac catheterization: _____

_____

_____

12. Describe selective angiography: _____

_____

13. Describe the implications of a low central venous pressure reading: _____

_____

14. Identify five possible complications of pulmonary artery monitoring: _____

_____

MATCHING

Match the anatomic term in column II with its associated function listed in column I.

Column I

1. _____ Separates the right and left atria

2. _____ Is located at the juncture of the superior vena cava and the right atrium

3. _____ Supports the heart in the mediastinum

4. _____ Sits between the right ventricle and the pulmonary artery

5. _____ Distributes venous blood to the lungs

6. _____ Is embedded in the right atrial wall near the tricuspid valve

Column II

a. Parietal pericardium

b. Pulmonary artery

c. Bicuspid valve

d. Pulmonic valve

e. Sinoatrial node

f. Atrioventricular node

CROSSWORD PUZZLE: TERMINOLOGY ASSOCIATED WITH CORONARY ATHEROSCLEROSIS

Complete the following crossword puzzle using terminology associated with coronary atherosclerosis.

DOWN

1. A principal blood lipid
2. A risk factor that causes pulmonary damage
4. The functional lesion of atherosclerosis
5. Biochemical substances, soluble in fat, that accumulate within a blood vessel
6. A risk factor that is endocrine in origin
9. A risk factor associated with a type A personality
10. A risk factor related to weight gain
14. A recommended dietary restriction

ACROSS

3. For persons of this sex, the incidence of coronary heart disease increases steadily with age
6. Influences amount of fat ingested
7. A symptom of myocardial ischemia
8. An unmodifiable risk factor
11. Myocardial manifestation of coronary artery disease
12. A risk factor related to patterns of daily activity
13. A part of blood vessels
15. A lifestyle habit that is considered a modifiable risk factor for heart disease

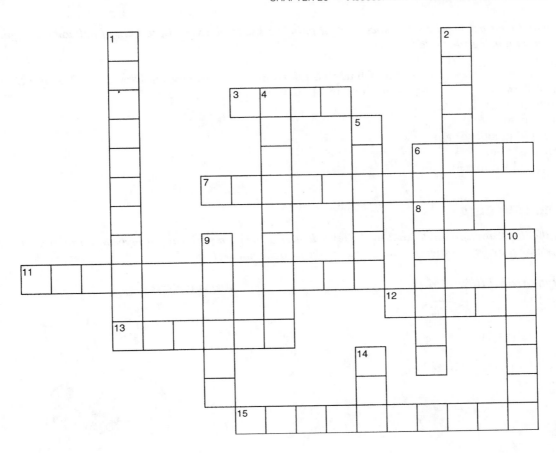

II. Critical Thinking Questions and Exercises

DISCUSSION AND ANALYSIS

Discuss the following topics with your classmates.

1. Describe the most common signs and symptoms of coronary vascular disease.
2. Compare and contrast the character, duration, aggravating factors, and precipitating events of cardiac and noncardiac chest pain.
3. Draft a detailed assessment guide that the nurse would use to evaluate various symptoms associated with chest pain, shortness of breath, palpitations, fatigue, and syncope.
4. Describe the classic "type A personality" and explain what is meant by "cardiac reactivity."
5. Describe the cause and significance of "gallop sounds."

EXAMINING ASSOCIATIONS

Read each analogy. Write the best response in the space provided.

1. The pulmonary artery : lungs :: Aorta : _____.
2. Epicardium : outer layer of cells lining the heart :: _____ : the heart muscle itself.
3. Apical area of the heart : fifth intercostal space :: Erb's point : _____.
4. The first heart sound : closure of the mitral and tricuspid valves :: The second heart sound : closure of _____.
5. Murmurs : malfunctioning valves :: Friction rubs : _____.

Compare and contrast the characteristics of chest pain specific to pericarditis, to pain of pulmonary origin, and to esophageal pain using the table below.

Type of Pain	Pain Character, Location, Duration, and Radiation	Precipitating Events	Nursing Measures
Pericarditis			
Pleuritic pain			
Pain of pulmonary origin			
Esophageal pain			
Pain caused by anxiety			

INTERPRETING DATA

Refer to the illustration in Table 26-2 in the text, depicting the pain pathways of myocardial infarction and angina pectoris, and the drawing below. Answer the associated questions.

Myocardial Infarction

Angina Pectoris

1. Name nursing assessment data that are relevant to record/report about the pain location, character, radiation, and duration.

_____

_____

_____

_____

_____

_____

_____

_____

2. Describe relevant precipitation events that would help with collaborative diagnosis.

_____

_____

_____

_____

_____

3. Describe relevant nursing interventions based on pain assessment.

_____

_____

_____

_____

_____

_____

CLINICAL APPLICATIONS

Read the following case studies. Circle the correct answer.

CASE STUDY: Cardiac Assessment for Chest Pain

Mr. Anderson is a 45-year-old executive with a major oil firm. Lately he has experienced frequent episodes of chest pressure that are relieved with rest. He has requested a complete physical examination. The nurse conducts an initial cardiac assessment.

1. The nurse immediately inspects the patient's skin. She observes a bluish tinge around the patient's lips. She knows that this is an indication of:

   a. central cyanosis.

   b. pallor.

   c. peripheral cyanosis.

   d. xanthelasma.

2. The nurse takes a baseline blood pressure measurement after the patient has rested for 10 minutes in a supine position. The reading that reflects a reduced pulse pressure is:

   a. 140/90 mm Hg.

   b. 140/100 mm Hg.

   c. 140/110 mm Hg.

   d. 140/120 mm Hg.

3. Five minutes after the initial blood pressure measurement is taken, the nurse assesses additional readings with the patient in a sitting and then in a standing position. The reading indicative of an abnormal postural response would be:

   a. lying, 140/110 mm Hg; sitting, 130/110 mm Hg; standing, 135/106 mm Hg.

   b. lying, 140/110 mm Hg; sitting, 135/112 mm Hg; standing, 130/115 mm Hg.

   c. lying, 140/110 mm Hg; sitting, 135/100 mm Hg; standing, 120/90 mm Hg.

   d. lying, 140/110 mm Hg; sitting, 130/108 mm Hg; standing, 125/108 mm Hg.

4. The nurse returns Mr. Anderson to the supine position and measures for jugular vein distention. The finding that would initially indicate an abnormal increase in the volume of the venous system would be obvious distention of the veins with the patient at what angle?

   a. 15 degrees

   b. 25 degrees

   c. 35 degrees

   d. 45 degrees

5. The nurse auscultates the apex of the heart by placing a stethoscope over:

   a. Erb's point.

   b. the fifth intercostal space.

   c. the pulmonic area.

   d. the tricuspid area.

CHAPTER 27

Management of Patients With Dysrhythmias and Conduction Problems

I. Interpretation, Completion, and Comparison

MULTIPLE CHOICE

Read each question carefully. Circle your answer.

1. The heart is under the control of the autonomic nervous system. Stimulation of the parasympathetic system results in all of the following *except:*

   a. slowed heart rate.

   b. lowered blood pressure.

   c. reduction in the force of contraction.

   d. positive inotropy.

2. The total time for ventricular depolarization and repolarization is represented on an electrocardiogram (ECG) reading as the:

   a. QRS complex.

   b. QT interval.

   c. ST segment.

   d. TP interval.

3. Ventricular rhythm can be determined by examining what interval on the ECG strip?

   a. PP interval

   b. QT interval

   c. RR interval

   d. TP interval

4. The PR interval on an ECG strip that reflects normal sinus rhythm would be between:

   a. 0.05 and 0.10 seconds.

   b. 0.12 and 0.20 seconds.

   c. 0.15 and 0.30 seconds.

   d. 0.25 and 0.40 seconds.

5. Characteristics of sinus bradycardia include all of the following *except:*

   a. a P wave precedes every QRS complex.

   b. every QRS complex is normal.

   c. the rate is 40 to 60 bpm.

   d. the rhythm is altered.

6. A dysrhythmia common in normal hearts and is described by patients as "my heart skipped a beat" is:

   a. premature atrial complex.

   b. atrial flutter.

   c. sinus tachycardia.

   d. ventricular fibrillation.

7. A "sawtooth" P wave is seen on an ECG strip with:

   a. sinus bradycardia.

   b. atrial flutter.

   c. atrioventricular nodal reentry.

   d. premature junctional complex.

8. Atrial fibrillation is associated with a heart rate up to:

   a. 300 bpm.

   b. 400 bpm.

   c. 500 bpm.

   d. 600 bpm.

9. Atrioventricular (AV) nodal reentry tachycardia is characterized by an atrial rate:
   a. of 100 bpm.
   b. between 100 and 150 bpm.
   c. between 150 and 250 bpm.
   d. greater than 250 bpm.

10. *Ventricular bigeminy* refers to a conduction defect in which:
    a. conduction is primarily from the AV node.
    b. every other beat is premature.
    c. rhythm is regular but fast.
    d. the rate is between 150 and 250 bpm.

11. With ventricular tachycardia:
    a. conduction originates in the ventricle.
    b. electrical defibrillation is used immediately.
    c. the P wave usually is normal.
    d. the ventricular rate is twice the normal atrial rate.

12. Ventricular fibrillation is associated with an absence of:
    a. heartbeat.
    b. palpable pulse.
    c. respirations.
    d. all of the above.

13. First-degree AV block is characterized by:
    a. a variable heart rate, usually slower than 60 bpm.
    b. an irregular rhythm.
    c. delayed conduction, producing a prolonged PR interval.
    d. P waves hidden with the QRS complex.

14. A conduction abnormality whereby no atrial impulse travels through the AV node is known as:
    a. first-degree AV block.
    b. second-degree AV block, type 1.
    c. second-degree AV block, type 2.
    d. third-degree AV block.

15. When assessing vital signs in a patient with a permanent pacemaker, the nurse needs to know the:
    a. date and time of insertion.
    b. location of the generator.
    c. model number.
    d. pacer rate.

16. Cardioversion is used to terminate dysrhythmias. With cardioversion, the:
    a. amount of voltage used should exceed 400 W-sec.
    b. electrical impulse can be discharged during the T wave.
    c. machine should be set to deliver a shock during the QRS complex.
    d. above statements are all true.

17. When electrical defibrillation is used:
    a. between 20 and 25 lb of pressure should be exerted on each paddle in order to ensure good skin contact.
    b. the defibrillator should discharge at 100 W-sec per kilogram of body weight.
    c. the discharge shock needs to be timed to the T wave.
    d. all of the above are necessary.

18. Candidates for an implantable cardioverter defibrillator (ICD) are patients at high risk who have:
    a. experienced syncope secondary to ventricular tachycardia.
    b. survived sudden cardiac death.
    c. sustained ventricular tachycardia.
    d. experienced one or more of the above.

19. The nurse needs to teach the patient with an automatic ICD that he or she must:
    a. avoid magnetic fields such as metal detection booths.
    b. call for emergency assistance if he or she feels dizzy.
    c. record events that trigger a shock sensation.
    d. be compliant with all of the above.

SHORT ANSWER

Read each statement carefully. Write your response in the space provided.

1. Name the four sites of origin of impulses that are used to name dysrhythmias.

    _____
    _____
    _____
    _____

2. Describe the normal electrical conduction through the heart: _____
    _____

3. Name five causes of sinus tachycardia.

    _____
    _____
    _____
    _____
    _____

4. Sinus tachycardia occurs when the ventricular and atrial rate are greater than _____.

5. A rate and rhythm characteristic that is necessary to diagnose ventricular tachycardia is
    _____ and _____.

6. List three potential collaborative problems that a nurse would choose for a patient with a dysrhythmia.

    _____
    _____
    _____

7. Name the one major difference between cardioversion and defibrillation: _____
    _____

8. Describe the placement of the electrode paddles used for defibrillation on a patient's chest:
    _____
    _____

9. Describe the difference between demand and fixed pacemakers: _____
    _____

SCRAMBLEGRAM

Unscramble the letters used to answer each statement, and write the word in the space provided.

1. A term used to describe an irregular or erratic heart rhythm: _____

S H R I C H M D T Y Y

2. The ability of the cardiac muscle to initiate an electrical impulse: _____

T A Y O I T A T I C M U

3. The ability of the cardiac muscle to transmit electrical impulses: _____

O U V T I C N Y I T D C

4. A term used to describe the electrical stimulation of the heart: _____

N O I P T R A D O L Z A E I

5. Stage of conduction in which the ventricles relax: _____

T S L D I A E O

6. Treatment of dysrhythmias by destroying causative cells: _____

N B A I A T L O

II. Critical Thinking Questions and Exercises

EXAMINING ASSOCIATIONS

Read each analogy and fill in the space provided with the best response.

1. The sinus node : night atrium :: Purkinje fibers : _____ .

2. Depolarization : systole :: _____ : diastole.

3. The _____ : ventricular repolarization :: The

_____ : repolarization of the Purkinje fibers.

4. Normal sinus rhythm : an atrial rate of 60 to 100 bpm :: _____ : an atrial rate of less than 60 bpm.

5. Cardizem : atrial flutter :: _____ : atrial fibrillation.

6. First-degree AV block : P : QRS ratio of 1:1 :: Second-degree AV block : P : QRS ratio of

_____ or _____ .

CLINICAL SITUATIONS

Graph Analysis

Analyze the following ECG graphs and answer the questions.

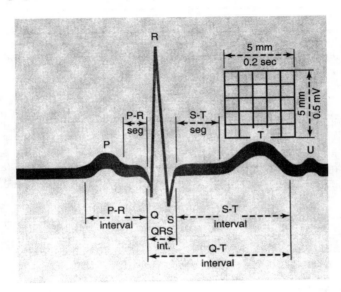

The first ECG graph shows commonly measured complex components. Each small box represents 0.04 seconds on the horizontal axis and 1 mm or 0.1 millivolt (mV) on the vertical axis. The PR interval is measured from the beginning of the P wave to the beginning of the QRS complex; the QRS complex is measured from the beginning of the Q wave to the end of the S wave; the QT interval is measured from the beginning of the Q wave to the end of the T wave.

1. Look at the above graphic recording of cardiac electrical activity. For each action, choose a wave deflection that corresponds to it, and write the appropriate letter or letters on the line provided.

   a. _____ ventricular muscle repolarization

   b. _____ time required for an impulse to travel through the atria and the conduction system to the Purkinje fibers

   c. _____ atrial muscle depolarization

   d. _____ ventricular muscle depolarization

   e. _____ early ventricular repolarization of the ventricles

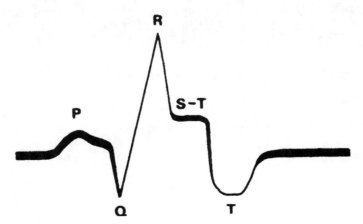

2. Consider the above graphic recording, and identify three alterations that are consistent with myocardial ischemia and infarction hours to days after the attack.

a. _____

b. _____

c. _____

Analyze the graphic recording for each of the following dysrhythmias and describe the altered deflection.

1.

| normal PP interval | shorter PP interval | longer PP interval | ★ = PAC |

noncompensatory pause

Premature atrial complexes (PACs): _____

_____

_____

2.

Multifocal premature ventricular contractions (PVCs) in quadrigeminy: _____

_____

_____

3.

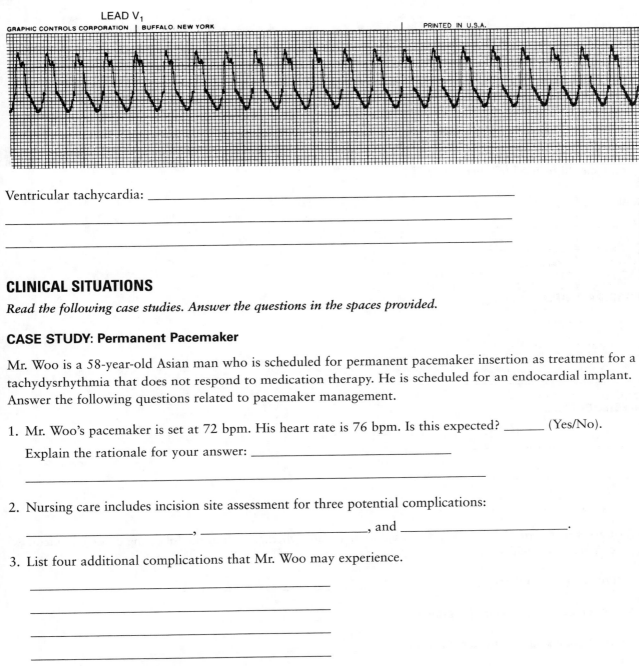

Ventricular tachycardia: _____

_____

_____

CLINICAL SITUATIONS

Read the following case studies. Answer the questions in the spaces provided.

CASE STUDY: Permanent Pacemaker

Mr. Woo is a 58-year-old Asian man who is scheduled for permanent pacemaker insertion as treatment for a tachydysrhythmia that does not respond to medication therapy. He is scheduled for an endocardial implant. Answer the following questions related to pacemaker management.

1. Mr. Woo's pacemaker is set at 72 bpm. His heart rate is 76 bpm. Is this expected? _____ (Yes/No).

   Explain the rationale for your answer: _____

   _____

2. Nursing care includes incision site assessment for three potential complications:

   _____, _____, and _____.

3. List four additional complications that Mr. Woo may experience.

   _____

   _____

   _____

   _____

4. The most common initial postoperative complication is _____.

5. List six things about the pacemaker that must be noted on a patient's chart.

   a. _____

   b. _____

   c. _____

   d. _____

   e. _____

   f. _____

6. List the three major goals of patient care and describe nursing interventions and expected patient outcomes that should be used to meet them.

GOAL

   a. _____

   b. _____

   c. _____

NURSING ACTIVITIES

   a. _____

   b. _____

   c. _____

EXPECTED OUTCOME

   a. _____

   b. _____

   c. _____

7. List assessment criteria that should be used to determine whether each of the following expected outcomes of care has been achieved.

   a. Freedom from infection _____

   b. Adherence to a self-care program _____

   c. Maintenance of pacemaker function _____

CHAPTER 28

Management of Patients With Coronary Vascular Disorders

I. Interpretation, Completion, and Comparison

MULTIPLE CHOICE

Read each question carefully. Circle your answer.

1. The most common heart disease for adults in the United States is:
   a. angina pectoris.
   b. coronary artery disease.
   c. myocardial infarction.
   d. valvular heart disease.

2. Lumen narrowing with atherosclerosis is caused by:
   a. atheroma formation on the intima.
   b. scarred endothelium.
   c. thrombus formation.
   d. all of the above.

3. A healthy level of serum cholesterol would be a reading of:
   a. 160 to 200 mg/dL.
   b. 210 to 240 mg/dL.
   c. 250 to 275 mg/dL.
   d. 280 to 300 mg/dL.

4. Which of the following findings is a strong negative risk factor for heart disease?
   a. cholesterol, 280 mg/dL
   b. low-density lipoproteins (LDL), 160 mg/dL
   c. high-density lipoproteins (HDL), 60 mg/dL
   d. ratio of LDL to HDL, 4.5 to 1.0

5. Hypertension is present with repeated blood pressure measurements exceeding:
   a. 110/80 mm Hg.
   b. 120/80 mm Hg.
   c. 130/90 mm Hg.
   d. 140/90 mm Hg.

6. The incidence of coronary artery disease (CAD) tends to be equal for men and women after the age of:
   a. 45 years.
   b. 50 years.
   c. 55 years.
   d. 65 years.

7. The pain of angina pectoris is produced primarily by:
   a. coronary vasoconstriction.
   b. movement of thromboemboli.
   c. myocardial ischemia.
   d. the presence of atheromas.

8. A common side effect of nitroglycerin is:
   a. musculoskeletal weakness.
   b. hypertension.
   c. bradycardia.
   d. headache.

9. The nurse advises a patient that sublingual nitroglycerin should alleviate angina pain within:
   a. 3 to 4 minutes.
   b. 10 to 15 minutes.
   c. 30 minutes.
   d. 60 minutes.

10. Patient education includes telling someone who takes nitroglycerin sublingually that he or she should call emergency services (#911) if no relief has been obtained after taking _____ tablets at 5-minute intervals:
    a. more than 1
    b. 2 or more
    c. 3 or more
    d. more than 4

11. The scientific rationale supporting the administration of beta-adrenergic blockers is the drugs' ability to:
    a. block sympathetic impulses to the heart.
    b. elevate blood pressure.
    c. increase myocardial contractility.
    d. induce bradycardia.

12. An antidote for propranolol hydrochloride (a beta-adrenergic blocker) that is used to treat bradycardia is:
    a. digoxin.
    b. atropine.
    c. protamine sulfate.
    d. sodium nitroprusside.

13. Calcium channel blockers act by:
    a. decreasing SA node automaticity.
    b. increasing AV node conduction.
    c. increasing the heart rate.
    d. creating a positive inotropic effect.

14. In the United States, about 1 million people will have an acute myocardial infarction (MI) each year. Of these 1 million, what percentage will die?
    a. 10% to 15%
    b. 25%
    c. 30% to 40%
    d. 60%

15. The classic ECG changes that occur with an MI include all of the following *except*:
    a. an absent P wave
    b. an abnormal Q wave
    c. T-wave inversion
    d. ST-segment elevation

16. The most common site of myocardial infarction is the:
    a. left atrium.
    b. left ventricle.
    c. right atrium.
    d. right ventricle.

17. Which of the following statements about myocardial infarction pain is *incorrect?*
    a. it is relieved by rest and inactivity.
    b. it is substernal in location.
    c. it is sudden in onset and prolonged in duration.
    d. it is viselike and radiates to the shoulders and arms.

18. Myocardial cell damage can be reflected by high levels of cardiac enzymes. The most specific index of all cardiac enzymes is:
    a. alkaline phosphatase.
    b. creatine kinase (CK-MB).
    c. myoglobin.
    d. troponin.

19. The most common vasodilator used to treat myocardial pain is:
    a. amyl nitrite.
    b. Inderal.
    c. nitroglycerin.
    d. Pavabid HCl.

20. A newer thrombolytic agent that increases plasminogen activator is:
    a. Activase.
    b. Urokinase.
    c. Tenecteplase.
    d. Retavase.

21. An intravenous analgesic frequently administered to relieve chest pain associated with myocardial infarction is:
    a. meperidine hydrochloride.
    b. hydromorphone hydrochloride.
    c. morphine sulfate.
    d. codeine sulfate.

22. The need for surgical intervention in CAD is determined by the:
    a. amount of stenosis in the coronary arteries.
    b. myocardial area served by the stenotic artery.
    c. occurrence of previous infarction related to the affected artery.
    d. all of the above.

23. A candidate for percutaneous transluminal coronary angioplasty (PTCA) is a patient with CAD who:
    a. has compromised left ventricular function.
    b. has had angina longer than 3 years.
    c. has at least 70% occlusion of a major coronary artery.
    d. has questionable left ventricular function.

24. A goal of dilation in PTCA is to increase the size of the artery's lumen to at least _____%.
    a. 20%
    b. 35%
    c. 60%
    d. 80%

25. The nurse expects a patient who has undergone PTCA to be discharged:
    a. the same day as surgery.
    b. within 24 hours after the procedure.
    c. 3 days later.
    d. after 1 week.

26. The nurse needs to be alert to assess for clinical symptoms of possible postoperative complications of PTCA, which include:
    a. abrupt closure of the artery.
    b. arterial dissection.
    c. coronary artery spasm.
    d. all of the above.

27. One of the most important and immediate postoperative PTCA complications for which the nurse needs to assess is:
    a. bleeding.
    b. depression.
    c. hypertension.
    d. hypoventilation.

28. A candidate for traditional coronary artery bypass grafting (CABG) must meet which of the following criteria?
    a. blockage that cannot be treated by PTCA.
    b. greater than 60% blockage in the left main coronary artery.
    c. unstable angina.
    d. all of the above.

29. According to the critical care pathway outlined for CABG, the nurse knows that postoperative teaching must occur before discharge on about which day after surgery?
    a. second
    b. fourth
    c. seventh
    d. tenth

30. The most common nursing diagnosis for patients awaiting cardiac surgery is:
    a. activity intolerance.
    b. fear related to the surgical procedure.
    c. decreased cardiac output.
    d. anginal pain.

31. Extremity paresthesia, dysrhythmias (peaked T waves), and mental confusion after cardiac surgery are signs of electrolyte imbalance related to the level of:
    a. calcium.
    b. magnesium.
    c. potassium.
    d. sodium.

32. A complication after cardiac surgery that is associated with an alteration in preload is:
    a. cardiac tamponade.
    b. elevated central venous pressure.
    c. hypertension.
    d. hypothermia.

33. The most common dysrhythmia seen after cardiac surgery is:
    a. bradycardia.
    b. ectopic beats.
    c. tachycardia.
    d. all of the above.

SHORT ANSWER

Read each statement carefully. Write your response in the space provided.

1. The leading cause of death in the United States for men and women of all ethnic and racial groups is

   _____.

2. The most common cause of cardiovascular disease is _____.

3. The most frequently occurring sign of myocardial ischemia is _____.

4. More than 50% of people with coronary artery disease have the risk factor of

   _____.

5. List four modifiable risk factors that are considered major causes of coronary artery disease.

   _____

   _____

   _____

   _____

6. Management of coronary heart disease requires a therapeutic range of cholesterol and lipoproteins. An acceptable blood level of cholesterol is _____, with an LDL/HDL ratio of _____. The desired level of LDL should be _____ mg/dL, and the HDL level should be greater than _____ mg/dL.

7. The American Heart Association recommends that an average American diet contain about _____% fat.

8. Intractable angina is chest pain described as _____.

9. Postpericardiotomy syndrome can be diagnosed by assessment of the following five symptoms:

   a. _____

   b. _____

   c. _____

   d. _____

   e. _____

II. Critical Thinking Questions and Exercises

DISCUSSION AND ANALYSIS

Discuss the following topics with your classmates.

1. Explain why atherosclerosis is such a damaging process.
2. Explain how cigarette smoking contributes to the development of coronary artery disease.

EXAMINING ASSOCIATIONS

Examine the association among the items in each cluster and identify the common factor.

1. Abdominal aortic aneurysm, carotid artery disease, diabetes, existing coronary artery disease, and peripheral arterial disease

   _____

2. Abdominal obesity, elevated triglycerides, low level of HDL, hypertension, and impaired function of insulin

   _____

3. Age, cholesterol level, systolic blood pressure, levels of LDL and HDL, and cigarette smoking

   _____

4. Cholesterol abnormalities, cigarette smoking, diabetes mellitus, and hypertension

   _____

5. Total cholesterol, LDL, HDL, and triglycerides

   _____

IDENTIFYING PATTERNS

Review the accompanying figure and answer the questions.

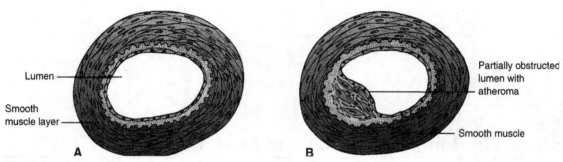

Normal and atherosclerotic arteries. **A,** Cross-section of normal artery in which the lumen is fully patent (open). **B,** Cross-section of artery with diminished patency resulting from atheroma.

1. Describe the underlying pathophysiology that causes a normal artery (**A**) to narrow because of atheroma deposits: _____

   _____

   _____

2. An atheroma is described as: _____

   _____

3. A possible complication of rupture or hemorrhage of the lipid core into the plaque is

   _____.

4. A thrombus is a dangerous complication of atherosclerosis because it can lead to

   _____ and _____.

SUPPORTING ARGUMENTS

Offer a supporting rationale for your response.

1. Explain, supported with a scientific base to your rationale, why cigarette smoking contributes to the severity of coronary heart disease for each of these three factors:

   a. increased CO levels: _____

   _____

   b. increased catecholamines: _____

   _____

   c. increased platelet adhesion: _____

   _____

2. Argue in support of using calcium channel blockers for treatment of angina: _____

   _____

   _____

CLINICAL SITUATIONS

Read the following case studies. Circle the correct answer.

CASE STUDY: Angina Pectoris

Ermelina, a 64-year-old retired secretary, is admitted to the medical-surgical area for management of chest pain caused by angina pectoris.

1. The nurse knows that the basic cause of angina pectoris is believed to be:
   a. dysrhythmias triggered by stress.
   b. insufficient coronary blood flow.
   c. minute emboli discharged through the narrowed lumens of the coronary vessels.
   d. spasms of the vessel walls owing to excessive secretion of epinephrine (adrenaline).

2. The medical record lists a probable diagnosis of chronic stable angina. The nurse knows that Ermelina's pain:
   a. has increased progressively in frequency and duration.
   b. is incapacitating.
   c. is relieved by rest and is predictable.
   d. usually occurs at night and may be relieved by sitting upright.

3. Ermelina has nitroglycerin at her bedside to take PRN. The nurse knows that nitroglycerin acts in all of the following ways *except:*
   a. causing venous pooling throughout the body.
   b. constricting arterioles to lessen peripheral blood flow.
   c. dilating the coronary arteries to increase the oxygen supply.
   d. lowering systemic blood pressure.

4. Ermelina took a nitroglycerin tablet at 10:00 AM, after her morning care. It did not relieve her pain, so she repeated the dose. Ten minutes later and still in pain, she calls the nurse, who should:
   a. administer a PRN dose of diazepam (Valium), try to calm her, and recommend that she rest in a chair with her legs dependent to encourage venous pooling.
   b. assist her to the supine position, give her oxygen at 6 L/min, and advise her to rest in bed.
   c. help her to a comfortable position, give her oxygen at 2 L/min, and call her physician.
   d. suggest that she take double her previous dose after 5 minutes and try to sleep to decrease her body's need for oxygen.

CASE STUDY: Decreased Myocardial Tissue Perfusion

Mr. Lillis, a 46-year-old bricklayer, is brought to the emergency department by ambulance with a suspected diagnosis of myocardial infarction. He appears ashen, is diaphoretic and tachycardiac, and has severe chest pain. The nursing diagnosis is decreased cardiac output, related to decreased myocardial tissue perfusion.

1. The nurse knows that the most critical time period for his diagnosis is:
   a. within the first hour after symptoms begin.
   b. within 24 hours after the onset of symptoms.
   c. within the first 48 hours after the attack.
   d. between the third and fifth day after the attack.

2. The nurse needs to look for symptoms associated with one of the major causes of sudden death during the first 48 hours, which is:
   a. cardiogenic shock.
   b. pulmonary edema.
   c. pulmonary embolism.
   d. ventricular rupture.

3. Mr. Lillis is transferred to a telemetry unit after 6 days in the cardiac care unit, where he was treated for an anterior wall myocardial infarction. The nurse expects Mr. Lillis to be able to do all of the following *except:*

   a. isometric exercises.

   b. self-care activities.

   c. sit in a chair several times a day.

   d. walk within his room.

4. The nurse is aware that ischemic tissue remains sensitive to oxygen demands, because scar formation is not seen until the:

   a. second week.

   b. third week.

   c. sixth week.

   d. eighth week.

5. Mr. Lillis needs to be advised that myocardial healing will not be complete for about:

   a. 2 months.

   b. 4 months.

   c. 6 months.

   d. 8 months.

6. For discharge planning, Mr. Lillis is advised to:

   a. avoid large meals.

   b. exercise daily.

   c. restrict caffeine-containing beverages.

   d. do all of the above.

Management of Patients With Structural, Infectious, and Inflammatory Cardiac Disorders

I. Interpretation, Comparison, and Completion

MULTIPLE CHOICE

Read each question carefully. Circle your answer.

1. Incomplete closure of the tricuspid valve results in a backward flow of blood from the:
   a. aorta to the left ventricle.
   b. left atrium to the left ventricle.
   c. right atrium to the right ventricle.
   d. right ventricle to the right atrium.

2. Backward flow of blood from the left ventricle to the left atrium is through the:
   a. aortic valve.
   b. mitral valve.
   c. pulmonic valve.
   d. tricuspid valve.

3. The pathophysiology of mitral stenosis is consistent with:
   a. aortic stenosis.
   b. left ventricular failure.
   c. right atrial hypertrophy.
   d. all of the above.

4. On auscultation, the nurse suspects a diagnosis of mitral valve regurgitation when which of the following is heard?
   a. mitral click
   b. high-pitched blowing sound at the apex
   c. low-pitched diastolic murmur at the apex
   d. diastolic murmur at the left sternal border

5. The presence of a water-hammer pulse (quick, sharp strokes that suddenly collapse) is diagnostic for:
   a. aortic regurgitation.
   b. mitral insufficiency.
   c. tricuspid insufficiency.
   d. tricuspid stenosis.

6. Severe aortic stenotic disease is consistent with all of the following *except*:
   a. increased cardiac output.
   b. left ventricular hypertrophy.
   c. pulmonary edema.
   d. right-sided heart failure.

7. The most common valvuloplasty procedure is the:
   a. balloon valvuloplasty.
   b. annuloplasty.
   c. chordoplasty.
   d. commissurotomy.

8. Xenografts, used for valve replacement, have a viability of about:
   a. 2 years.
   b. 4 years.
   c. 8 years.
   d. 12 years.

9. The nurse knows that a patient who is to receive a xenograft from a pig or cow will be receiving:
   a. an allograft.
   b. an autograft.
   c. a heterograft.
   d. a homograft.

10. The most commonly occurring cardiomyopathy is:
    a. dilated.
    b. hypertrophic.
    c. idiopathic.
    d. restrictive.

11. Probably the most helpful diagnostic test to identify cardiomyopathy is:
    a. serial enzyme studies.
    b. cardiac catheterization.
    c. the echocardiogram.
    d. the phonocardiogram.

12. An immunosuppressant that allowed heart transplantation to become a therapeutic option for end-stage heart disease is:
    a. Procardia.
    b. cyclosporine.
    c. Calan.
    d. Vancocin.

13. Rheumatic endocarditis is an inflammatory reaction to:
    a. group A streptococcus.
    b. *Pseudomonas aeruginosa.*
    c. *Serratia marcescens.*
    d. *Staphylococcus aureus.*

14. The causative microorganism for rheumatic endocarditis can be accurately identified only by:
    a. a throat culture.
    b. an echocardiogram.
    c. roentgenography.
    d. serum analysis.

15. Clinical manifestations of infective endocarditis may include:
    a. embolization.
    b. focal neurologic lesions.
    c. heart murmurs.
    d. all of the above.

16. The most characteristic symptom of pericarditis is:
    a. dyspnea.
    b. constant chest pain.
    c. fatigue lasting longer than 1 month.
    d. uncontrolled restlessness.

17. The characteristic sign of pericarditis is:
    a. a friction rub.
    b. dyspnea.
    c. fever.
    d. hypoxia.

18. Which of the following medications would *not* be used to treat pericarditis because it can decrease blood flow?
    a. colchicine
    b. Indocin
    c. Motrin
    d. prednisone

19. A serious consequence of pericarditis is:
    a. cardiac tamponade.
    b. decreased venous pressure.
    c. hypertension.
    d. left ventricular hypertrophy.

SHORT ANSWER

Read each statement carefully. Write your response in the space provided.

1. Describe the basic dysfunction of mitral valve prolapse: _____

   _____

2. If dysrhythmias occur with mitral valve prolapse syndrome, the nurse advises the patient to avoid

   _____, _____, and _____.

3. A nurse, using auscultation to identify aortic regurgitation, would place the stethoscope

   _____ and would expect to hear _____.

4. With aortic stenosis, the patient should receive _____ to prevent endocarditis.

5. List four potential complications or collaborative problems for patients with cardiomyopathy.

   _____

   _____

   _____

   _____

6. Identify five common indicators for heart transplantation.

   _____

   _____

   _____

   _____

   _____

7. Prompt treatment of streptococcal pharyngitis with _____ can prevent almost all

   attacks of _____.

8. Briefly describe the pathophysiology of endocarditis, beginning with the formation of a vegetation:

   _____

   _____

9. Infective endocarditis is usually caused by the following bacteria: _____,

   _____, _____, and _____.

10. Briefly describe the pathophysiology of myocarditis: _____

    _____

    _____

11. Describe the anatomic landmark for auscultation of a pericardial friction rub: _____

    _____

MATCHING

Match the pathophysiology in column II with the valvular disorder listed in column I.

Column I

1. _____ Mitral valve prolapse
2. _____ Mitral stenosis
3. _____ Mitral regurgitation
4. _____ Aortic valve stenosis
5. _____ Aortic regurgitation

Column II

a. Leaflet malformation prevents complete closure
b. Can be caused by rheumatic endocarditis
c. Characterized by a significantly widened pulse pressure
d. Blood seeps backward into left atrium
e. Thickening and contracture of mitral valve cusps

II. Critical Thinking Questions and Exercises

DISCUSSION AND ANALYSIS

Discuss the following topics with your classmates.

1. Describe what a nurse would expect to hear when using auscultation to listen to the heart of a patient with mitral valve prolapse.
2. Explain how left ventricular hypertrophy develops from mitral valve insufficiency.
3. Describe the pathophysiology of aortic regurgitation.
4. Describe the characteristic sound of the murmur heard with aortic stenosis.
5. Explain the purpose and process of a balloon valvuloplasty.
6. Explain the purpose and process of valve replacement.
7. Describe the management of a patient who has undergone a valvuloplasty and replacement.
8. Explain the pathophysiology of all cardiomyopathies.
9. Discuss at least five nursing diagnoses and collaborative problems for a patient with cardiomyopathy.
10. Describe the pathophysiology of pericarditis and list at least six underlying causes.

IDENTIFYING PATTERNS

Outline on the flow chart the pathophysiologic sequence of events that occurs when mitral valve stenosis leads to right ventricular failure.

Mitral Valve Stenosis

Right Ventricular Failure

CLINICAL SITUATIONS

Read the following case studies. Fill in the blanks below or circle the correct answer.

CASE STUDY: Infective Endocarditis

Mr. Fontana, a 60-year-old executive, is admitted to the hospital with a diagnosis of infective endocarditis. Pertinent history includes a previous diagnosis of mitral valve prolapse. A physical examination at his physician's office before admission revealed complaints of anorexia, joint pain, intermittent fever, and a 10-lb weight loss in the past 2 months.

1. The nurse knows, before assessment, that Mr. Fontana's vague clinical symptoms are characteristic of an insidious disease onset that develops from one of three conditions:

   _____, _____, or _____.

2. While examining Mr. Fontana's eyes during the admission assessment, the nurse notes conjunctival hemorrhages with pale centers caused by emboli in the nerve fiber of the eye. These are known as:
   a. Roth's spots.
   b. Osler's nodes.
   c. Janeway's lesions.
   d. Heberden's nodes.

3. The nurse also assesses for central nervous system manifestations of the infectious disease. She looks for

   symptoms such as _____, _____, _____,

   and _____.

4. The primary objective of medical management in this case is: _____.

5. Serial blood cultures identified *Streptococcus viridans* as the causative organism, and parenteral antibiotic treatment was initiated. The nurse expects that Mr. Fontana will probably remain on the antibiotic intravenous infusion for:
   a. 5 days.
   b. 1 week.
   c. 2 to 6 weeks.
   d. 8 to 10 weeks.

6. Even with successful treatment, organ damage can occur. Cardiac complications may include

   _____, _____, _____, and

   _____.

7. Mr. Fontana needs to be advised that prophylactic antibiotic therapy is also recommended for:
   a. tooth extraction.
   b. bronchoscopy.
   c. cystoscopy.
   d. all of the above.

CASE STUDY: Acute Pericarditis

Mrs. Russell is a 46-year-old Caucasian man who developed symptoms of acute pericarditis secondary to a viral infection. Diagnosis was based on the characteristic sign of a friction rub and pain over the pericardium.

1. Based on knowledge of pericardial pain, the nurse suggests the following body position to relieve the pain symptoms:
   a. flat in bed with feet slightly higher than the head
   b. Fowler's
   c. right side-lying
   d. semi-Fowler's

2. Based on assessment data, the major nursing diagnosis is _____.

3. Initial nursing intervention includes maintenance of bed rest until the following symptom disappears:
   a. fever
   b. friction rub
   c. pain
   d. all of the above

4. Identify three drug classifications that are commonly prescribed for management or treatment.

   _____

   _____

   _____

5. Name the anatomic landmarks used to auscultate for a pericardial friction rub:

   _____

6. List the two major expected patient outcomes for nursing management of a patient with pericarditis.

   _____

   _____

CHAPTER 30

Management of Patients With Complications From Heart Disease

I. Interpretation, Completion, and Comparison

MULTIPLE CHOICE

Read each question carefully. Circle your answer.

1. The multilumen pulmonary artery catheter allows the nurse to measure hemodynamic pressures at various points in the heart. When the tip enters the small branches of the pulmonary artery, the nurse can assess all of the following measurements *except:*
   a. central venous pressure (CVP).
   b. pulmonary artery capillary pressure (PACP).
   c. pulmonary artery obstructive pressure (PAOP).
   d. pulmonary artery wedge pressure (PAWP).

2. Hemodynamic monitoring by means of a multilumen pulmonary artery catheter can provide detailed information about:
   a. preload.
   b. afterload.
   c. cardiac output.
   d. all of the above.

3. Nursing measures in hemodynamic monitoring include assessing for localized ischemia caused by inadequate arterial flow. The nurse should:
   a. assess the involved extremity for color temperature.
   b. check for capillary filling.
   c. evaluate pulse rate.
   d. do all of the above.

4. The most frequent cause for hospitalization among people older than 65 years of age is:
   a. angina pectoris.
   b. heart failure.
   c. hypertension.
   d. pulmonary edema.

5. The primary cause of heart failure (HF) is:
   a. arterial hypertension.
   b. coronary atherosclerosis.
   c. myocardial dysfunction.
   d. valvular dysfunction.

6. The dominant function in cardiac failure is:
   a. ascites.
   b. hepatomegaly.
   c. inadequate tissue perfusion.
   d. nocturia.

7. On assessment, the nurse knows that a patient who reports no symptoms of heart failure at rest but is symptomatic with increased physical activity would have a heart failure classification of:
   a. I.
   b. II.
   c. III.
   d. IV.

8. On assessment, the nurse knows that the presence of pitting edema indicates fluid retention of at least:
   a. 4 lb.
   b. 6 lb.
   c. 8 lb.
   d. 10 lb.

9. The diagnosis of heart failure is usually confirmed by:
   a. a chest x-ray.
   b. an echocardiogram.
   c. an electrocardiogram.
   d. ventriculogram.

10. A key diagnostic laboratory test for heart failure is the:
    a. blood urea nitrogen (BUN).
    b. complete blood cell count.
    c. B-type natriuretic peptide.
    d. serum electrolyte counts.

11. The treatment for cardiac failure is directed at:
    a. decreasing oxygen needs of the heart.
    b. increasing the cardiac output by strengthening muscle contraction or decreasing peripheral resistance.
    c. reducing the amount of circulating blood volume.
    d. all of the above.

12. A primary classification of medications used in the treatment of systolic heart failure is:
    a. angiotensin-converting enzyme (ACE) inhibitors.
    b. beta-blockers.
    c. diuretics.
    d. calcium channel blockers.

13. The nurse knows that the following ACE inhibitor ordered by the physician has a rapid onset of action, within 15 minutes.
    a. Altace
    b. Capoten
    c. Lotensin
    d. Vasotec

14. An example of a potassium-sparing diuretic that might be prescribed for a person with congestive heart failure is:
    a. Aldactone.
    b. Mykrox.
    c. Zaroxolyn.
    d. Lasix.

15. Digitalis toxicity can occur when serum digitalis levels are in the range of:
    a. 0.25 to 0.50 mg/dL.
    b. 0.50 to 1.0 mg/dL.
    c. 1.0 to 2.0 mg/dL.
    d. 2.5 to 3.5 mg/dL.

16. The primary underlying disorder of pulmonary edema is:
    a. decreased left ventricular pumping.
    b. decreased right ventricular elasticity.
    c. increased left atrial contractility.
    d. increased right atrial resistance.

17. Pulmonary edema is characterized by:
    a. elevated left ventricular end-diastolic pressure.
    b. a rise in pulmonary venous pressure.
    c. increased hydrostatic pressure.
    d. all of the above alterations.

18. With pulmonary edema, there is usually an alteration in:
    a. afterload.
    b. contractility.
    c. preload.
    d. all of the above.

19. A commonly prescribed diuretic that is given intravenously to produce a rapid diuretic effect is:
    a. Bumex.
    b. Lasix.
    c. Mykrox.
    d. Zaroxolyn.

20. A popular catecholamine that when given intravenously can rapidly increase cardiac contractility is:
    a. Bumex.
    b. Dobutrex.
    c. Primacor.
    d. Natrecor.

21. Morphine is given in acute pulmonary edema to redistribute the pulmonary circulation to the periphery by decreasing:
    a. peripheral resistance.
    b. pulmonary capillary pressure.
    c. transudation of fluid.
    d. all of the above.

22. A recommended position for a patient in acute pulmonary edema is:
    a. prone, to encourage maximum rest, thereby decreasing respiratory and cardiac rates.
    b. semi-Fowler's, to facilitate breathing and promote pooling of blood in the sacral area.
    c. Trendelenburg, to drain the upper airways of congestion.
    d. upright with the legs down, to decrease venous return.

23. Cardiogenic shock is pump failure that occurs primarily as the result of:
    a. coronary artery stenosis.
    b. left ventricular damage.
    c. myocardial ischemia.
    d. right atrial flutter.

24. Classic signs of cardiogenic shock include all of the following *except*:
    a. bradycardia.
    b. cerebral hypoxia.
    c. hypotension.
    d. oliguria.

25. The nurse expects that positive inotropic medications would be administered to treat cardiogenic shock, with the exception of:
    a. Adrenalin.
    b. Dobutrex.
    c. Intropin.
    d. Levophed.

26. A clinical manifestation of pericardial effusion is:
    a. widening pulse pressure.
    b. a decrease in venous pressure.
    c. shortness of breath.
    d. an increase in blood pressure.

27. The most reliable sign of cardiac arrest is:
    a. absence of a pulse.
    b. cessation of respirations.
    c. dilation of the pupils.
    d. inaudible heart sounds.

28. Brain damage occurs with cessation of circulation after an approximate interval of:
    a. 2 minutes.
    b. 4 minutes.
    c. 6 minutes.
    d. 8 minutes.

29. The drug of choice during cardiopulmonary resuscitation to suppress ventricular dysrhythmias is:
    a. atropine.
    b. epinephrine.
    c. lidocaine.
    d. morphine.

MATCHING

Match the type of ventricular heart failure in column II with its associated pathophysiology listed in column I.

Column I

1. _____ Fatigability
2. _____ Dependent edema
3. _____ Pulmonary congestion predominates
4. _____ Distended neck veins
5. _____ Ascites
6. _____ Dyspnea from fluid in alveoli
7. _____ Orthopnea
8. _____ Hepatomegaly
9. _____ Cough that may be blood-tinged
10. _____ Nocturia

Column II

a. Left-sided heart failure
b. Right-sided heart failure

SHORT ANSWER

Read each statement carefully. Write your response in the space provided.

1. Decipher the following formula: CO = HR × SV

   _____

   _____

2. Distinguish between the terms *preload* and *afterload*: _____

   _____

   _____

3. Two factors that determine preload are _____ and _____,
   and two factors that determine afterload are _____ and _____
   _____.

4. Three noninvasive tests are used to assess cardiac hemodynamics: _____ for right
   ventricular preload, _____ for left ventricular afterload, and
   _____ for left ventricular preload.

5. List four common etiologic factors that cause myocardial dysfunction.

   _____

   _____

   _____

   _____

6. Coronary atherosclerosis results in tissue ischemia that causes myocardial dysfunction because

_____

_____.

7. Three types of cardiomyopathy are _____, _____, and

_____; of these, _____ is the most common.

8. The primary clinical manifestations of pulmonary congestion in left-sided heart failure are

_____, _____, _____,

_____, and a probable _____.

9. The primary systemic clinical manifestations of right-sided heart failure are _____,

_____, _____, _____,

_____, _____, and _____.

10. Name four drug classifications normally prescribed for systolic heart failure.

_____

_____

_____

_____

11. List four common side effects of diuretics.

_____

_____

_____

_____

12. List six symptoms indicative of hypokalemia.

_____

_____

_____

_____

_____

_____

13. The most common thrombohemolytic problem among patients with heart failure is

_____.

II. Critical Thinking Questions and Exercises

DISCUSSION AND ANALYSIS

Discuss the following topics with your classmates.

1. Explain how the ejection factor, as a test to determine the type of heart failure present, is calculated.
2. Describe in detail the pathophysiologic events that occur in systolic heart failure, especially the fluid dynamic alterations that occur as a result of the conversion of angiotensin I to angiotensin II.
3. Distinguish between the pathophysiology of left-sided and right-sided heart failure.
4. Describe cardiac resynchronization therapy (CRT), a treatment for heart failure.
5. Explain the pathophysiology of cardiogenic shock.
6. Explain and demonstrate the process of cardiopulmonary resuscitation (CPR).

IDENTIFYING PATTERNS

Complete the following flow chart to depict the pathophysiology of pulmonary edema.

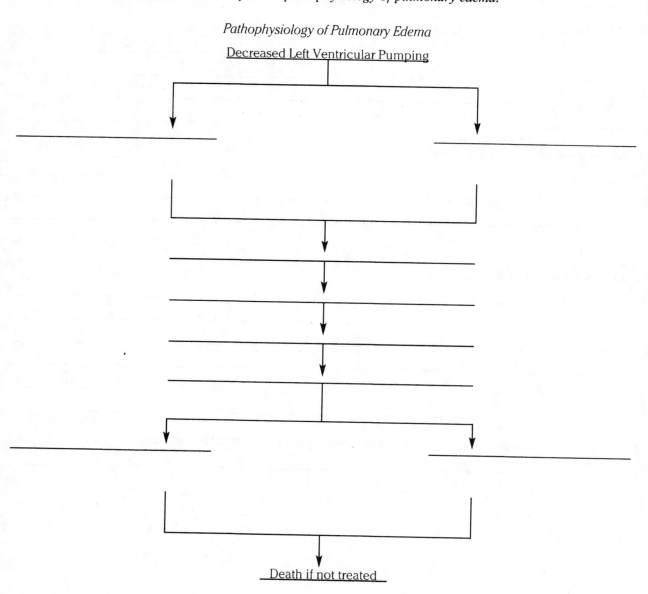

Pathophysiology of Pulmonary Edema

Decreased Left Ventricular Pumping

Death if not treated

CLINICAL SITUATIONS

Read the following case study. Fill in the blanks or circle the correct answer.

CASE STUDY: Pulmonary Edema

Mr. Wolman is to be discharged from the hospital to home. He is 79 years old, lives with his wife, and has just recovered from mild pulmonary edema secondary to congestive heart failure.

1. The most common cause of pulmonary edema is _____.

2. The sequence of pathophysiologic events is triggered by:
   a. elevated left ventricular end-diastolic pressure.
   b. elevated pulmonary venous pressure.
   c. increased hydrostatic pressure.
   d. impaired lymphatic drainage.

3. The nurse advises Mr. Wolman to rest frequently at home. This advice is based on the knowledge that rest:
   a. decreases blood pressure.
   b. increases the heart reserve.
   c. reduces the work of the heart.
   d. does all of the above.

4. The nurse reminds Mr. Wolman to sleep with two pillows to elevate his head about 10 inches. This position is recommended because:
   a. preload can be increased, thus enhancing cardiac output.
   b. pulmonary congestion can be reduced.
   c. venous return to the lungs can be improved, thus reducing peripheral edema.
   d. all of the above can help relieve his symptoms.

5. Mr. Wolman takes 0.25 mg of digoxin once a day. The nurse should tell him about signs of digitalis toxicity, which include:
   a. anorexia.
   b. bradycardia and tachycardia.
   c. nausea and vomiting.
   d. all of the above.

6. Mr. Wolman also takes Lasix (40 mg) twice a day. He is aware of signs related to hypokalemia and supplements his diet with foods high in potassium, such as:
   a. bananas.
   b. raisins.
   c. orange juice.
   d. all of the above.

Assessment and Management of Patients With Vascular Disorders and Problems of Peripheral Circulation

I. Interpretation, Completion, and Comparison

MULTIPLE CHOICE

Read each question carefully. Circle your answer.

1. The most important factor in regulating the caliber of blood vessels, which determines resistance to flow, is:
   a. hormonal secretion.
   b. independent arterial wall activity.
   c. the influence of circulating chemicals.
   d. the sympathetic nervous system.

2. Clinical manifestations of acute venous insufficiency include all of the following *except:*
   a. cool and cyanotic skin.
   b. initial absence of edema.
   c. sharp pain that may be relieved by the elevation of the extremity.
   d. full superficial veins.

3. With peripheral arterial insufficiency, leg pain during rest can be reduced by:
   a. elevating the limb above heart level.
   b. lowering the limb so that it is dependent.
   c. massaging the limb after application of cold compresses.
   d. placing the limb in a plane horizontal to the body.

4. Probably the strongest risk factor for the development of atherosclerotic lesions is:
   a. cigarette smoking.
   b. lack of exercise.
   c. obesity.
   d. stress.

5. Saturated fats are strongly implicated in the causation of atherosclerosis. Saturated fats include all of the following *except:*
   a. corn oil.
   b. eggs and milk.
   c. meat and butter.
   d. solid vegetable oil.

6. The American diet is known to be high in fat. About what percentage of the total caloric intake is typically supplied by fat in most diets?

    a. 20%

    b. 40%

    c. 60%

    d. 80%

7. Buerger's disease is characterized by all of the following *except*:

    a. arterial thrombus formation and occlusion.

    b. lipid deposits in the arteries.

    c. redness or cyanosis in the limb when it is dependent.

    d. venous inflammation and occlusion.

8. The most outstanding symptom of Buerger's disease is:

    a. a burning sensation.

    b. cramping in the feet.

    c. pain.

    d. paresthesia.

9. The most common cause of all thoracic aortic aneurysms is:

    a. a congenital defect in the vessel wall.

    b. atherosclerosis.

    c. infection.

    d. trauma.

10. Diagnosis of a thoracic aortic aneurysm is done primarily by:

    a. computed tomography.

    b. sonography.

    c. radiography.

    d. all of the above.

11. A nurse who suspects the presence of an abdominal aortic aneurysm should look for the presence of:

    a. a pulsatile abdominal mass.

    b. low back pain.

    c. lower abdominal pain.

    d. all of the above.

12. To save a limb that is affected by occlusion of a major artery, surgery must be initiated before necrosis develops, which is usually:

    a. within the first 4 hours.

    b. between 6 and 10 hours.

    c. between 12 and 24 hours.

    d. within 1 to 2 days.

13. Raynaud's disease is a form of:

    a. arterial vessel occlusion caused by multiple emboli that develop in the heart and are transported through the systemic circulation.

    b. arteriolar vasoconstriction, usually on the fingertips, that results in coldness, pain, pallor.

    c. peripheral venospasm in the lower extremities owing to valve damage resulting from prolonged venous stasis.

    d. phlebothrombosis related to prolonged vasoconstriction resulting from overexposure to the cold.

14. A significant cause of venous thrombosis is:

    a. altered blood coagulation.

    b. stasis of blood.

    c. vessel wall injury.

    d. all of the above.

15. Clinical manifestations of deep vein obstruction include:
    a. edema and pain.
    b. pigmentation changes.
    c. ulcerations.
    d. all of the above.

16. When administering anticoagulant therapy, the nurse needs to monitor the clotting time to make certain that it is within the therapeutic range of:
    a. 1 to 2 times the normal control.
    b. 2 to 3 times the normal control.
    c. 3.5 times the normal control.
    d. 4.5 times the normal control.

17. When caring for a patient who has started anticoagulant therapy with warfarin (Coumadin), the nurse knows not to expect therapeutic benefits for:
    a. at least 12 hours.
    b. the first 24 hours.
    c. 2 to 3 days.
    d. 3 to 5 days.

18. Knowing the most serious complication of venous insufficiency, the nurse would assess the patient's lower extremities for signs of:
    a. rubor.
    b. cellulitis.
    c. dermatitis.
    d. ulceration.

19. A nurse should teach a patient with chronic venous insufficiency to do all of the following *except*:
    a. avoid constricting garments.
    b. elevate the legs above the heart level for 30 minutes every 2 hours.
    c. sit as much as possible to rest the valves in the legs.
    d. sleep with the foot of the bed elevated about 6 inches.

20. Nursing measures to promote a clean leg ulcer include:
    a. applying wet-to-dry saline solution dressings, which would remove necrotic debris when changed.
    b. flushing out necrotic material with hydrogen peroxide.
    c. using an ointment that would treat the ulcer by enzymatic débridement.
    d. all of the above.

21. The physician prescribed a Tegapore dressing to treat a venous ulcer. What must the ankle-brachial index (ABI) be for the circulatory status to be adequate?
    a. 0.10
    b. 0.25
    c. 0.35
    d. 0.50

22. A varicose vein is caused by:
    a. phlebothrombosis.
    b. an incompetent venous valve.
    c. venospasm.
    d. venous occlusion.

23. Postoperative nursing management for vein ligation and stripping include all of the following *except*:
    a. dangling the legs over the side of the bed for 10 minutes every 4 hours for the first 24 hours.
    b. elevating the foot of the bed to promote venous blood return.
    c. maintaining elastic compression of the leg continuously for about 1 week.
    d. starting the patient ambulating 24 to 48 hours after surgery.

MATCHING

Match the type of vessel insufficiency in column II with its associated symptoms listed in column I.

Column I

1. _____ Intermittent claudication

2. _____ Paresthesia

3. _____ Dependent rubor

4. _____ Cold, pale extremity

5. _____ Ulcers of lower legs and ankles

6. _____ Muscle fatigue and cramping

7. _____ Diminished or absent pulses

8. _____ Reddish blue discoloration with dependency

Column II

a. Arterial insufficiency

b. Venous insufficiency

II. Critical Thinking Questions and Exercises

DISCUSSION AND ANALYSIS

Discuss the following topics with your classmates.

1. Explain what is meant by the following formula: Flow rate = $\Delta P/R$.
2. Explain the etiology of pain associated with the condition known as "intermittent claudication."
3. Describe the steps required for a nurse to take an accurate ankle-brachial index (ABI) calculation.
4. Discuss four nursing diagnoses and related goals for a patient with peripheral vascular problems.
5. Compare and contrast the etiology, clinical manifestations and nursing and medical interventions for a thoracic and abdominal aortic aneurysm.
6. Discuss the four major complications of venous thrombosis and associated nursing interventions.
7. Distinguish between the pathophysiology and clinical manifestations of arterial and venous leg ulcers.
8. Compare and contrast the three treatments used for varicose veins: ligation and stripping, thermal ablation and sclerotherapy.

EXAMINING ASSOCIATIONS

Read each analogy. Fill in the space provided with the best response.

1. Arteriosclerosis : hardening of the arteries :: _____ : the accumulation of plaque and atheromas.

2. Rubor : reddish-blue discoloration :: _____ : cramp-like pain in the extremities with exercise.

3. International normalized ratio (INR) : the measurement of anticoagulant levels :: Ankle-brachial index (ABI) : _____.

4. The intima : inner layer of the arterial wall :: _____ : outer layer of connective tissue.

5. The right lymphatic duct : lymphatic fluid delivery to the right side of the head and neck :: The thoracic duct : _____.

6. Arterial pressure : 100 mm Hg :: Venous pressure : _____.

7. Hydrostatic pressure : force generated by blood pressure :: Osmotic pressure :

   _____.

8. Turner's syndrome : congenital arterial aneurysm :: Lupus erythematosus : _____.

9. Cellulitis : infectious limb swelling :: _____ : lymphatic channel inflammation.

CLINICAL APPLICATIONS

Read the following case study. Circle the correct answer.

CASE STUDY: Peripheral Arterial Occlusive Disease

Fred, a 43-year-old construction worker, has a history of hypertension. He smokes two packs of cigarettes a day, is nervous about the possibility of being unemployed, and has difficulty coping with stress. His current concern is calf pain during minimal exercise, which decreases with rest.

1. The nurse assesses Fred's symptoms as being associated with peripheral arterial occlusive disease. The nursing diagnosis is probably:

   a. alteration in tissue perfusion related to compromised circulation.

   b. dysfunctional use of extremities related to muscle spasms.

   c. impaired mobility related to stress associated with pain.

   d. impairment in muscle use associated with pain on exertion.

2. The nurse knows that the hallmark symptom of peripheral arterial occlusion disease is:

   a. intermittent claudication.

   b. phlebothrombosis.

   c. postphlebitis syndrome.

   d. thrombophlebitis.

3. Additional symptoms to support the nurse's diagnosis include all of the following *except:*

   a. blanched skin appearance when the limb is dependent.

   b. diminished distal pulsations.

   c. reddish-blue discoloration of the limb when it is elevated.

   d. warm and rosy coloration of the extremity after exercise.

4. The pain associated with this condition commonly occurs in muscle groups _____ (location).

5. The pain is due to the irritation of nerve endings by the build-up of _____ and

   _____.

6. Pain is experienced when the arterial lumen narrows to about:
   a. 15%.
   b. 25%.
   c. 35%.
   d. 50%.

7. The nurse notices that several minutes after Jack's leg is dependent, the vessels remain dilated. This is evidenced by the coloring of the skin, which the nurse describes as:
   a. rosy.
   b. rubor.
   c. pallor.
   d. cyanotic.

8. The nurse is asked to determine ABI. The right posterior tibial reading is 75 mm Hg, and the brachial systolic pressure is 150 mm Hg. The ABI would be:
   a. 0.25.
   b. 0.50.
   c. 0.65.
   d. 0.80.

9. In health teaching, the nurse should suggest methods to increase arterial blood supply, which include:
   a. a planned program involving systematic lowering of the extremity below heart level.
   b. Buerger-Allen exercises.
   c. graded extremity exercises.
   d. all of the above.

APPLYING CONCEPTS

Refer to Figure 31-1 in the textbook and document the physiologic function of specific components of the vascular system.

1. Superior vena cava _____

2. Pulmonary circulation _____

3. Aorta _____

4. Right and left pulmonary veins _____

5. Hepatic circulation _____

6. Systemic circulation _____

7. Right and left ventricle _____

8. Right and left atrium _____

9. Inferior vena cava _____

10. Renal circulation _____

CHAPTER 32

Assessment and Management of Patients With Hypertension

I. Interpretation, Completion, and Comparison

MULTIPLE CHOICE

Read each question carefully. Circle your answer.

1. Prehypertension, a precursor to hypertension, can be diagnosed when the diastolic reading is:
   a. between 60 and 70 mm Hg.
   b. at 75 mm Hg.
   c. at 80 mm Hg.
   d. between 85 and 90 mm Hg.

2. Stage 1 hypertension is defined as persistent blood pressure levels in which the systolic pressure is higher than _____ and the diastolic is higher than _____.
   a. 110/60 mm Hg
   b. 120/70 mm Hg
   c. 130/80 mm Hg
   d. 140/90 mm Hg

3. The percentage of adults in the United States who have hypertension is approximately:
   a. 10%.
   b. 15%.
   c. 30%.
   d. 40%.

4. The incidence of hypertension is highest in which section of the United States?
   a. northeastern
   b. southeastern
   c. northwestern
   d. southwestern

5. The desired systolic reading for a person with diabetes mellitus receiving antihypertensive treatment is:
   a. 120 mm Hg.
   b. 130 mm Hg.
   c. 140 mm Hg.
   d. 150 mm Hg.

6. Pharmacologic therapy for patients with uncomplicated hypertension would include the administration of:
   a. ACE inhibitors.
   b. alpha-blockers.
   c. beta-blockers.
   d. calcium antagonists.

7. A characteristic symptom of damage to the vital organs as a result of hypertension is:
   a. angina.
   b. dyspnea.
   c. epistaxis.
   d. all of the above.

8. An expected nursing diagnosis for a patient with hypertension is:
   a. heart failure.
   b. knowledge deficit.
   c. myocardial infarction.
   d. renal insufficiency.

9. The percentage of patients with hypertension who discontinue their drug therapy within 1 year after its initiation is estimated to be:
   a. 15%.
   b. 30%.
   c. 50%.
   d. 75%.

10. One of the most significant concerns for medical and nursing management of hypertension is:
   a. complications from medications.
   b. insufficient information.
   c. noncompliance with recommended therapy.
   d. uncontrolled dietary management.

11. Blood pressure control is initially achieved by approximately what percentage of patients when they actively participate in their care?
   a. 10%
   b. 25%
   c. 45%
   d. 70%

SHORT ANSWER

Read each statement carefully. Write your response in the space provided.

1. Blood pressure is the product of _____ multiplied by _____.

2. Cardiac output is the product of _____ multiplied by _____.

3. Approximately _____% of the population has primary hypertension, a class of hypertension with an unidentified cause.

4. Prolonged hypertension can cause significant damage to blood vessels in four "target organs":
   _____, _____, _____, and
   _____.

5. List six consequences of prolonged, uncontrolled hypertension on the body and its systems.

   _____

   _____

   _____

   _____

   _____

   _____

6. Structural and functional changes in the heart and blood vessels that occur with aging and cause hypertension are _____, _____, _____, and _____.

7. Give four examples of conditions that can trigger a hypertensive emergency in which blood pressure must be immediately lowered.

   _____

   _____

   _____

   _____

MATCHING

Match the hypertension medication in column II with its associated action listed in column I.

Column I

1. _____ Blocks reabsorption of sodium and water in kidneys
2. _____ Stimulates alpha$_2$-adrenergic receptors
3. _____ Decreases blood volume, renal blood flow, and cardiac output
4. _____ Blocks beta-adrenergic receptors
5. _____ Inhibits aldosterone
6. _____ Impairs synthesis of norepinephrine

Column II

a. Inderal

b. Tenex

c. Aldactone

d. Lasix

e. Serpasil

f. Hygroton

II. Critical Thinking Questions and Exercises

DISCUSSION AND ANALYSIS

Discuss the following topics with your classmates.

1. Discuss in detail several hypotheses about the pathophysiologic basis for elevated blood pressure.
2. Explain how lifestyle changes and medications can control, not cure, hypertension.
3. Discuss the implications for morbidity and mortality for eight risk factors associated with hypertension.
4. Discuss the rationale for and advantages of lifestyle and dietary modifications to prevent/manage hypertension.

IDENTIFYING PATTERNS

Complete the following diagram describing the pathophysiology of hypertension secondary to renal dysfunction.

Pathophysiology of Essential Hypertension

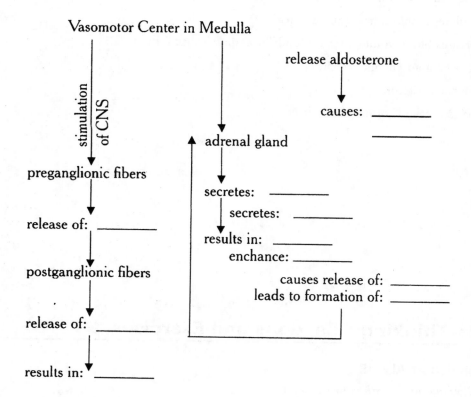

Vasomotor Center in Medulla

stimulation of CNS

preganglionic fibers

release of: _____

postganglionic fibers

release of: _____

results in: _____

release aldosterone

causes: _____
_____

adrenal gland

secretes: _____

secretes: _____

results in: _____

enchance: _____

causes release of: _____

leads to formation of: _____

CLINICAL APPLICATIONS

Read the following case study. Circle the correct answers.

CASE STUDY: Secondary Hypertension

Georgia, 30 years old, is diagnosed as having secondary hypertension when serial blood pressure recordings show her average reading to be 170/100 mm Hg. Her hypertension is the result of renal dysfunction.

1. The kidneys help maintain the hypertensive state in essential hypertension by:

   a. increasing their elimination of sodium in response to aldosterone secretion.

   b. releasing renin in response to decreased renal perfusion.

   c. secreting acetylcholine, which stimulates the sympathetic nervous system to constrict major vessels.

   d. doing all of the above.

2. Renal pathology associated with essential hypertension can be identified by:

   a. a urine output greater than 2000 mL in 24 hours.

   b. a urine specific gravity of 1.005.

   c. hyponatremia and decreased urine osmolality.

   d. increased blood urea nitrogen and creatinine levels.

3. Georgia is prescribed spironolactone (Aldactone), 50 mg once every day. The nurse knows that spironolactone:

   a. blocks the reabsorption of sodium, thereby increasing urinary output.

   b. inhibits renal vasoconstriction, which prevents the release of renin.

   c. interferes with fluid retention by inhibiting aldosterone.

   d. prevents the secretion of epinephrine from the adrenal medulla.

4. Health education for Georgia includes advising her to:

   a. adhere to her dietary regimen.

   b. become involved in a regular program of exercise.

   c. take her medication as prescribed.

   d. do all of the above.

Assessment and Management of Patients With Hematologic Disorders

I. Interpretation, Completion, and Comparison

MULTIPLE CHOICE

Read each question carefully. Circle your answer.

1. The physician expects that the patient has a deficiency in the leukocyte responsible for cell-mediated immunity. The nurse knows to check the white blood cell count for:

   a. basophils.

   b. monocytes.

   c. plasma cells.

   d. T lymphocytes.

2. Myeloid and lymphoid stem cells produce specific types of blood cells. The nurse knows, when evaluating blood tests, that myeloid stem cells differentiate into all of the following types of blood cells *except:*

   a. erythrocytes. RBC

   b. leukocytes. WBC

   c. lymphocytes.

   d. platelets.

3. The nurse notes that a patient, who is a vegetarian, has an abnormal number of megaloblasts. The nurse suspects a deficiency in:

   a. iron.

   b. zinc.

   c. vitamin C.

   d. vitamin B_{12}.

4. An elderly patient presents to the physician's office with a complaint of exhaustion. The nurse, aware of the most common hematologic condition affecting the elderly, knows to check the patient's:

   a. white blood cell count.

   b. red blood cell count.

   c. thrombocyte count.

   d. levels of plasma proteins.

5. A nurse who cares for a patient who has experienced bone marrow aspiration or biopsy should be aware of the most serious hazard, which is:

   a. hemorrhage.

   b. infection.

   c. shock.

   d. splintering of bone fragments.

6. A person can usually tolerate a gradual reduction in hemoglobin until the level reaches:

   a. 5.0 to 5.5 g/dL.

   b. 4.0 to 4.5 g/dL.

   c. 3.0 to 3.5 g/dL.

   d. 2.0 to 2.5 g/dL.

7. The nurse begins to design a nutritional packet of information for a patient diagnosed with iron deficiency anemia. The nurse would recommend an increased intake of:

   a. fresh citrus fruits.

   b. milk and cheese.

   c. organ meats.

   d. whole-grain breads.

8. A physician prescribes one tablet of ferrous sulfate daily for a 15-year-old girl who experiences heavy flow during her menstrual cycle. The nurse advises the patient and her mother that this over-the-counter preparation must be taken for how many months for iron replenishment to occur?

    a. 1 to 2

    b. 3 to 5

    c. 6 to 12

    d. longer than 12

9. A patient with chronic renal failure is being examined by the nurse practitioner for anemia. The nurse knows to review the laboratory data for a decreased hemoglobin level, decreased red blood cell count, and:

    a. decreased level of erythropoietin.

    b. decreased total iron-binding capacity.

    c. increased mean corpuscular volume.

    d. increased reticulocyte count.

10. The most frequent symptom and complication of anemia is:

    a. bleeding gums.

    b. ecchymosis.

    c. fatigue.

    d. jaundice.

11. The cause of aplastic anemia may:

    a. be related to drugs, chemicals, or radiation damage.

    b. be idiopathic.

    c. result from certain infections.

    d. be related to all of the above.

12. During a routine assessment of a patient diagnosed with anemia, the nurse notes the patient's beefy red tongue. The nurse knows that this is a sign of what kind of anemia?

    a. autoimmune

    b. folate deficiency

    c. iron deficiency

    d. megaloblastic

13. A nurse should know that a diagnosis of hemolytic anemia is associated with all of the following *except*:

    a. abnormality in the circulation of plasma.

    b. decrease in the reticulocyte count.

    c. defect in the erythrocyte.

    d. elevated indirect bilirubin.

14. Absence of intrinsic factor is associated with a vitamin B_{12} deficiency, because the vitamin cannot bind to be transported for absorption in the:

    a. duodenum.

    b. ileum.

    c. jejunum.

    d. stomach.

15. A diagnostic sign of pernicious anemia is:

    a. a smooth, sore, red tongue.

    b. exertional dyspnea.

    c. pale mucous membranes.

    d. weakness.

16. The Schilling test is used to diagnose:

    a. aplastic anemia.

    b. iron deficiency anemia.

    c. megaloblastic anemia.

    d. pernicious anemia.

17. All of the following are inherited forms of sickle cell anemia *except*:

    a. autoimmune hemolytic.

    b. G6PD deficiency.

    c. thalassemia.

    d. sickle cell anemia.

18. A nurse expects an adult patient with sickle cell anemia to have a hemoglobin value of:

    a. approximately 3 g/dL.

    b. approximately 5 g/dL.

    c. between 5 and 7 g/dL.

    d. between 7 and 10 g/dL.

19. Sickle-shaped erythrocytes cause:
    a. cellular blockage in small vessels.
    b. decreased organ perfusion.
    c. tissue ischemia and infarction.
    d. all of the above.

20. A person with sickle cell trait would:
    a. be advised to avoid fluid loss and dehydration.
    b. be protected from crisis under ordinary circumstances.
    c. experience hemolytic jaundice.
    d. have chronic anemia.

21. Polycythemia vera is characterized by bone marrow overactivity, resulting in the clinical manifestations of:
    a. angina.
    b. claudication.
    c. thrombophlebitis.
    d. all of the above.

22. A patient diagnosed with neutropenia resulting from increased destruction of neutrophils would most likely have:
    a. aplastic anemia.
    b. infectious hepatitis.
    c. leukemia.
    d. a lymphoma.

23. The common feature of the leukemias is:
    a. a compensatory polycythemia stimulated by thrombocytopenia.
    b. an unregulated accumulation of white cells in the bone marrow, which replace normal marrow elements.
    c. increased blood viscosity, resulting from an overproduction of white cells.
    d. reduced plasma volume in response to a reduced production of cellular elements.

24. Nursing assessment for a patient with leukemia should include observation for:
    a. fever and infection.
    b. dehydration.
    c. petechiae and ecchymoses.
    d. all of the above.

25. The major cause of death in patients with acute myeloid leukemia is believed to be:
    a. anemia.
    b. dehydration.
    c. embolus.
    d. infection.

26. Multiple myeloma:
    a. can be diagnosed by roentgenograms that show bone lesion destruction.
    b. is a malignant disease of plasma cells that affects bone and soft tissue.
    c. is suspected in any person who evidences albuminuria.
    d. is associated with all of the above.

27. The classic presenting symptom of multiple myeloma is:
    a. debilitating fatigue.
    b. bone pain in the back of the ribs.
    c. gradual muscle paralysis.
    d. severe thrombocytopenia.

28. A patient is admitted with thrombocytopenia caused by decreased platelet production. The nurse knows that the diagnosis is most likely:
    a. disseminated intravascular coagulation (DIC)
    b. aplastic anemia
    c. lupus erythematosus
    d. malignant lymphoma

29. In the normal blood-clotting cycle, the final formation of a clot occurs:

    a. during the platelet phase.

    b. during the vascular phase.

    c. when fibrin reinforces the platelet plug.

    d. when the plasmin system produces fibrinolysis.

30. Bleeding and petechiae do not usually occur with thrombocytopenia until the platelet count falls below 50,000/mm³. The normal value for blood platelets is:

    a. 50,000 to 100,000/mm³.

    b. 100,000 to 150,000/mm³.

    c. between 150,000 and 350,000/mm³.

    d. greater than 350,000/mm³.

31. Hemophilia is a hereditary bleeding disorder that:

    a. has a higher incidence among males.

    b. is associated with joint bleeding, swelling, and damage.

    c. is related to a genetic deficiency of a specific blood-clotting factor.

    d. is associated with all of the above.

32. Hypoprothrombinemia, in the absence of gastrointestinal or biliary dysfunction, may be caused by a deficiency in:

    a. vitamin A.

    b. vitamin B_{12}.

    c. vitamin C.

    d. vitamin K.

33. A potential blood donor would be rejected if he or she:

    a. had a history of infectious disease exposure within the past 2 to 4 months.

    b. had close contact with a hemodialysis patient within the past 6 months.

    c. had donated blood within the past 3 to 6 months.

    d. had received a blood transfusion within the past 9 to 12 months.

34. The recommended minimum hemoglobin level for a woman to donate blood is:

    a. 8.0 g/dL.

    b. 10.5 g/dL.

    c. 12.5 g/dL.

    d. 14 g/dL.

SHORT ANSWER

Read each statement carefully. Write your response in the space provided.

1. The volume of blood in humans is about _5-6_ liters.

2. Blood cell formation (hematopoiesis) occurs in the _bone marrow_.

3. Red bone marrow activity is confined in adults to the _ribs_, _vertebrae_, _sternum_, and _pelvic_.

4. The principal function of the erythrocyte, which is composed primarily of _hemoglobin_, is to _transport oxygen between_ the lungs and the tissue

5. Each 100 mL of blood should normally contain _15_ grams of hemoglobin.

6. Women of childbearing years need an additional _2mg_ daily of iron to replace that loss during menstruation.

7. The nurse advises a patient who is iron deficient to take extra vitamin _C_, which is known for increasing iron absorption.

8. The major function of leukocytes is to: _protect the body from invasion by bacteria and other foreign entities_

9. Plasma proteins consist primarily of _Albumin_ and _globulins_.

10. The two most common areas used for bone marrow aspirations in an adult are _Sternum_ and _iliac Crest_.

11. Distinguish between *primary* and *secondary* polycythemia: _____

_____

12. The thalassemias (hereditary anemias) are characterized by _hypochromia_, _microcytosis_, _anemia_, and _hemolysis_.

13. Secondary polycythemia is caused by _erythropoietin_, which may be in response to _reduced oxygen_.

SCRAMBLEGRAM

Complete the following scramblegram by circling the word or words that answer each statement below. Answers may read horizontally or vertically.

F	I	B	R	I	N	O	G	E	N	A	N	O	E	L
B	D	H	E	M	O	S	T	A	S	I	S	P	R	M
F	R	S	S	C	M	P	R	H	S	G	T	H	Y	I
I	E	W	C	V	R	T	C	E	L	L	S	A	T	P
B	E	A	B	B	T	L	D	E	F	I	J	G	H	R
R	S	W	A	O	H	O	A	S	V	T	S	O	R	K
I	F	T	P	N	R	K	L	B	J	N	M	C	O	L
N	E	U	T	R	O	P	H	I	L	S	K	Y	C	B
F	W	O	D	C	M	F	N	K	G	H	A	T	Y	O
A	H	B	E	R	B	S	J	C	T	C	B	O	T	N
H	E	M	A	T	O	P	O	I	E	S	I	S	E	E
E	M	N	E	E	C	F	M	F	G	P	S	I	S	M
M	O	N	O	C	Y	T	E	S	P	L	A	S	M	A
O	S	C	G	D	T	K	L	A	I	E	L	K	A	R
G	T	O	A	H	E	E	I	J	B	E	B	A	J	R
L	A	G	P	E	S	F	R	M	C	N	U	L	B	O
O	S	G	T	I	J	D	S	A	N	M	M	S	L	W
B	I	H	E	O	A	G	H	H	D	O	I	I	T	L
I	S	D	A	U	O	U	L	M	E	S	N	P	U	M
N	A	S	E	L	Y	M	P	H	O	C	Y	T	E	S

DEFINITION OF TERMS

1. The fluid portion of blood
2. Another term for platelets
3. The mature form of white blood cells
4. The process of continually replacing blood cells
5. The site of blood cell formation
6. Makes up 95% of the mass of the red blood cell
7. The ingestion and digestion of bacteria by neutrophils
8. The largest classification of leukocytes
9. A clotting factor present in plasma
10. A plasma protein primarily responsible for the maintenance of fluid balance
11. The site of activity for most macrophages
12. The process of stopping bleeding from a severed blood vessel
13. A protein that forms the basis of blood clotting
14. Integral component of the immune system
15. The term for red blood cell
16. The letters used for the term reticuloendothelial system
17. The balance between clot formation and clot dissolution
18. A term used to describe T lymphocytes

II. Critical Thinking Questions and Exercises

DISCUSSION AND ANALYSIS

Discuss the following topics with your classmates.

1. Distinguish among the following anemias in terms of etiology, clinical manifestations, and nursing interventions: hypoproliferative, bleeding, and hemolytic.
2. Compare the various causes of inherited and acquired hemolytic anemias.
3. Describe the pathophysiology, clinical manifestations, and nursing interventions for a patient with sickle cell anemia.
4. Distinguish the pathophysiology of acute lymphocytic leukemia from that of chronic lymphocytic leukemia, and compare nursing interventions for each disease.
5. Discuss nursing diagnoses and interventions for a patient with disseminated intravascular coagulation (DIC).
6. Explain what the term *international normalized ratio* (INR) refers to.

CLINICAL SITUATIONS

Read the following case studies. Fill in the blanks or circle the correct answer.

CASE STUDY: Sickle Cell Crises

Tonika, a 15-year-old girl with sickle cell disease, is admitted to the hospital for treatment of sickle cell crisis.

1. Based on knowledge of the inheritance of the sickle cell gene (*HBS*), the nurse expects the patient to be of what descent?

   a. African   c. Middle Eastern
   b. Indian   d. Mediterranean

2. The nurse understands that the shape of the red blood cell is altered with this disease. Instead of being round, biconcave, and disc-like in appearance, it can be described as ___deformed, rigid___, and ___sickle-shaped___; the hemoglobin value is usually ___7-10___ g/dL.

3. On assessment, the nurse notes that the patient's face and skull bones are enlarged. She knows this is a compensatory response to _____.

4. The severe pain that occurs during sickle cell crises is the result of _____.

5. The nurse understands that Tonika's abdominal pain is probably caused by involvement the organ most commonly responsible for sequestration crises in young adults, which is the:

   a. kidney.

   b. liver.

   c. pancreas.

   d. spleen.

6. A cardiac response to chronic anemia includes _heart murmurs_, _cardiac megaly_, and _Tachycardia_.

7. List three complications of sickle cell crises.

   Stroke, infection, renal failure, heart failure, impotence and pulmonary hypertension

8. Nursing interventions are focused on five goals: _managing pain_, _promoting coping Skills_, _preventing + managing_, _minimizing knowledge deficient_, and _monitoring/managing potential_ _Infection_ _complications_

CASE STUDY: Leukemia

John is a 51-year-old accountant recently diagnosed with acute myeloid leukemia.

1. Acute myeloid leukemia affects the _hematopoietic Stem_ _Cell_ and has a peak incidence at _60_ years, with a survival prognosis of about _1_ year(s).

2. A bone marrow specimen is diagnostic if it shows an excess of _immature blastcells_.

3. A characteristic symptom that results from insufficient red blood cell production is:

   a. bleeding tendencies.

   b. fatigue.

   c. susceptibility to infection.

   d. all of the above.

4. Survival time for those who receive treatment averages:

   a. 6 months.

   b. 1 year.

   c. 2 years.

   d. 5 years.

5. The major form of therapy that frequently results in remission is:

   a. bone marrow transplantation.

   b. chemotherapy.

   c. radiation.

   d. surgical intervention.

CASE STUDY: Hodgkin Disease

Ian, a 24-year-old graduate student, was recently diagnosed as having Hodgkin disease. He sought medical attention because of an annoying pruritus and a small enlargement on the right side of his neck.

1. Ian's disease is classified as Hodgkin paragranuloma. The nurse knows that this classification is associated with:
   - a. a minimal degree of cellular differentiation in the affected nodes.
   - b. an excessive production of the Reed-Sternberg cell, the diagnostic atypical cell of Hodgkin disease.
   - c. nodular sclerosis, which reflects advanced malignancy.
   - d. replacement of the involved lymph nodes by tumor cells.

2. A positive diagnosis of Hodgkin disease depends on:
   - a. enlarged, firm, and painful lymph nodes.
   - b. histologic analysis of an enlarged lymph node.
   - c. progressive anemia.
   - d. the presence of generalized pruritus.

3. Ian's diagnosis of stage I Hodgkin disease implies that the disease:
   - a. has disseminated diffusely to one or more extrahepatic sites.
   - b. involves multiple nodes and is confined to one side of the diaphragm.
   - c. is limited to a single node or a single intralymphatic organ or site.
   - d. is present above and below the diaphragm and may include spleen involvement.

4. The nurse expects that Ian's course of treatment will involve:
   - a. a combination of chemotherapy and radiation.
   - b. a drug regimen of nitrogen mustard, vincristine, and a steroid.
   - c. chemotherapy with vincristine alone.
   - d. radiotherapy to the specific node over a space of 4 weeks.

CASE STUDY: Transfusion

Jerry is to receive 1 unit of packed red cells because he has a hemoglobin level of 8 g/dL and a diagnosis of gastrointestinal bleeding.

1. Before initiating the transfusion, the nurse needs to check:
   - a. for the abnormal presence of gas bubbles and cloudiness in the blood bag.
   - b. that the blood has been typed and cross-matched.
   - c. that the recipient's blood numbers match the donor's blood numbers.
   - d. all of the above.

2. Administration technique should include all of the following *except*:
   - a. adding 50 to 100 mL of 0.9% NaCl to the packed cells to dilute the solution and speed up delivery of the transfusion.
   - b. administering the unit in combination with dextrose in water if the patient needs additional carbohydrates.
   - c. administering the unit of blood over 1 to 2 hours.
   - d. squeezing the bag of blood every 20 to 30 minutes during administration to mix the cells.

3. The nurse is aware that a transfusion reaction, if it occurs, will probably happen:
   - a. 1 to 2 minutes after the infusion begins.
   - b. during the first 15 to 30 minutes of the transfusion.
   - c. after half the solution has been infused.
   - d. several hours after the infusion, when the body has assimilated the new blood components into the general circulation.

4. If a transfusion reaction occurs, the nurse should:

a. call the physician and wait for directions based on the specific type of reaction.

b. stop the transfusion immediately and keep the vein patent with a saline or dextrose solution.

c. slow the infusion rate and observe for an increase in the severity of the reaction.

d. slow the infusion and request a venipuncture for retyping to start a second transfusion.

CHAPTER 34

Assessment of Digestive and Gastrointestinal Function

I. Interpretation, Completion, and Comparison

MULTIPLE CHOICE

Read each question carefully. Circle your answer.

1. Reflux of food into the esophagus from the stomach is prevented by contraction of the:
   a. ampulla of Vater.
   b. cardiac sphincter.
   c. ileocecal valve.
   d. pyloric sphincter.

2. The digestion of starches begins in the mouth with the secretion of the enzyme:
   a. lipase.
   b. pepsin.
   c. ptyalin.
   d. trypsin.

3. The stomach, which derives its acidity from hydrochloric acid, has a pH of approximately:
   a. 1.0.
   b. 3.5.
   c. 5.0.
   d. 7.5.

4. Intrinsic factor is a gastric secretion that is necessary for the intestinal absorption of the vitamin that prevents pernicious anemia, which is:
   a. Vitamin B_1.
   b. Vitamin B_{12}.
   c. Vitamin C.
   d. Vitamin K.

5. A hormonal regulatory substance that inhibits stomach contraction is:
   a. acetylcholine.
   b. gastrin.
   c. norepinephrine.
   d. secretin.

6. An enzyme, secreted by the gallbladder, that is responsible for fat emulsification is:
   a. amylase.
   b. bile.
   c. maltase.
   d. steapsin.

7. During the initial assessment of a patient complaining of increased stomach acid related to stress, the nurse knows that the physician will want to consider the influence of the neuroregulator:
   a. gastrin.
   b. cholecystokinin.
   c. norepinephrine.
   d. secretin.

8. Pancreatic secretions into the duodenum:

   a. are stimulated by hormones released in the presence of chyme as it passes through the duodenum.

   b. have an alkaline effect on intestinal contents.

   c. increase the pH of the food contents.

   d. accomplish all of the above.

9. Bile, which emulsifies fat, enters the duodenum through the:

   a. cystic duct.

   b. common bile duct.

   c. common hepatic duct.

   d. pancreatic duct.

10. Secretin is a gastrointestinal hormone that:

    a. causes the gallbladder to contract.

    b. influences contraction of the esophageal and pyloric sphincters.

    c. regulates the secretion of gastric acid.

    d. stimulates the production of bicarbonate in pancreatic juice.

11. The major carbohydrate that tissues use for fuel is:

    a. fructose.

    b. galactose.

    c. glucose.

    d. sucrose.

12. It usually takes how long for food to enter the colon?

    a. 2 or 3 hours after a meal is eaten

    b. 4 or 5 hours after a meal is eaten

    c. 6 or 7 hours after a meal is eaten

    d. 8 or 9 hours after a meal is eaten

13. During a nursing assessment, the nurse knows that the most common symptom of patients with gastrointestinal dysfunction is:

    a. diffuse pain.

    b. dyspepsia.

    c. constipation.

    d. abdominal bloating.

14. When completing a nutritional assessment of a patient who is admitted for a gastrointestinal disorder, the nurse notes a recent history of dietary intake. This is based on the knowledge that a portion of digested waste products can remain in the rectum for how many days after a meal is digested?

    a. 1

    b. 2

    c. 3

    d. 4

15. Obstruction of the gastrointestinal tract leads to:

    a. increased force of intestinal contraction.

    b. distention above the point of obstruction.

    c. pain and a sense of bloating.

    d. all of the above.

16. A nurse who is investigating a patient's statement about duodenal pain should assess the:

    a. epigastric area and consider possible radiation of pain to the right subscapular region.

    b. hypogastrium in the right or left lower quadrant.

    c. left lower quadrant.

    d. periumbilical area, followed by the right lower quadrant.

17. Abdominal pain associated with indigestion is usually:

    a. described as crampy or burning.

    b. in the left lower quadrant.

    c. less severe after an intake of fatty foods.

    d. relieved by the intake of coarse vegetables, which stimulate peristalsis.

18. On examination of a patient's stool, the nurse suspects the presence of an upper gastrointestinal bleed when she observes a stool that is:
    a. clay-colored.
    b. greasy and foamy.
    c. tarry and black.
    d. threaded with mucus.

19. Consequences of diarrhea include all of the following *except:*
    a. acidosis.
    b. decreased bicarbonate.
    c. electrolyte imbalance.
    d. hyperkalemia.

20. The nurse has been directed to position a patient for an examination of the abdomen. She knows to place the patient in the:
    a. prone position with pillows positioned to alleviate pressure on the abdomen.
    b. semi-Fowler's position with the left leg bent to minimize pressure on the abdomen.
    c. supine position with the knees flexed to relax the abdominal muscles.
    d. reverse Trendelenburg position to facilitate the natural propulsion of intestinal contents.

21. The nurse auscultates the abdomen to assess bowel sounds. She documents five to six sounds heard in less than 30 seconds. She documents that the patient's bowel sounds are:
    a. normal.
    b. hypoactive.
    c. hyperactive.
    d. none of the above.

22. A gastric analysis with stimulation that results in an excess of gastric acid being secreted could be diagnostic of:
    a. chronic atrophic gastritis.
    b. a duodenal ulcer.
    c. gastric carcinoma.
    d. pernicious anemia.

23. Before a gastroscopy, the nurse should inform the patient that:
    a. he or she must fast for 6 to 12 hours before the examination.
    b. his or her throat will be sprayed with a local anesthetic.
    c. he or she cannot eat or drink after the surgery until the gag reflex returns (1–2 hours).
    d. all of the above will be necessary.

24. A flexible sigmoidoscope permits examination of the lower bowel for:
    a. 5 to 10 inches.
    b. 10 to 15 inches.
    c. 16 to 20 inches.
    d. 25 to 35 inches.

25. A fiberoptic colonoscopy is most frequently used for a diagnosis of:
    a. bowel disease of unknown origin.
    b. cancer.
    c. inflammatory bowel disease.
    d. occult bleeding.

26. For adults who are older than 50 years of age and at low risk for colorectal cancer, the recommended screening is a:
    a. flexible sigmoidoscopy every 3 years.
    b. colonoscopy every 10 years.
    c. fecal occult blood test annually.
    d. colonoscopy every 2 years.

27. Magnetic resonance imaging (MRI) is contraindicated for patients who have:
    a. permanent pacemakers.
    b. artificial heart valves.
    c. implanted insulin pumps.
    d. all of the above.

28. Patient preparation for esophageal manometry requires the withholding of specific medications such as:
    a. anticholinergics.
    b. calcium channel blockers.
    c. sedatives.
    d. all of the above.

29. The results of a gastric analysis can be used to diagnose various disease states. An excess amount of acid can indicate the presence of:
    a. a duodenal ulcer.
    b. gastric cancer.
    c. a peptic ulcer.
    d. pernicious anemia.

MATCHING

Match the major digestive enzyme in column II with its associated digestive action listed in column I.

Column I

1. _____ Helps convert protein into amino acids
2. _____ Facilitates the production of dextrins and maltose
3. _____ Digests protein and helps form polypeptides
4. _____ Digests carbohydrates and helps form fructose
5. _____ Glucose is a product of this enzyme's action
6. _____ Helps form galactose

Column II

a. Amylase
b. Maltase
c. Sucrase
d. Lactase
e. Pepsin
f. Trypsin

FILL-IN

For each diagnostic test, list one or more patient preparation activities that the nurse must monitor and/or document.

Diagnostic Test	*Patient Preparation*
1. Barium enema	a. _____
	b. _____
	c. _____
	d. _____
	e. _____
2. Gastric analysis	a. _____
	b. _____
	c. _____

3. Upper gastrointestinal fiberscopic examination

a. _____

b. _____

c. _____

4. Fiberoptic colonoscopy

a. _____

b. _____

c. _____

d. _____

Critical Thinking Questions and Exercises

IDENTIFYING PATTERNS

Accurate documentation of a pain's location by the nurse is essential to help with a diagnosis. Examine Figure 34-3 in the text. For each site of referred abdominal pain identified, name the quadrant and the region of the pain's location. Begin clockwise with the first site (referred heart pain) and end with the ninth site (referred liver pain). Use Figure 34-5 in the text as a reference for the names of the quadrants and the regions. An example is given.

SITE OF REFERRED PAIN

1. Heart (Example)

2. Renal colic

3. Small intestine

4. Ureteral colic

5. Colon

6. Appendicitis

7. Cholecystitis

8. Biliary colic

9. Liver

QUADRANT

Left upper (LUQ) (Example)

_____

_____

_____

_____

_____

_____

REGION

Left hypochondriac region (LHR) (Example)

_____

_____

_____

_____

_____

_____

CHAPTER 35

Management of Patients With Oral and Esophageal Disorders

I. Interpretation, Completion, and Comparison

MULTIPLE CHOICE

Read each question carefully. Circle your answer.

1. A nurse knows that adequate nutrition is related to good dental health. As part of health assessment, a nurse also knows that about what percentage of adults 45 to 64 years of age have severe periodontal disease?
   a. 5%
   b. 10%
   c. 15%
   d. 25%

2. Actinic cheilitis is a lip lesion that results from sun exposure and can lead to squamous cell carcinoma. It is evidenced by:
   a. erythema.
   b. fissuring.
   c. white hyperkeratosis.
   d. all of the above.

3. A common disease of oral tissue characterized by painful, inflamed, and swollen gums is:
   a. candidiasis.
   b. gingivitis.
   c. herpes simplex.
   d. periodontitis.

4. A common lesion of the mouth that is also referred to as a "canker sore" is:
   a. aphthous stomatitis.
   b. candidiasis.
   c. leukoplakia buccalis.
   d. lichen planus.

5. The incidence of most dental caries is directly related to too high a dietary intake of:
   a. fat.
   b. protein.
   c. salt.
   d. sugar.

6. Postoperative nursing care for drainage of a dentoalveolar or periapical abscess includes all of the following *except*:
   a. soft diet after 24 hours.
   b. fluid restriction for the first 48 hours because the gums are swollen and painful.
   c. external heat by pad or compress to hasten the resolution of the inflammatory swelling.
   d. warm saline mouthwashes every 2 hours while awake.

7. Preventive orthodontics for malocclusion can start as early as age:
   a. 3 years.
   b. 5 years.
   c. 7 years.
   d. 9 years.

8. A patient complains about an inflamed salivary gland below his right ear. The nurse documents probable inflammation of which gland(s)?

   a. buccal

   b. parotid

   c. sublingual

   d. submandibular

9. Mumps, a viral infection affecting children, is an inflammation of which gland(s)?

   a. buccal

   b. parotid

   c. sublingual

   d. submaxillary

10. Parotitis, frequently seen in the elderly or debilitated patient, is usually caused by:

    a. Methicillin-resistant *Staphylococcus aureus* (MRSA).

    b. *Pneumococcus*.

    c. *Staphylococcus aureus*.

    d. *Streptococcus viridans*.

11. Neoplasms of the salivary glands:

    a. are normally malignant and are treated by surgical excision.

    b. commonly recur, and recurrences are more malignant than the original tumor.

    c. are usually treated with radiation.

    d. are characterized by all of the above.

12. If detected early, before lymph node involvement, the 5-year survival rate for oral cancer is about what percent?

    a. 50%

    b. 70%

    c. 80%

    d. 100%

13. The most common site for cancer of the oral cavity is the:

    a. lip.

    b. mouth.

    c. pharynx.

    d. tongue.

14. The typical lesion in oral cancer can be described as:

    a. an indurated ulcer.

    b. a warty growth.

    c. a white or red plaque.

    d. a painful sore.

15. A nurse inspects the Stensen duct of the parotid gland to determine inflammation and possible obstruction. The nurse would examine the oral cavity in the area of the:

    a. buccal mucosa next to the upper molars.

    b. dorsum of the tongue.

    c. roof of the mouth next to the incisors.

    d. posterior segment of the tongue near the uvula.

16. Usually the first symptom associated with esophageal disease is:

    a. dysphagia.

    b. malnutrition.

    c. pain.

    d. regurgitation of food.

17. The nurse suspects that a patient who presents with the symptom of food "sticking" in the lower portion of the esophagus may have the motility disorder known as:

    a. achalasia.

    b. diffuse spasm.

    c. gastroesophageal reflex.

    d. hiatal hernia.

18. A hiatal hernia involves:
   a. an extension of the esophagus through the diaphragm.
   b. an involution of the esophagus, which causes a severe stricture.
   c. a protrusion of the upper stomach into the lower portion of the thorax.
   d. a twisting of the duodenum through an opening in the diaphragm.

19. Intervention for a person who has swallowed strong acid includes all of the following *except:*
   a. administering an irritant that will stimulate vomiting.
   b. aspirating secretions from the pharynx if respirations are affected.
   c. neutralizing the chemical.
   d. washing the esophagus with large volumes of water.

20. The most common symptom that patients with gastroesophageal reflux disease (GERD) mention is:
   a. dyspepsia.
   b. odynophagia.
   c. pyrosis.
   d. regurgitation.

21. Cancer of the esophagus occurs primarily in:
   a. black men older than 50 years of age.
   b. black women after menopause.
   c. white men 30 to 40 years old.
   d. white women older than 60 years of age.

22. A common postoperative complication of esophageal surgery for cancer is:
   a. aspiration pneumonia.
   b. hemorrhage.
   c. incompetence of the suture line, resulting in fluid seepage.
   d. the dumping syndrome.

MATCHING

Match the abnormality in column II with its associated symptomatology of the lip, mouth, or gums listed in column I.

Column I

1. _____ Ulcerated and painful, white papules

2. _____ Reddened area or rash associated with itching

3. _____ Painful, inflamed, swollen gums

4. _____ White overgrowth of horny layer of epidermis

5. _____ Shallow ulcer with a red border and white or yellow center

6. _____ Hyperkeratotic white patches, usually in buccal mucosa

7. _____ Reddened, circumscribed lesion that ulcerates and becomes encrusted

8. _____ White patches with rough, hairlike projections, usually found on the tongue

Column II

a. Actinic cheilitis

b. Leukoplakia

c. Chancre

d. Canker sore

e. Gingivitis

f. Lichen planus

g. Contact dermatitis

h. Hairy leukoplakia

I. Critical Thinking Questions and Exercises

DISCUSSION AND ANALYSIS

Discuss the following topics with your classmates.

1. Discuss at least eight healthy oral hygiene habits that have been found to promote good dental health.
2. Explain the infectious process, clinical manifestations, and medical/ nursing management associated with a periapical abscess.
3. Distinguish between sialadenitis and sialolithiasis.
4. Distinguish between the three types of neck dissection: radical, modified radical, and selective.
5. Discuss about nine major nursing diagnoses related to the surgical process of neck dissection.

APPLYING CONCEPTS

Refer to the accompanying figure and answer the following questions related to a neck dissection procedure.

Intact
sternocleidomastoid
muscle

A   B   C

(**A**) A classic radical neck dissection in which the sternocleidomastoid and smaller muscles are removed. All tissue is removed, from the ramus of the jaw to the clavicle. The jugular vein has also been removed. The functional neck dissection (**B**) is similar but preserves the sternocleidomastoid muscle, internal jugular vein, and the spinal accessory nerve. The wound is closed (**C**), and portable suction drainage tubes are in place.

Read each question carefully. Either circle the correct answer or write the best response in the space provided.

1. A radical neck dissection (see figure) is often performed to help prevent _____, the primary reason for death from neck malignancies.

2. Two common morbidities associated with a radical neck dissection are _____ and _____.

3. Reconstructive techniques involve grafts that normally use the _____ muscle.

4. List three postoperative complications expected when someone has surgery to the neck area (see parts A and B of the figure).

   _____

   _____

   _____

   _____

5. Two collaborative, postoperative nursing problems may be _____ and

   _____.

6. After a radical neck dissection, a patient is placed in Fowler's position to:

   a. decrease venous pressure on the skin flaps.   c. increase lymphatic drainage.

   b. facilitate swallowing.   d. accomplish all of the above.

7. Postoperatively, a finding that should be immediately reported is:

   a. temperature of 99°F.   c. stridor.

   b. pain.   d. localized wound tenderness.

8. A nurse who is caring for a patient who has had radical neck surgery notices an abnormal amount of serosanguineous secretions in the wound suction unit during the first postoperative day. An expected normal amount of drainage is:

   a. between 40 and 80 mL.   c. between 120 and 160 mL.

   b. approximately 80 to 120 mL.   d. greater than 160 mL.

9. A major potential complication is hemorrhage from the:

   a. brachial artery.   c. innominate artery.

   b. carotid artery.   d. vertebral artery.

10. Postoperatively, the nurse observes excessive drooling. She assesses for damage to the:

    a. facial nerve.   c. spinal accessory nerve.

    b. hypoglossal nerve.   d. auditory nerve.

CLINICAL SITUATIONS

Read the following case studies. Fill in the blanks or circle the correct answer.

Case Study: Mandibular Fracture

William, a 17-year-old student, suffered a mandibular fracture while playing football. He is scheduled for jaw repositioning surgery.

1. Preoperatively, the nurse explains the surgical procedure for treatment of a mandibular fracture. Describe

   the procedure that would be used: _____

   _____

2. Postoperatively, the nurse should immediately position William:

   a. flat on his back to facilitate lung expansion during inspiration.

   b. on his side with his head slightly elevated to prevent aspiration.

   c. supine with his head to the side to promote the drainage of secretions.

   d. with his head lower than his trunk to prevent aspiration of fluids.

3. Postoperatively, the nurse's primary goal is to maintain:

   a. adequate nutrition.

   b. an open airway.

   c. jaw immobilization.

   d. oral hygiene.

4. What would you tell the patient to explain why nasogastric suctioning is needed?

   _____

   _____

5. For emergency use, which of the following should be available at the head of the bed?

   a. a nasogastric suction tube

   b. a nasopharyngeal suction catheter

   c. a wire cutter or scissors

   d. an oxygen cannula

6. A recommended initial postoperative diet for William would be:

   a. bland pureed.

   b. clear liquid.

   c. full liquid.

   d. semisoft.

7. William must be instructed not to chew food until which postoperative week?

   a. third

   b. fourth

   c. fifth

   d. eighth

8. What essential item must be sent home with William when he is discharged?

   _____

   _____

CASE STUDY: Cancer of the Mouth

Edith, a 64-year-old mother of two, has been a chain smoker for 20 years. During the past month she noticed a dryness in her mouth and a roughened area that is irritating. She mentioned her symptoms to her dentist, who referred her to a medical internist.

1. Based on the patient's health history, the nurse suspects oral cancer. Describe what the nurse would expect the lesion to look like: _____

   _____

2. During the health history the nurse noted that Edith did not mention a late-occurring symptom of mouth cancer, which is:

   a. drainage.

   b. fever.

   c. odor.

   d. pain.

3. On physical examination, Edith evidenced changes associated with cancer of the mouth, such as:

    a. a sore, roughened area that has not healed in 3 weeks.

    b. minor swelling in an area adjacent to the lesion.

    c. numbness in the affected area of the mouth.

    d. all of the above.

4. To confirm a diagnosis of carcinoma of the mouth, a physician would order:

    a. a biopsy.

    b. a staining procedure.

    c. exfoliative cytology.

    d. roentgenography.

5. List three therapies that are considered effective for treatment.

    a. _____

    b. _____

    c. _____

CHAPTER 36

Gastrointestinal Intubation and Special Nutritional Modalities

I. Interpretation, Completion, and Comparison

MULTIPLE CHOICE

Read each question carefully. Circle your answer.

1. The physician ordered a nasoenteric feeding tube with a tungsten-weighted tip. The nurse knows to obtain what kind of tube?
   a. Dobbhoff
   b. Levin
   c. Salem
   d. Sengstaken- Blakemore

2. The Levin tube, a commonly used nasogastric tube, has circular markings at specific points. The tube should be inserted to:
   a. a length of 50 cm (20 in).
   b. a point that equals the distance from the nose to the xiphoid process.
   c. the midpoint between a 50-cm marking and the distance measured from the tip of the nose to the xiphoid process.
   d. the distance determined by measuring from the tragus of the ear to the xiphoid process.

3. When continuous or intermittent suction is used with a nasogastric tube, the goal is to have the amount of suction in the gastric mucosa reduced to:
   a. 30 to 40 mm Hg.
   b. 60 mm Hg.
   c. 70 to 80 mm Hg.
   d. 100 to 120 mm Hg.

4. To confirm placement of a nasogastric tube, the nurse tests the pH of the tube aspirate. The nurse knows that tube placement in the lungs is indicated by what pH?
   a. 3
   b. 5
   c. 6
   d. 7

5. A nurse prepares a patient for insertion of a nasoenteric tube. The nurse positions the patient:
   a. in high Fowler's position.
   b. flat in bed.
   c. on his or her right side.
   d. in semi-Fowler's position with his or her head turned to the left.

6. It is essential for the nurse who is managing a gastric sump tube to:
   a. maintain intermittent or continuous suction at a rate greater than 120 mm Hg.
   b. keep the vent lumen above the patient's midline to prevent gastric content reflux.
   c. irrigate only through the vent lumen.
   d. do all of the above.

7. A nasoenteric-decompression tube can be safely advanced 2 to 3 inches every:

a. 1 hour.

b. 2 hours.

c. 4 hours.

d. 8 hours.

8. Nasoenteric tubes usually remain in place until:

a. bowel sounds are present.

b. flatus is passed.

c. peristalsis is resumed.

d. all of the above mechanisms occur.

9. Symptoms of oliguria, lethargy, and hypothermia in a patient would indicate to the nurse that the patient may be experiencing the initial common potential complication of nasoenteric intubation, which is:

a. a cardiac dysrhythmia.

b. fluid volume deficit.

c. mucous membrane irritation.

d. pulmonary complications.

10. Osmosis is the process whereby:

a. particles disperse throughout a liquid medium to achieve an equal concentration throughout.

b. particles move from an area of greater concentration to an area of lesser concentration to establish equilibrium.

c. water moves through a membrane from a dilute solution to a more concentrated solution to achieve equal osmolality.

d. water moves through a membrane from an area of higher osmolality to an area of lesser osmolality to establish equilibrium.

11. Residual content is checked before each tube feeding. A feeding would be delayed and the patient reassessed if the residual were:

a. about 50 mL.

b. between 50 and 80 mL.

c. about 100 mL.

d. greater than 200 mL.

12. The dumping syndrome occurs when high-carbohydrate foods are administered over a period of less than 20 minutes. A nursing measure to prevent or minimize the dumping syndrome is to administer the feeding:

a. at a warm temperature to decrease peristalsis.

b. by bolus to prevent continuous intestinal distention.

c. with about 100 mL of fluid to dilute the high carbohydrate concentration.

d. with the patient in semi-Fowler's position to decrease transit time influenced by gravity.

13. Gastrostomy feedings are preferred to nasogastric feedings in the comatose patient, because the:

a. gastroesophageal sphincter is intact, lessening the possibility of regurgitation.

b. digestive process occurs more rapidly as a result of the feeding's not having to pass through the esophagus.

c. feedings can be administered with the patient in the recumbent position.

d. the patient cannot experience the deprivational stress of not swallowing.

14. Initial fluid nourishment after a gastrostomy usually consists of:

a. distilled water.

b. 10% glucose and tap water.

c. milk.

d. high-calorie liquids.

15. When administering a bolus gastrostomy feeding, the receptacle should be held no higher than:

a. 9 inches.

b. 18 inches.

c. 27 inches.

d. 36 inches.

16. The basic hyperalimentation solution contains what percentage of glucose?

    a. 10%   c. 35%

    (b.) 25%   d. 50%

17. The preferred route for infusion of parenteral nutrition is the:

    a. brachial vein.   (c.) subclavian vein.

    b. jugular vein.   d. superior vena cava.

18. The most common infectious fungal organism for patients receiving parenteral nutrition is:

    (a.) *Candida albicans.*   c. *Staphylococcus aureus.*

    b. *Klebsiella pneumoniae.*   d. *Staphylococcus epidermidis.*

19. Patients who are receiving total parenteral nutrition should be observed for signs of hyperglycemia, which would include:

    a. diuresis.   c. stupor.

    b. lethargy.   (d.) all of the above.

MATCHING

Match the description of the nasogastric, nasoenteric, or regular feeding tube in column II with its appropriate name listed in column I.

Column I

1. _____ Sengstaken-Blakemore

2. _____ Levin

3. _____ Gastric-Sump Salem

4. _____ Moss

5. _____ Dobbhoff or Keofeed II

Column II

a. Triple-lumen nasogastric tube that also has a duodenal lumen for postoperative feedings

b. Nasoenteric feeding tube about 4 feet in length

c. Single-lumen, plastic or rubber nasogastric tube about 4 feet in length

d. Double-lumen, plastic nasogastric tube about 120 cm in length

e. Triple-lumen, rubber nasogastric tube (two lumens are used to inflate the gastric and esophageal balloons)

II. Critical Thinking Questions and Exercises

Read the following case studies. Fill in the blanks or circle the correct answer.

CASE STUDY: Dumping Syndrome

Nancy is 37 years old, 5 feet 7 inches tall, and weighs 140 lb. She receives 250 mL of Osmolite (liquid nutrition) over a 15-minute period every 4 hours through a nasogastric tube. Nancy has had esophageal surgery for carcinoma.

1. Nancy tells the nurse that she has diarrhea. The nurse suspects Nancy is experiencing the dumping syndrome. The nurse also knows that other possible causes need to be eliminated, such as

_____, _____, _____, and

_____.

2. The nurse reviews Nancy's chart to see what medications she is receiving, because certain drugs increase the frequency of the syndrome in some patients. List several of these medications:

_____

_____

_____

3. Because of the dumping syndrome, the physician reduces Nancy's current rate of infusion by 50%. The nurse should adjust the rate of the gastrostomy feeding to:
   a. 8 mL/min.
   b. 10 mL/min.
   c. 12 mL/min.
   d. 16 mL/min.

4. The nurse notes a residual gastric content of 50 mL. She should:
   a. delay the feeding for 2 hours and reassess.
   b. discard the 50 mL and administer the next feeding.
   c. notify the physician.
   d. return the solution through the tube and administer the next feeding.

CASE STUDY: Total Parenteral Nutrition

Penny is 30 years old and single. She is 5 feet 7 inches tall, weighs 150 pounds, and is receiving parenteral nutrition solution at the rate of 3 L/day. Her postoperative condition warrants receiving nutrients by the intravenous route.

1. The nurse knows that, to spare body protein, Penny's daily calorie intake must be:
   a. approximately 500 calories per day.
   b. approximately 1500 calories per day.
   c. approximately 800 calories per day.
   d. 1000 calories per day.

2. The nurse estimates Penny's caloric intake for each 1000 mL of total parenteral nutrition to yield a glucose concentration of:
   a. 500 calories.
   b. 800 calories.
   c. 1000 calories.
   d. 1500 calories.

3. Penny's infusion rate is 120 mL/hour. Her rate has slowed because of positional body changes. To compensate, the nurse could safely increase Penny's rate for 8 hours to:
   a. 100 mL/hour.
   b. 125 mL/hour.
   c. 138 mL/hour.
   d. 146 mL/hour.

4. The nurse should observe Penny for signs of rapid fluid intake, which may include:
   a. chills.
   b. fever.
   c. nausea.
   d. all of the above.

5. The nurse weighs Penny daily. After 7 days, Penny's weight gain is abnormal at:
   a. 3.5 lb.
   b. 5.0 lb.
   c. 7.0 lb.
   d. 12 lb.

APPLYING CONCEPTS

Refer to the accompanying figure and answer the following questions.

Gastrostomy feeding by gravity. (**A**) Feeding is instilled at an angle so that air does not enter the stomach. (**B**) Syringe is raised perpendicular to the stomach so that feeding can enter by gravity.

1. List three nursing diagnoses for a postoperative patient that address nursing care for a gastrotomy tube.

   a. _____

   b. _____

   c. _____

2. List three possible collaborative problems for a patient with a gastrostomy tube.

   a. _____

   b. _____

   c. _____

3. When giving an initial tube feeding, the nurse would be looking for what around the tube site on the abdomen? _____

4. A dressing over the tube outlet and the gastrostomy tube protects the skin around the incision from _____ and _____.

5. The syringe, filled with feeding solution, is raised perpendicular to the abdomen so that the solution can enter by gravity. How long should it take for 100 mL to instill? _____.

6. If the solution fails to instill, the nurse could _____

   _____

7. The syringe should not be elevated higher than 18 inches above the abdominal wall, because:_____

   _____

8. Explain why the patient in the figure is sitting upright: _____

   _____

   _____

CHAPTER 37

Management of Patients With Gastric and Duodenal Disorders

1. Interpretation, Completion, and Comparison

MULTIPLE CHOICE

Read each question carefully. Circle your answer.

1. Acute gastritis is often caused by:
   a. ingestion of strong acids.
   b. irritating foods.
   c. overuse of aspirin.
   d. all of the above.

2. To promote fluid balance when treating gastritis, the nurse knows that the minimal daily intake of fluids should be:
   a. 1.0 L.
   b. 1.5 L.
   c. 2.0 L.
   d. 2.5 L.

3. The most common site for peptic ulcer formation is the:
   a. duodenum.
   b. esophagus.
   c. pylorus.
   d. stomach.

4. A symptom that distinguishes a chronic gastric ulcer from a chronic duodenal ulcer is the:
   a. absence of any correlation between the presence of the ulcer and a malignancy.
   b. normal to below-normal secretion of acid.
   c. relief of pain after food ingestion.
   d. uncommon incidence of vomiting.

5. The blood group that seems most susceptible to peptic ulcer disease is group:
   a. A.
   b. B.
   c. AB.
   d. O.

6. Peptic ulcers occur with the most frequency in those between the ages of:
   a. 15 and 25 years.
   b. 20 and 30 years.
   c. 40 and 60 years.
   d. 60 and 80 years.

7. A frequently prescribed proton pump inhibitor of gastric acid is:
   a. Nexium.
   b. Pepcid.
   c. Tagamet.
   d. Zantac.

8. Gastrinomas present in Zollinger-Ellison syndrome have a malignancy rate of approximately:
   a. 10%.
   b. 30%.
   c. 50%.
   d. 80%.

9. A characteristic associated with peptic ulcer pain is a:
   a. burning sensation localized in the back or midepigastrium.
   b. feeling of emptiness that precedes meals from 1 to 3 hours.
   c. severe gnawing pain that increases in severity as the day progresses.
   d. combination of all of the above.

10. The best time to administer an antacid is:
    a. with the meal.
    b. 30 minutes before the meal.
    c. 1 to 3 hours after the meal.
    d. immediately after the meal.

11. A Billroth I procedure is a surgical approach to ulcer management whereby:
    a. a partial gastrectomy is done with anastomosis of the stomach segment to the duodenum.
    b. a sectioned portion of the stomach is joined to the jejunum.
    c. the antral portion of the stomach is removed and a vagotomy is performed.
    d. the vagus nerve is cut and gastric drainage is established.

12. The most common complication of peptic ulcer disease is:
    a. hemorrhage.
    b. intractable ulcer.
    c. perforation.
    d. pyloric obstruction.

13. Nursing interventions associated with peptic ulcers include:
    a. checking the blood pressure and pulse rate every 15 to 20 minutes.
    b. frequently monitoring hemoglobin and hematocrit levels.
    c. observing stools and vomitus for color, consistency, and volume.
    d. all of the above.

14. If peptic ulcer hemorrhage were suspected, an immediate nursing action would be to:
    a. place the patient in a recumbent position with his or her legs elevated.
    b. prepare a peripheral and central line for intravenous infusion.
    c. assess vital signs.
    d. accomplish all of the above.

15. Pyloric obstruction can occur when the area distal to the pyloric sphincter becomes stenosed by:
    a. edema.
    b. scar tissue.
    c. spasm.
    d. all of the above.

16. Symptoms associated with pyloric obstruction include all of the following *except*:
    a. anorexia.
    b. diarrhea.
    c. nausea and vomiting.
    d. epigastric fullness.

17. Morbid obesity is a term applied to people who are more than:
    a. 20 lb above ideal body weight.
    b. 50 lb above ideal body weight.
    c. 75 to 80 lb above ideal body weight.
    d. 100 lb above ideal body weight.

18. The average weight loss after bariatric surgery is about what percent of previous body weight?
    a. 25%
    b. 40%
    c. 60%
    d. 80%

19. Pulmonary complications frequently follow upper-abdominal incisions, because:
    a. aspiration is a common occurrence associated with postoperative injury to the pyloric sphincter or the cardiac sphincter.
    b. pneumothorax is a common complication of abdominal surgery when the chest cavity has been entered.
    c. the patient tends to have shallow respirations in an attempt to minimize incisional pain.
    d. all of the above.

20. Teaching points to help a patient with total gastric resection avoid the dumping syndrome include all of the following *except*:
    a. eating small, frequent meals.
    b. increasing the carbohydrate content of the diet to supply needed calories for energy.
    c. lying down after meals.
    d. taking fluids between meals to decrease the total volume in the stomach at one time.

SHORT ANSWER

Read each statement carefully. Write your response in the space provided.

1. Describe the immediate intervention that should be used to treat the ingestion of a corrosive acid:

   _____

   _____

2. Explain why patients with gastritis due to a vitamin deficiency usually have malabsorption of vitamin B_{12}:

   _____

   _____

3. Name two conditions specifically related to peptic ulcer development: _____ and

   _____ .

4. The bacillus that is commonly associated with gastric and possibly duodenal ulcers is

   _____ .

5. List several findings characteristic of Zollinger-Ellison syndrome: _____

   _____

   _____

6. Define the term stress ulcer: _____

   _____

7. Distinguish between Cushing's and Curling's ulcer in terms of cause and location:

   _____

   _____

   _____

8. Explain the current theory about diet modification for peptic ulcer disease: _____

   _____

   _____

9. Name three major complications of a peptic ulcer:

_____

_____

_____

10. Describe the clinical manifestations associated with peptic ulcer perforation: _____

_____

_____

11. The stomach pouches created by gastric bypass or bonding surgery can hold up to _____ mL of food and fluids.

12. The most common malignant tumor of the duodenum is _____.

SCRAMBLEGRAM

Unscramble the letters used to answer each statement, and write the word in the space provided.

1. Lack of hydrochloric acid in digestive secretions of the stomach: _____

L H O D H I A R C Y R A

2. Inflammation of the stomach: _____

A R T S G T I I S

3. Vomiting of blood: _____

M T E S E H S A I M E

4. Term used to describe black and tarry stools: _____

L N E A M E

5. Opening between the stomach and duodenum: _____

L R P U S O Y

6. Medical term to describe heartburn: _____

Y O S P I S R

II. Critical Thinking Questions and Exercises

DISCUSSION AND ANALYSIS

Discuss the following topics with your classmates.

1. Compare the etiology of chronic and acute gastritis.
2. Describe the pathophysiology of gastritis.
3. Chronic gastritis can be caused by the bacteria *Helicobacter pylori*. Name four diagnostic tests that can be used to determine the presence of the bacteria.

4. Discuss the dietary guidelines for a patient who has had bariatric surgery.
5. Describe the vasomotor and gastrointestinal symptoms found in the dumping syndrome.

EXTRACTING INFERENCES

Examine the accompanying figure. Outline in detail the pathophysiology of peptic ulcer formation. Explain why specific sites are more common and what contributes to common inflammatory sites.

Peptic lesions may occur in the esophagus (esophagitis), stomach (gastritis), or duodenum (duodenitis). Note peptic ulcer sites and common inflammatory sites. Hydrochloric acid is formed by parietal cells in the fundus; gastrin is secreted by G cells in the antrum. The duodenal glands secrete an alkaline mucous solution.

Clinical Situations

Read the following case study. Fill in the blanks or circle the correct answer.

CASE STUDY: Gastric Cancer

Mr. Jackson, a 66-year-old African American, has recently been seen by a physician to confirm a diagnosis of gastric cancer. He has a history of tobacco use and was diagnosed 10 years ago with pernicious anemia. He and his family are shocked about the possibility of this diagnosis because he was asymptomatic before recent complaints of pain and multiple gastrointestinal symptoms.

1. Based on knowledge of disease progression, the nurse assumes that organs adjacent to the stomach are also affected, such as the _____, _____, _____, and _____.

2. On palpation, the nurse notes two signs that confirm metastasis to the liver: _____ and _____.

3. The nurses advises the patient that one diagnostic procedure, _____, will be conducted to confirm a diagnosis of cancer and another procedure, _____, will be done to determine surgical resectability of the probable tumor.

4. The surgical team has decided that a Billroth II would be the best approach to treatment. The nurse explains to the family that this procedure involves a:
   a. limited resection in the distal portion of the stomach.
   b. wide resection of the middle and distal portions of the stomach.
   c. proximal subtotal gastrectomy.
   d. total gastrectomy and esophagogastrectomy.

5. The nurse explains that combination chemotherapy frequently follows surgery. The primary agent used would most likely be _____.

CHAPTER 38

Management of Patients With Intestinal and Rectal Disorders

I. Interpretation, Completion, and Comparison

MULTIPLE CHOICE

Read each question carefully. Circle your answer.

1. The pathophysiology of constipation may be related to interference with:
   a. myoelectric activity of the colon.
   b. mucosal transport.
   c. processes involved in defecation.
   d. all of the above mechanisms.

2. Nursing suggestions to help a person break the constipation habit include all of the following *except*:
   a. a fluid intake of at least 2 L/day.
   b. a low-residue, bland diet.
   c. establishing a regular schedule of exercise.
   d. establishing a regular time for daily elimination.

3. An example of a stimulant laxative that works in 6 to 8 hours is:
   a. Colace.
   b. Colyte.
   c. Dulcolax.
   d. Milk of Magnesia.

4. The classification of *moderate diarrhea* refers to the quantity of daily unformed stools described as:
   a. more than two bowel movements a day.
   b. between two and four bowel movements a day.
   c. between three and six bowel movements a day.
   d. more than six bowel movements a day.

5. In assessing stool characteristics associated with diarrhea, the nurse knows that the presence of greasy stools suggests:
   a. disorders of the colon.
   b. inflammatory enteritis.
   c. intestinal malabsorption.
   d. small-bowel disorders.

6. Hypokalemia can occur rapidly in an elderly person who experiences diarrhea. The nurse should immediately report to the physician a critical potassium level of:
   a. 3.0 mEq/L.
   b. 4.0 mEq/L.
   c. 4.5 mEq/L.
   d. 5.0 mEq/L.

7. A disorder of malabsorption that inactivates pancreatic enzymes is:
   a. celiac disease.
   b. cystic fibrosis.
   c. Whipple's disease.
   d. Zollinger-Ellison syndrome.

8. Malabsorption diseases may affect the ability of the digestive system to absorb which major water-soluble vitamin?
   a. vitamin A
   b. vitamin B
   c. vitamin D
   d. vitamin K

9. A positive Rovsing's sign is indicative of appendicitis. The nurse knows to assess for this indicator by palpating the:
   a. right lower quadrant.
   b. left lower quadrant.
   c. right upper quadrant.
   d. left upper quadrant.

10. The most common site for diverticulitis is the:
    a. duodenum.
    b. ileum.
    c. jejunum.
    d. sigmoid.

11. The incidence of diverticulitis among those older than 60 years of age is about:
    a. 15%.
    b. 35%.
    c. 60%.
    d. 80%.

12. Diverticulitis is clinically manifested by:
    a. a low-grade fever.
    b. a change in bowel habits.
    c. left lower quadrant pain.
    d. all of the above.

13. Common clinical manifestations of Crohn's disease are:
    a. abdominal pain and diarrhea.
    b. edema and weight gain.
    c. nausea and vomiting.
    d. obstruction and ileus.

14. A nurse suspects a diagnosis of regional enteritis when she assesses the symptoms of:
    a. abdominal distention and rebound tenderness.
    b. hyperactive bowel sounds in the right lower quadrant.
    c. intermittent pain associated with diarrhea.
    d. all of the above.

15. Nutritional management for regional enteritis consists of diet therapy that is:
    a. high in fats.
    b. high in fiber.
    c. low in protein.
    d. low in residue.

16. Remission of inflammation in ulcerative colitis is possible with:
    a. antidiarrheal medication.
    b. periods of rest after meals.
    c. steroid therapy.
    d. all of the above.

17. A problem unique to the patient with an ileostomy is that:
    a. regular bowel habits cannot be established.
    b. sexual activity is restricted.
    c. skin excoriation can occur.
    d. the collecting appliance is bulky and large.

18. Postoperative nursing management for a patient with a continent ileostomy includes all of the following *except*:
    a. checking to make certain that the rectal packing is in place.
    b. irrigating the ileostomy catheter every 3 hours.
    c. nasogastric tube feedings, 30 to 50 mL, every 4 to 6 hours.
    d. perineal irrigations after the dressings are removed.

19. Clinical manifestations associated with small-bowel obstruction include all of the following *except*:
    a. dehydration.
    b. pain that is wavelike.
    c. the passage of blood-tinged stool.
    d. vomiting.

20. The 5-year survival rate for cancer of the colon that is detected early is:
    a. less than 20%.
    b. 25% to 35%.
    c. 50% to 60%.
    d. 90%.

21. Preoperatively, intestinal antibiotics are given for colon surgery to:
    a. decrease the bulk of colon contents.
    b. reduce the bacteria content of the colon.
    c. soften the stool.
    d. do all of the above.

22. For colostomy irrigation, the enema catheter should be inserted into the stoma:
    a. 1 inch.
    b. 2 to 3 inches.
    c. 4 to 6 inches.
    d. 8 inches.

23. For colostomy irrigation, the patient should be directed to hold the enema can or bag at shoulder level, approximately how far above the stoma?
    a. 6 inches.
    b. 8 to 16 inches.
    c. 18 to 20 inches.
    d. 30 inches.

24. The total quantity of irrigating solution that can be instilled at one session is:
    a. 1000 mL.
    b. 1500 mL.
    c. 2500 mL.
    d. 3000 mL.

CROSSWORD PUZZLE

Complete the following crossword puzzle using common terms associated with intestinal and rectal disorders.

DOWN

1. A tubular fibrous tract that extends from an opening beside the anus into the anal canal
2. Dilated and atonic colon caused by a fecal mass
3. A chemotherapeutic agent used to treat colon cancer
4. A food to avoid for a patient with an ileostomy
6. Straining at stool
8. Another name for regional enteritis
12. A highly reliable blood study used to diagnose appendicitis
13. Painful straining at stool
14. The most common bacteria associated with peritonitis

ACROSS

5. Another term for fecal matter
7. An ileal outlet on the abdomen
9. Intestinal rumbling
10. Another food to avoid for a patient with an ileostomy
11. The most popular "over-the-counter" medication purchased in the United States
15. Intravenous nutrition used for inflammatory bowel disease
16. The most common complication of colon cancer

MATCHING

First, match each type of laxative in column III with the appropriate classification listed in column II; write the Roman numeral in the space provided. Then, match the classification in column II with its action listed in column I; write the small letter in the space provided.

Column I

1._____ Magnesium ions alter stool consistency

2._____ Surfactant action hydrates stool

3._____ Electrolytes induce diarrhea

4._____ Polysaccharides and cellulose mix with intestinal contents

5._____ Colon is irritated and sensory nerve endings stimulated

6._____ Hydrocarbons soften fecal matter

Column II

a. _____ Bulk-forming

b. _____ Stimulant

c. _____ Fecal softener

d. _____ Lubricant

e. _____ Saline agent

f. _____ Osmotic agent

Column III

 I. Mineral oil

II. Metamucil

III. Milk of Magnesia

IV. Dulcolax

 V. Colace

VI. Colyte

SHORT ANSWER

Read each statement carefully. Write your response in the space provided.

1. The three most common changes in the gastrointestinal tract that are symptoms of functional disorders or diseases are: _____, _____, and _____.

2. Name two diseases of the colon commonly associated with constipation.

   _____

   _____

3. List the four common bacteria found in peritonitis.

   _____

   _____

   _____

   _____

4. The most common cause of small bowel obstruction is _____, followed by _____ and _____.

5. The majority of large bowel obstructions are caused by _____.

6. List the six risk factors for colorectal cancer.

   _____

   _____

   _____

   _____

   _____

   _____

II. Critical Thinking Questions and Exercises

DISCUSSION AND ANALYSIS

Discuss the following topics with your classmates.

1. Discuss the physiologic processes that result in the urge to defecate.
2. Explain the Valsalva maneuver that can occur as a complication of constipation.

3. For each of these three diseases, explain the pathophysiology of malabsorption:

   Pancreatic insufficiency: _____

   Zollinger-Ellison syndrome: _____

   Celiac disease: _____

4. Describe the nursing care management for a patient with inflammatory bowel disease (IBD).
5. Discuss seven nursing diagnoses for patients undergoing ostomy surgery.
6. Explain the steps involved in changing an ostomy appliance.

7. Compare and contrast the five different surgical procedures used in colorectal cancer surgery.
8. Explain the differences between the etiology and clinical manifestations of five mechanical causes of intestinal obstruction: adhesions, intussusception, a volvulus, hernia and tumor.
9. Compare and contrast the clinical manifestations and nursing interventions for eight potential complications of intestinal surgery.
10. Describe the steps for irrigating a colostomy.

RECOGNIZING CONTRADICTIONS

Rewrite each statement correctly. Underline the key concepts.

1. Diarrhea is a condition in which there is an increased frequency of bowel movements (more than six per day) associated with increased amount and consistency.

_____

2. Peritonitis, the most common reason for emergency abdominal surgery, occurs in about 10% of the population.

_____

3. The most serious complication of appendicitis is strangulation of adjacent bowel tissue, which occurs in 5% of the cases.

_____

4. The major cause of death from peritonitis is hypovolemia.

_____

5. The most common areas affected in Crohn's disease are the sigmoid colon and the cecum.

_____

6. Surgery is rarely necessary for the treatment of regional enteritis.

_____

7. Rectal bleeding is the most common symptom of colon cancer.

_____

CLINICAL SITUATIONS

Read the following case studies. Fill in the blanks or circle the correct answer.

CASE STUDY: Appendicitis

Rory, an 18-year-old girl, is admitted to the hospital with a possible diagnosis of appendicitis. She had been symptomatic for several days before admission.

1. During assessment, the nurse is looking for positive indicators of appendicitis, which include all of the following *except:*
   a. a low-grade fever.
   b. abdominal tenderness on palpation.
   c. thrombocytopenia.
   d. vomiting.

2. On physical examination, the nurse should be looking for tenderness on palpation at McBurney's point, which is located in the:

a. left lower quadrant.

b. left upper quadrant.

c. right lower quadrant.

d. right upper quadrant.

3. Symptoms suggestive of acute appendicitis include:

a. a positive Rovsing's sign.

b. increased abdominal pain with coughing.

c. tenderness around the umbilicus.

d. all of the above.

4. Preparation for an appendectomy includes:

a. an intravenous infusion.

b. prophylactic antibiotic therapy.

c. salicylates to lower an elevated temperature.

d. all of the above.

CASE STUDY: Peritonitis

Sharon has peritonitis subsequent to ambulatory peritoneal dialysis. Her presenting symptoms are pain, abdominal tenderness, and nausea.

1. On assessment, the nurse should be looking for additional symptoms diagnostic of peritonitis, which include:

a. abdominal rigidity.

b. diminished peristalsis.

c. leukocytosis.

d. all of the above.

2. A central venous pressure (CVP) catheter is inserted to monitor fluid balance. The nurse's readings indicate low circulatory volume. The reading is probably between:

a. 2 and 4 cm HO.

b. 6 and 8 cm HO.

c. 10 and 12 cm HO.

d. 14 and 16 cm HO.

3. Given Sharon's CVP reading indicating hypovolemia, the nurse should assess for all of the following *except*:

a. bradycardia.

b. hypotension.

c. oliguria.

d. tachypnea.

4. With treatment, Sharon's peritonitis subsides. However, the nurse continues to assess for the common complication of:

a. abscess formation.

b. respiratory arrest owing to excessive pressure on the diaphragm.

c. umbilical hernia.

d. urinary tract infection.

IDENTIFYING PATTERNS

Review Figure 38-1 in the text and answer the following questions about irritable bowel syndrome (IBS).

1. List at least five etiologic factors associated with the change in intestinal motility in IBS.

_____

_____

_____

_____

_____

2. The primary symptom in IBS is _____.

3. Based on the figure, describe the pathophysiologic changes that result in IBS:

_____

_____

4. Standard diagnostic tests used in IBS are _____, _____,

_____, and _____.

5. Goals of medical management include _____, _____,

_____, and _____.

6. A popular drug, _____, is prescribed when the chief complaint is chronic constipation.

7. Discuss the nurse's role in providing patient and family education: _____

_____

_____

CHAPTER 39

Assessment and Management of Patients With Hepatic Disorders

I. Interpretation, Completion, and Comparison

MULTIPLE CHOICE

Read each question carefully. Circle your answer.

1. The majority of blood supply to the liver, which is rich in nutrients from the gastrointestinal tract, comes from the:
   a. hepatic artery.
   b. hepatic vein.
   c. portal artery.
   d. portal vein.

2. The liver plays a major role in glucose metabolism by:
   a. producing ketone bodies.
   b. synthesizing albumin.
   c. participating in gluconeogenesis.
   d. doing all of the above.

3. The liver synthesizes prothrombin only if there is enough:
   a. vitamin A.
   b. vitamin B_{12}.
   c. vitamin D.
   d. vitamin K.

4. The substance necessary for the manufacture of bile salts by hepatocytes is:
   a. albumin.
   b. bilirubin.
   c. cholesterol.
   d. vitamin D.

5. The main function of bile salts is:
   a. albumin synthesis.
   b. fat emulsification in the intestines.
   c. lipid manufacture for the transport of proteins.
   d. urea synthesis from ammonia.

6. Hepatocellular dysfunction results in all of the following *except*:
   a. decreased serum albumin.
   b. elevated serum bilirubin.
   c. increased blood ammonia levels.
   d. increased levels of urea.

7. Jaundice becomes evident when serum bilirubin levels exceed:
   a. 0.5 mg/dL.
   b. 1.0 mg/dL.
   c. 1.5 mg/dL.
   d. 2.5 mg/dL.

8. The liver converts ammonia to urea. What level of ammonia would suggest liver failure?
   a. 40 µg/dL
   b. 100 mg/dL
   c. 200 µg/dL
   d. 300 mg/dL

9. The most common cause of parenchymal cell damage and hepatocellular dysfunction is:
   a. infectious agents.
   b. malnutrition.
   c. metabolic disorders.
   d. toxins.

10. Negative sodium balance is important for a patient with ascites. An example of food permitted on a low-sodium diet is:
    a. 1/4 cup of peanut butter.
    b. 1 cup of powdered milk.
    c. one frankfurter.
    d. two slices of cold cuts.

11. The nurse expects that the diuretic of choice for a patient with ascites would be:
    a. Aldactone.
    b. Ammonium chloride.
    c. Diamox.
    d. Lasix.

12. An indicator of probable esophageal varices is:
    a. hematemesis.
    b. a positive guaiac test.
    c. melena.
    d. all of the above.

13. The mortality rate from bleeding esophageal varices is about:
    a. 10%.
    b. 20%.
    c. 50%.
    d. 80%.

14. Bleeding esophageal varices result in a decrease in:
    a. nitrogen load from bleeding.
    b. renal perfusion.
    c. serum ammonia.
    d. all of the above.

15. The initial model of therapy to treat variceal hemorrhage that decreases portal pressure is:
    a. Corgard.
    b. Isordil.
    c. Pitressin.
    d. Somatostatin.

16. A person who consumes contaminated shellfish would probably develop:
    a. hepatitis B.
    b. hepatitis C.
    c. hepatitis D.
    d. hepatitis E.

17. The hepatitis virus that is transmitted via the fecal-oral route is:
    a. hepatitis A virus.
    b. hepatitis B virus.
    c. hepatitis C virus.
    d. hepatitis D virus.

18. Immune serum globulin provides passive immunity against type A hepatitis in those not vaccinated if it is administered within 2 weeks of exposure. Immunity is effective for about:
    a. 1 month.
    b. 2 months.
    c. 3 months.
    d. 4 months.

19. Choose the correct statement about hepatitis B vaccine.
    a. All persons at risk should receive active immunization.
    b. Evidence suggests that the human immunodeficiency virus (HIV) may be harbored in the vaccine.
    c. Booster doses are recommended every 5 years.
    d. One dose in the dorsogluteal muscle is recommended.

20. Indications for postexposure vaccination with hepatitis B immune globulin include:
    a. accidental exposure to HBsAg-positive blood.
    b. perinatal exposure.
    c. sexual contact with those who are positive for HBsAg.
    d. all of the above exposures.

21. The hepatitis virus caused by contaminated needles shared by drug users is expected to increase fourfold over the next 10 years. This type of hepatitis, which is also the most common cause for liver transplantation, is:
    a. hepatitis A.
    b. hepatitis B.
    c. hepatitis C.
    d. hepatitis D.

22. The chemical most commonly implicated in toxic hepatitis is:
    a. chloroform.
    b. gold compounds.
    c. phosphorus.
    d. all of the above hepatotoxins.

23. Acetaminophen, found in over-the-counter (OTC) drugs, is the leading cause of acute liver failure. A popular drug containing acetaminophen is:
    a. Advil.
    b. Aleve.
    c. Motrin.
    d. Tylenol.

24. Fulminant hepatic failure may progress to hepatic encephalopathy about how many weeks after disease onset?
    a. 2
    b. 4
    c. 6
    d. 8

25. The major causative factor in the etiology of cirrhosis is:
    a. acute viral hepatitis.
    b. chronic alcoholism.
    c. chronic biliary obstruction.
    d. infection (cholangitis).

26. Late symptoms of hepatic cirrhosis include all of the following *except*:
    a. edema.
    b. hypoalbuminemia.
    c. hypokalemia.
    d. hyponatremia.

27. Cirrhosis results in shunting of portal system blood into collateral blood vessels in the gastrointestinal tract. The most common site is:
    a. the esophagus.
    b. the lower rectum.
    c. the stomach.
    d. a combination of all of the above.

28. Signs of advanced liver disease include:
    a. ascites.
    b. jaundice.
    c. portal hypertension.
    d. all of the above.

29. The most common single cause of death in patients with cirrhosis is:
    a. congestive heart failure.
    b. hepatic encephalopathy.
    c. hypovolemic shock.
    d. ruptured esophageal varices.

30. Hepatic lobectomy for cancer can be successful if the primary site is localized. Because of the regenerative capacity of the liver, a surgeon can remove up to what percentage of liver tissue?
    a. 25%
    b. 50%
    c. 75%
    d. 90%

MATCHING

Match the vitamin column II with the signs of deficiency due to severe chronic liver disease listed in Column I.

Column I

1. _____ Hypoprothrombinemia

2. _____ Beriberi and polyneuritis

3. _____ Hemorrhagic lesions of scurvy

4. _____ Night blindness

5. _____ Macrocytic anemia

6. _____ Skin and neurologic changes

7. _____ Mucous membrane lesions

Column II

a. Vitamin A

b. Vitamin C

c. Vitamin K

d. Folic acid

e. Thiamine

f. Riboflavin

g. Pyridoxine

II. Critical Thinking Questions and Exercises

DISCUSSION AND ANALYSIS

Discuss the following topics with your classmates.

1. Discuss the age-related changes of the hepatobiliary system.
2. Distinguish among hemolytic, hepatocellular, and obstructive jaundice in regard to cause.
3. Describe the pathophysiology of ascites.
4. Distinguish among three types of portal system shunts used to surgically bypass variceal bleeding sites.
5. Explain the pathophysiology of hepatic encephalopathy.
6. Explain the pathophysiology of alcoholic cirrhosis.

CLINICAL SITUATIONS

Read the following case studies. Circle the correct answer.

CASE STUDY: Liver Biopsy

Veronica is scheduled for a liver biopsy. The staff nurse assigned to care for Veronica is to accompany her to the treatment room.

1. Before a liver biopsy, the nurse should check to see that:
    a. a compatible donor blood is available.
    b. hemostasis tests have been completed.
    c. vital signs have been assessed.
    d. all of the above have been done.

2. The nurse begins preparing Veronica for the biopsy by assisting her to the correct position, which is:

a. jackknife, with her entire back exposed.

b. recumbent, with her right upper abdomen exposed.

c. lying on her right side, with the left upper thoracic area exposed.

d. supine, with the left lateral chest wall exposed.

3. The nurse knows that the biopsy needle will be inserted into the liver between the:

a. third and fourth ribs.

b. fourth and fifth ribs.

c. sixth and seventh ribs.

d. eighth and ninth ribs.

4. Immediately before needle insertion, Veronica needs to be instructed to:

a. breathe slowly and deeply so that rib cage expansion will be minimized during needle insertion.

b. inhale and exhale deeply and then hold her breath at the end of expiration until the needle is inserted.

c. pant deeply and continue panting during needle insertion so pain perception will be minimized.

d. take a deep inspiration and not breathe for 30 to 40 seconds so that the area for needle insertion can be determined; she should then resume normal breathing for the remainder of the procedure.

5. After the biopsy, the nurse assists Veronica to:

a. high Fowler's position, in which she can effectively take deep breaths and cough.

b. ambulate while splinting her incision.

c. assume the Trendelenburg position to prevent postbiopsy shock.

d. the right side-lying position with a pillow placed under the right costal margin.

CASE STUDY: Paracentesis

Wendy is scheduled for a paracentesis because of ascites formation subsequent to cirrhosis of the liver.

1. Before the procedure, the nurse obtains several drainage bottles. She knows that the maximum amount of fluid to be aspirated at one time is:

a. 1 L.

b. 2 L.

c. 3 L.

d. 4 L.

2. The nurse helps Wendy to assume the proper position for a paracentesis, which is:

a. recumbent so that the fluid will pool to the lower abdomen.

b. lying on her left side so that fluid will not exert pressure on the liver.

c. semi-Fowler's to avoid shock and provide the most comfort.

d. upright with her feet resting on a support so that the puncture site will be readily visible.

3. After the paracentesis, Wendy should be observed for signs of vascular collapse, which include all of the following *except:*

a. bradycardia.

b. hypotension.

c. oliguria.

d. pallor.

CASE STUDY: Alcoholic or Nutritional Cirrhosis

Nathan, a 50-year-old physically disabled veteran, has lived alone for 30 years. He has maintained his independence despite chronic back pain resulting from a war injury. He has a long history of depression and limited food intake. He drinks 6 to 10 bottles of beer daily. He was recently admitted to a veteran's hospital with a diagnosis of alcoholic or nutritional cirrhosis. He was asymptomatic for ascites.

1. On assessment, the nurse notes early clinical manifestations of alcoholic or nutritional cirrhosis, which include all of the following *except:*
   a. pain caused by liver enlargement.
   b. a sharp edge to the periphery of the liver.
   c. a liver decreased in size and nodular.
   d. a firm liver.

2. An abnormal laboratory finding for Nathan is a:
   a. blood ammonia level of 35 mg/dL.
   b. serum albumin concentration of 4.0 g/dL.
   c. total serum bilirubin level of 0.9 mg/dL.
   d. total serum protein level of 5.5 g/dL.

3. Nathan is 5 feet 10 inches tall and weighs 140 lb. The physician recommends 50 cal/kg for weight gain. Nathan's daily caloric intake would be approximately:
   a. 2200 cal.
   b. 2800 cal.
   c. 3200 cal.
   d. 3800 cal.

4. A recommended daily protein intake for Nathan to gain weight is:
   a. 31 to 44 g.
   b. 41 to 54 g.
   c. 51 to 64 g.
   d. 61 to 74 g.

5. The physician recommends a sodium-restricted diet. The nurse expects the suggested sodium intake to be approximately:
   a. 250 to 500 mg/24 hours.
   b. 500 to 1000 mg/24 hours.
   c. 2000 to 2500 mg/24 hours.
   d. 3000 to 3500 mg/24 hours.

CASE STUDY: Liver Transplantation

Denise, a 54-year-old mother of three, is scheduled for a liver transplantation subsequent to an extensive hepatic malignancy with multifocal tumors greater than 8 cm in diameter.

1. Denise is hopeful that her surgery will be successful. She is aware, however, that her chance of survival at 5 years is about:
   a. 10%.
   b. 30%.
   c. 50%.
   d. 70%.

2. Denise knows that a successful outcome to transplantation will be compromised by:
   a. fluid and electrolyte disturbances.
   b. malnutrition.
   c. immunosuppressive therapy.
   d. all of the above.

3. The nurse is aware that, postoperatively, the leading cause of death after liver transplantation is:
   a. bleeding.
   b. hypotension.
   c. infection.
   d. portal hypertension.

4. The nurse knows that a patient receiving cyclosporine to prevent rejection of a transplanted liver may develop a drug side effect of:
   a. nephrotoxicity.
   b. septicemia.
   c. thrombocytopenia.
   d. all of the above reactions.

CHAPTER 40

Assessment and Management of Patients With Biliary Disorders

I. Interpretation, Completion, and Comparison

MULTIPLE CHOICE

Read each question carefully. Circle your answer.

1. Bile is stored in the:
   a. cystic duct.
   b. duodenum.
   c. gallbladder.
   d. common bile duct.

2. A patient is diagnosed with gallstones in the bile ducts. The nurse knows to review the results of blood work for a:
   a. serum ammonia concentration of 90 mg/dL.
   b. serum albumin concentration of 4.0 g/dL.
   c. serum bilirubin level greater than 1.0 mg/dL.
   d. serum globulin concentration of 2.0 g/dL.

3. The major stimulus for increased bicarbonate secretion from the pancreas is:
   a. amylase.
   b. lipase.
   c. secretin.
   d. trypsin.

4. An action *not* associated with insulin is the:
   a. conversion of glycogen to glucose in the liver.
   b. lowering of blood glucose.
   c. promotion of fat storage.
   d. synthesis of proteins.

5. The nurse knows that a patient with low blood sugar would have a blood glucose level of:
   a. 55 to 75 mg/dL.
   b. 80 to 120 mg/dL.
   c. 130 to 150 mg/dL.
   d. 160 to 180 mg/dL.

6. A patient with calculi in the gallbladder is said to have:
   a. cholecystitis.
   b. cholelithiasis.
   c. choledocholithiasis.
   d. choledochotomy.

7. Statistics show that there is a greater incidence of gallbladder disease for women who are:
   a. multiparous.
   b. obese.
   c. older than 40 years of age.
   d. characterized by all of the above.

8. The obstruction of bile flow due to cholelithiasis can interfere with the absorption of:
   a. vitamin A.
   b. vitamin B_6.
   c. vitamin B_{12}.
   d. vitamin C.

9. Clinical manifestations of obstruction of the common bile duct include all of the following *except*:

   a. amber-colored urine.

   b. clay-colored feces.

   c. pruritus.

   d. jaundice.

10. The diagnostic procedure of choice for cholelithiasis is:

    a. radiography.

    b. oral cholecystography.

    c. cholecystography.

    d. ultrasonography.

11. Pharmacologic therapy is frequently used to dissolve small gallstones. It takes about how many months of medication with UDCA or CDCA for stones to dissolve?

    a. 1 to 2

    b. 3 to 5

    c. 6 to 8

    d. 6 to 12

12. Chronic pancreatitis, commonly described as autodigestion of the pancreas, is often not detected until what percentage of the exocrine and endocrine tissue is destroyed?

    a. 10% to 25%

    b. 30% to 50%

    c. 60% to 75%

    d. 80% to 90%

13. Mild acute pancreatitis is characterized by:

    a. edema and inflammation.

    b. pleural effusion.

    c. sepsis.

    d. disseminated intravascular coagulopathy.

14. A major symptom of pancreatitis that brings the patient to medical care is:

    a. severe abdominal pain.

    b. fever.

    c. jaundice.

    d. mental agitation.

15. The nurse should assess for an important early indicator of acute pancreatitis, which is an increased:

    a. serum calcium level.

    b. serum lipase level.

    c. white cell count.

    d. urine amylase level.

16. Nursing measures for pain relief for acute pancreatitis include:

    a. encouraging bed rest to decrease the metabolic rate.

    b. teaching the patient about the correlation between alcohol intake and pain.

    c. withholding oral feedings to limit the release of secretin.

    d. all of the above.

17. The analgesic of choice for severe pancreatic pain is:

    a. codeine.

    b. Demerol.

    c. Percodan.

    d. morphine.

18. The risk for pancreatic cancer is directly proportional to:

    a. age.

    b. dietary intake of fat.

    c. cigarette smoking.

    d. presence of diabetes mellitus.

19. With pancreatic carcinoma, insulin deficiency is suspected when the patient evidences:

    a. an abnormal glucose tolerance.

    b. glucosuria.

    c. hyperglycemia.

    d. all of the above.

20. Clinical manifestations associated with a tumor of the head of the pancreas include:
    a. clay-colored stools.
    b. dark urine.
    c. jaundice.
    d. all of the above

21. A nurse should monitor blood glucose levels for a patient who is diagnosed as having hyperinsulinism. A value inadequate to sustain normal brain function is:
    a. 30 mg/dL.
    b. 50 mg/dL..
    c. 70 mg/dL.
    d. 90 mg/dL.

22. Zollinger-Ellison tumors are associated with hypersecretion of:
    a. aldosterone.
    b. gastric acid.
    c. insulin.
    d. vasopressin.

SHORT ANSWER

Read each statement carefully. Write your response in the space provided.

1. The capacity of the gallbladder for bile storage is _____ mL.

2. The endocrine secretions of the pancreas are _____, _____, and _____.

3. Digestive enzymes are secreted by the pancreas; _____ aids in the digestion of carbohydrates, _____ aids protein digestion, and _____ aids the digestion of fats.

4. The primary cause of acute cholecystitis is _____.

5. The severity of pancreatitis and associated mortality is directly related to the presence of six or more clinical signs such as: _____, _____, _____, _____, _____, and _____.

II. CRITICAL THINKING QUESTIONS AND EXERCISES

Clinical Situations

Read the following case studies. Circle the correct answer or fill in the blank space.

CASE STUDY: Cholecystectomy

Brenda, a 33-year-old obese mother of four, is diagnosed as having acute gallbladder inflammation. She is 5 feet 4 inches tall and weighs 190 lb. The physician decides to delay surgical intervention until Brenda's acute symptoms subside.

1. Brenda's initial course of treatment would probably consist of:
    a. analgesics and antibiotics.
    b. intravenous fluids.
    c. nasogastric suctioning.
    d. all of the above.

2. After her acute attack, Brenda was limited to low-fat liquids. As foods are added to her diet, she needs to know that she should avoid:
    a. cooked fruits.
    b. eggs and cheese.
    c. lean meats.
    d. rice and tapioca.

3. Brenda is being medicated with chenodeoxycholic acid. The nurse needs to tell Brenda that the drug may not be effective if it is taken in conjunction with:

   a. dietary cholesterol.

   b. estrogens.

   c. oral contraceptives.

   d. any of the above.

Because Brenda's symptoms continue to recur, she is scheduled for gallbladder surgery.

1. Brenda has signed a consent form for removal of her gallbladder and ligation of the cystic duct and artery. She is scheduled to undergo a:

   a. cholecystectomy.

   b. cholecystostomy.

   c. choledochostomy.

   d. choledocholithotomy.

2. Postoperative nursing observation includes assessing for:

   a. indicators of infection.

   b. leakage of bile into the peritoneal cavity.

   c. obstruction of bile drainage.

   d. all of the above.

3. Brenda needs to know that fat restriction is usually lifted after the biliary ducts dilate to accommodate bile once held by the gallbladder. This takes about:

   a. 1 week.

   b. 2 to 3 weeks.

   c. 4 to 6 weeks.

   d. 2 months.

CASE STUDY: Chronic Pancreatitis

Carl, a 56-year-old traveling salesman, has recently been diagnosed with chronic pancreatitis.

1. The nurse knows that the major cause of chronic pancreatitis is _long-Term Alcohol Consumption_

2. Describe the pathophysiologic sequence of the inflammatory process: _The inflammatory process causes the replacement of cells by fibrous tissues. This results in mechanical obstruction of the pancreatic and common bile ducts and the duodenum_

3. Dysfunction of the pancreatic islet cells leads to a diagnosis of _diabetes mellitus_.

4. A recommended surgical procedure that allows drainage of pancreatic secretions into the jejunum is _pancreaticojejunostomy_.

5. Long-term management requires two dietary modifications: _Avoidance of Alcohol_ and _avoidance of foods found to cause abd. pain and discomfort_

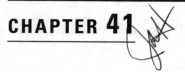
Assessment and Management of Patients With Diabetes Mellitus

I. Interpretation, Completion, and Comparison

MULTIPLE CHOICE

Read each question carefully. Circle your answer.

1. Glucose intolerance increases with age. The incidence in those older than 65 years is:
   a. 20%.
   b. 40%.
   c. 50%.
   d. 80%.

2. The ethnic group with the *lowest* incidence of diabetes mellitus in the United States is the:
   a. African Americans.
   b. Caucasians.
   c. Hispanics.
   d. Native Americans.

3. As a cause of death by disease in the United States, diabetes mellitus ranks:
   a. first.
   b. second.
   c. third.
   d. fourth.

4. A patient is diagnosed with type 1 diabetes. The nurse knows that all of the following are probable clinical characteristics *except:*
   a. ketosis-prone.
   b. little endogenous insulin.
   c. obesity at diagnosis.
   d. younger than 30 years of age.

5. A patient who is diagnosed with type 1 diabetes mellitus would be expected to:
   a. be restricted to an American Diabetic Association diet.
   b. have no damage to the islet cells of the pancreas.
   c. need exogenous insulin.
   d. need to receive daily doses of a hypoglycemic agent.

6. Possible risk factors associated with type 1 diabetes mellitus include:
   a. an autoimmune susceptibility to diabetogenic viruses.
   b. environmental factors.
   c. the presence of human leukocyte antigen (HLA).
   d. all of the above.

7. Clinical manifestations associated with a diagnosis of type 1 diabetes mellitus include all of the following *except:*
   a. hypoglycemia.
   b. hyponatremia.
   c. ketonuria.
   d. polyphagia.

8. The nurse is asked to assess a patient for glucosuria. The nurse would secure a specimen of:
   a. blood.
   b. sputum.
   c. stool.
   d. urine.

9. Knowing that gluconeogenesis helps to maintain blood levels, a nurse should:
   a. document weight changes because of fatty acid mobilization.
   b. evaluate the patient's sensitivity to low room temperatures because of decreased adipose tissue insulation.
   c. protect the patient from sources of infection because of decreased cellular protein deposits.
   d. do all of the above.

10. A nurse is assigned to care for a patient who is suspected of having type 2 diabetes mellitus. Clinical manifestations for which the nurse should assess include:
    a. blurred or deteriorating vision.
    b. fatigue and muscle cramping.
    c. wounds that heal slowly or respond poorly to treatment.
    d. all of the above.

11. There seems to be a strong positive correlation between type 2 diabetes mellitus and:
    a. hypotension.
    b. kidney dysfunction.
    c. obesity.
    d. sex.

12. The lowest fasting plasma glucose level suggestive of a diagnosis of diabetes is:
    a. 90 mg/dL.
    b. 115 mg/dL.
    c. 126 mg/dL.
    d. 180 mg/dL.

13. The most sensitive test for diabetes mellitus is the:
    a. fasting plasma glucose.
    b. two-hour post load glucose.
    c. intravenous glucose.
    d. urine glucose.

14. A female diabetic who weighs 130 lb has an ideal body weight of 116 lb. For weight reduction, her daily caloric intake should be approximately:
    a. 1000 cal.
    b. 1200 cal.
    c. 1500 cal.
    d. 1800 cal.

15. The nurse should encourage exercise in the management of diabetes, because it:
    a. decreases total triglyceride levels.
    b. improves insulin utilization.
    c. lowers blood glucose.
    d. accomplishes all of the above.

16. Self-monitoring of blood glucose is recommended for patients with:
    a. abnormal renal glucose thresholds.
    b. hypoglycemia without warning symptoms.
    c. unstable diabetes.
    d. all of the above conditions.

17. An example of a commonly administered intermediate-acting insulin is:
    a. NPH.
    b. Iletin II.
    c. Humalog.
    d. Humulin U.

18. The nurse knows that an intermediate-acting insulin should reach its "peak" in:
    a. 1 to 2 hours.
    b. 3 to 4 hours.
    c. 4 to 12 hours.
    d. 16 to 20 hours.

19. Insulin pumps in use today:
    a. can deliver a premeal dose (bolus) of insulin before each meal.
    b. deliver a continuous basal rate of insulin at 0.5 to 2.0 units/hour.
    c. prevent unexpected savings in blood glucose measurements.
    d. are capable of doing all of the above.

20. A probable candidate for diabetic management with oral antidiabetic agents is the patient who is:
    a. non–insulin dependent.
    b. stable and not prone to ketosis.
    c. unable to be managed by diet alone.
    d. characterized by all of the above.

21. An example of a first-generation sulfonylurea used in type 2 diabetes is:
    a. Dia-Beta.
    b. Glyset.
    c. Starlix.
    d. Tolinase.

22. The nurse should expect that insulin therapy will be temporarily substituted for oral antidiabetic therapy if the diabetic:
    a. develops an infection with fever.
    b. suffers trauma.
    c. undergoes major surgery.
    d. develops any of the above conditions.

23. The tissue area that provides the fastest absorption rate for regular insulin is believed to be the:
    a. abdominal area.
    b. anterior thigh.
    c. deltoid area.
    d. gluteal site.

24. Rotation sites for insulin injection should be separated from one another by 2.5 cm (1 inch) and should be used only once every:
    a. third day.
    b. week.
    c. 2 to 3 weeks.
    d. 2 to 4 weeks.

25. Hypoglycemia, an abnormally low blood glucose concentration, occurs with a glucose level that is:
    a. lower than 50 to 60 mg/dL.
    b. between 60 and 80 mg/dL.
    c. between 75 and 90 mg/dL.
    d. 95 mg/dL.

26. A clinical feature that distinguishes a hypoglycemic reaction from a ketoacidosis reaction is:
    a. blurred vision.
    b. diaphoresis.
    c. nausea.
    d. weakness.

27. The nurse knows that treatment modalities for diabetic ketoacidosis should focus on management of:
    a. acidosis.
    b. dehydration.
    c. hyperglycemia
    d. all of the above.

28. The major electrolyte of concern in the treatment of diabetic ketoacidosis is:
    a. calcium.
    b. magnesium.
    c. potassium.
    d. sodium.

29. Mortality rates for patients with diabetes are positively correlated with atherosclerotic complications, especially in the coronary arteries, which account for about what percentage of all deaths in these patients?
    a. 10%
    b. 30%
    c. 40%
    d. 60%

30. Macrovascular disease has a direct link with:
    a. hypertension.
    b. increased triglyceride levels.
    c. obesity.
    d. all of the above.

31. Clinical nursing assessment for a patient with microangiopathy who has manifested impaired peripheral arterial circulation includes all of the following *except*:
    a. integumentary inspection for the presence of brown spots on the lower extremities.
    b. observation for paleness of the lower extremities.
    c. observation for blanching of the feet after the legs are elevated for 60 seconds.
    d. palpation for increased pulse volume in the arteries of the lower extremities.

32. With nonproliferative (background) retinopathy, examination of the retina may reveal:
    a. leakage of fluid or serum (exudates).
    b. microaneurysms.
    c. focal capillary single closure.
    d. all of the above pathologic changes.

33. A diagnostic manifestation of proliferative retinopathy is:
    a. decreased capillary permeability.
    b. microaneurysm formation.
    c. neovascularization into the vitreous humor.
    d. the leakage of capillary wall fragments into surrounding areas.

34. A nurse caring for a diabetic with a diagnosis of nephropathy would expect the urinalysis report to indicate the presence of:
    a. albumin.
    b. bacteria.
    c. red blood cells.
    d. white blood cells.

35. With peripheral neuropathy, a diabetic has limited sensitivity to:
    a. heat.
    b. pain.
    c. pressure.
    d. all of the above.

36. Nursing care for a diabetic with peripheral neuropathy includes:
    a. assessing pain patterns to rule out peripheral vascular insufficiency.
    b. inspecting the feet for breaks in skin integrity.
    c. palpating the lower extremities for temperature variations.
    d. all of the above.

37. During surgery, glucose levels will rise, because there is an increased secretion of:
    a. cortisol.
    b. epinephrine.
    c. glucagon.
    d. all of the above.

38. The nurse expects that a type 1 diabetic may receive what percentage of his or her usual morning dose of insulin preoperatively?
    a. 10% to 20%
    b. 25% to 40%
    c. 50% to 60%
    d. 85% to 90%

MATCHING

Match the physiologic change in column II with its associated term listed in column I.

Column I

1. __C__ Gluconeogenesis
2. __A__ Glucosuria
3. __B__ Glycogenolysis
4. __E__ Nephropathy
5. __D__ Retinopathy

Column II

a. Filtered glucose that the kidney cannot absorb spills over into urine
b. Glycogen breaks down in the liver through the action of glucagon
c. New glucose is produced from amino acids
d. Microvascular changes develop in the eyes
e. Small vessel disease affects the kidneys

SHORT ANSWER

Read each statement carefully. Write your response in the space provided.

1. In the United States, diabetes mellitus is the leading cause of three pathologic conditions: __nontraumatic Amputation__, __blindness among working age adults__, and __end-stage renal disease__.

2. The renal threshold for glucose is __180 - 200 mg/dl__.

3. Gestational diabetes occurs in __14__ % of pregnant women.

4. The main goal of diabetes treatment is to: __normalize insulin activity and blood glucose levels__

5. List the five major components of management for diabetes.
   __nutrition management, exercise, monitoring, pharmacologic therapy, and education__

6. A person is overweight when the body mass index (BMI) is __25 - 29__; obesity is diagnosed with a BMI of __> 30__.

7. The current recommended distribution of calories for a diabetic meal plan is __50-60__% carbohydrates, __20-30__% fat, and __10-20__% protein.

8. The recommended amount of daily fiber intake is __25-30__ grams.

9. Two examples of rapid-acting insulin are __Humolog__ and __Novolog__.

10. The most common risk of insulin pump therapy is _Ketoacidosis_ .

11. The sulfonylureas act by _directly stimulating the_ _pancreas to secrete insulin_ .

12. List the four main areas for insulin injection.
Abdomen, leg/thigh, back of arm, lower back/hips

13. List three major acute complications of diabetes.
hypoglycemia, DKA, HHNS

14. Clinical manifestations characteristic of hyperglycemic, hyperosmolar, nonketotic syndrome would include _HTN_ , _profound dehydration_ , _tachycardia_ , and _Altered Neurologic Status_ .

15. Identify five possible collaborative problems that a nurse should be aware of for a patient newly diagnosed with diabetes mellitus.
hypokalemia, hyperglycemia, fluid overload, cerebral edema, ketoacidosis, hypoglycemia

16. The leading cause of blindness in the United States among those between the ages of 40 and 75 years of age is _diabetic Retinopathy_ .

II. Critical Thinking Questions and Exercises

DISCUSSION AND ANALYSIS

Discuss the following topics with your classmates.

1. Discuss the eight risk factors associated with diabetes mellitus and the nurse's role in health education.
2. Explain how insulin regulation is altered in the diabetic state.
3. Describe the pathophysiologic difference between type 1 and type 2 diabetes.
4. Explain the primary cause of gestational diabetes mellitus.
5. Explain the term *glycemic index*.
6. Describe the major complications of insulin therapy.
7. Distinguish between the *dawn phenomenon* and the *Somogyi effect*.

EXAMINING ASSOCIATIONS

For each of the clinical characteristics listed, choose the associated classification of diabetes mellitus. Enter "1" for type 1 diabetes mellitus or "2" for type 2 diabetes mellitus.

1. __2__ Etiology includes obesity
2. __2__ Ketosis is rare
3. __1__ Patient usually thin at diagnosis
4. __1__ Patient needs insulin to preserve life
5. __1__ Patient often has islet cell antibodies
6. __2__ Patient has no islet cell antibodies
7. __1__ Onset can occur at any age
8. __2__ Usually is diagnosed after age 30 years
9. __2__ Hyperosmolar nonketotic syndrome is a complication
10. __1__ There is little or no endogenous insulin

IDENTIFYING PATTERNS

In diagram format, illustrate the pathophysiologic sequence of changes that occurs with type 1 diabetes, from "decreased insulin production by beta cells" to "ketoacidosis." Any outline format is acceptable as long as a cause-and-effect sequence can be seen.

APPLYING CONCEPTS

Examine the accompanying figure and answer the following questions.

Neuropathic ulcers occur on pressure points in areas with diminished sensation in diabetic polyneuropathy. Because pain is absent, the ulcer may go unnoticed.

1. Explain how each of the following diabetic complications leads to the formation of neuropathic ulcers and foot infections.

    a. Sensory neuropathy causes: _loss of sensation to pain + pressure_

    b. Autonomic neuropathy causes: _increase in skin dryness + formation of skin fissure_

    c. Motor neuropathy causes: _muscular Atrophy_

2. Appropriate foot care could prevent up to __50__ % of lower extremity amputations as a result of foot infections and complications.

3. Explain how peripheral vascular disease affects the progression of a foot infection and ulcer formation:

prevents nutrients from getting to local wound.

4. Explain how hyperglycemia affects the spread of a foot infection: _impairs_
the ability of specialized leukocytes to destroy bacteria

5. The three events that typically occur in sequence and lead to the development of a diabetic foot ulcer are _soft tissue damage_, _formation of fissure_, and _formation of callus_.

6. List five daily activities related to foot care that a nurse should instruct a diabetic to complete.

Bathe, dry, + lubricate feet, inspect both feet, report redness,
swelling or drainage, wear well-fitting, closed toe shoes

7. Foot infections and ulcers may progress to the point that amputation is necessary, because:

PVD may prevent oxygen, nutrients and antibiotics from reaching the
injured tissue

CLINICAL SITUATIONS

Read the following case studies. Circle the correct answer.

CASE STUDY: Type 1 Diabetes

Albert, a 35-year-old insulin-dependent diabetic, is admitted to the hospital with a diagnosis of pneumonia. He has been febrile since admission. His daily insulin requirement is 24 units of NPH.

1. Every morning Albert is given NPH insulin at 7:30 AM. Meals are served at 8:30 AM, 12:30 PM, and 6:30 PM. The nurse expects that the NPH insulin will reach its maximum effect (peak) between the hours of:
   a. 11:30 AM and 1:30 PM.
   b. 11:30 AM and 7:30 PM.
   c. 3:30 PM and 9:30 PM.
   d. 5:30 PM and 11:30 PM.

2. A bedtime snack is provided for Albert. This is based on the knowledge that intermediate-acting insulins are effective for an approximate duration of:
   a. 6 to 8 hours.
   b. 10 to 14 hours.
   c. 16 to 20 hours.
   d. 24 to 28 hours.

3. Albert refuses his bedtime snack. This should alert the nurse to assess for:
   a. an elevated serum bicarbonate and a decreased blood pH.
   b. signs of hypoglycemia earlier than expected.
   c. symptoms of hyperglycemia during the peak time of NPH insulin.
   d. sugar in the urine.

CASE STUDY: Hypoglycemia

Betty, an 18-year-old type 1 diabetic, is unconscious when admitted to the hospital. Her daily dose of insulin has been 32 units of NPH each morning.

1. Based on knowledge of hypoglycemia, the nurse would expect that Betty's serum glucose level on admission is approximately:

   a. 50 mg/dL.

   b. 70 mg/dL.

   c. 90 mg/dL.

   d. 110 mg/dL.

2. Betty is given 1 mg of glucagon hydrochloride, subcutaneously, in the emergency department. Knowledge about the action of this drug alerts the nurse to observe for latent symptoms associated with:

   a. glucosuria.

   b. hyperglycemia.

   c. ketoacidosis.

   d. rebound hypoglycemia.

3. After Betty is medically stabilized, she is admitted to the clinical area for observation and health teaching. The nurse should make sure that Betty is aware of warning symptoms associated with hypoglycemia, such as:

   a. emotional changes.

   b. slurred speech and double vision.

   c. staggering gait and incoordination.

   d. all of the above.

4. Betty should also be taught that hypoglycemia may be prevented by:

   a. eating regularly scheduled meals.

   b. eating snacks to cover the peak time of insulin.

   c. increasing food intake when engaging in increased levels of physical exercise.

   d. doing all of the above.

CASE STUDY: Diabetic Ketoacidosis

Christine, a 64-year-old woman, is admitted to the clinical area with a diagnosis of diabetic ketoacidosis. On admission, she is drowsy yet responsive.

1. Nursing actions for a diagnosis of ketoacidosis include:

   a. monitoring urinary output by means of an indwelling catheter.

   b. evaluating serum electrolytes.

   c. testing for glucosuria and acetonuria.

   d. all of the above.

2. The nurse should expect that the rehydrating intravenous solution used will be:

   a. 0.9% saline solution.

   b. 5% dextrose in water.

   c. 10% dextrose in water.

   d. sterile water.

3. In evaluating the laboratory results, the nurse expects all of the following to indicate ketoacidosis *except*:

   a. a decreased serum bicarbonate level.

   b. an elevated blood glucose.

   c. an increased blood urea.

   d. an increased blood pH.

4. The physician notes a change in Christine's respirations. Her breathing is described as Kussmaul respirations. The nurse knows that these respirations are:

   a. deep.

   b. labored.

   c. rapid.

   d. shallow.

5. Christine is started on low-dose intravenous insulin therapy. Nursing assessment includes all of the following *except* frequent:

   a. blood pressure measurements to monitor the degree of hypotension.

   b. estimates of serum potassium, because increased blood glucose levels are correlated with elevated potassium levels.

   c. evaluation of blood glucose levels, because glucose levels should decline as insulin levels increase.

   d. elevation of serum ketones to monitor the course of ketosis.

6. As blood glucose levels approach normal, the nurse should assess for signs of electrolyte imbalance associated with:

   a. hypernatremia.

   b. hypercapnia.

   c. hypocalcemia.

   d. hypokalemia.

CHAPTER 42

Assessment and Management of Patients With Endocrine Disorders

I. Interpretation, Completion, and Comparison

MULTIPLE CHOICE

Read each question carefully. Circle your answer.

1. An example of exocrine glands are the:
   a. adrenals.
   b. ovaries.
   c. parathyroids.
   d. sweat glands.

2. The nurse knows that the anterior pituitary gland is responsible for secreting all of the following *except*:
   a. adrenocorticotropic hormone (ACTH).
   b. antidiuretic hormone (ADH).
   c. follicle-stimulating hormone (FSH).
   d. thyroid-stimulating hormone (TSH).

3. The major structure balancing the rapid action of the nervous system with slower hormonal action is the:
   a. hypothalamus.
   b. pineal gland.
   c. hypophysis.
   d. thyroid gland.

4. Diabetes insipidus is a disorder related to a deficiency of:
   a. growth hormone.
   b. prolactin.
   c. oxytocin.
   d. vasopressin.

5. When thyroid hormone is administered for prolonged hypothyroidism, the nurse knows to monitor the patient for:
   a. angina.
   b. depression.
   c. mental confusion.
   d. hypoglycemia.

6. The preferred medication for treating hypothyroidism is:
   a. lithium.
   b. proprandol.
   c. propylthiouracil.
   d. Synthroid.

7. A clinical manifestation *not* usually associated with hyperthyroidism is:
   a. a pulse rate slower than 90 bpm.
   b. an elevated systolic blood pressure.
   c. muscular fatigability.
   d. weight loss.

8. Patients with hyperthyroidism are characteristically:
   a. apathetic and anorexic.
   b. calm.
   c. emotionally stable.
   d. insensitive to heat.

9. Iodine or iodide compounds are used for hyperthyroidism because they do all of the following *except:*
   a. decrease the basal metabolic rate.
   b. increase the vascularity of the gland.
   c. lessen the release of thyroid hormones.
   d. reduce the size of the gland.

10. The objectives of pharmacotherapy for hyperthyroidism include:
    a. destroying overreactive thyroid cells.
    b. preventing thyroid hormonal synthesis.
    c. increasing the amount of thyroid tissue.
    d. all of the above.

11. Signs of thyroid storm include all of the following *except:*
    a. bradycardia.
    b. delirium or somnolence.
    c. dyspnea and chest pain.
    d. hyperpyrexia.

12. Medical management for thyroid crisis includes:
    a. intravenous dextrose fluids.
    b. hypothermia measures.
    c. oxygen therapy.
    d. all of the above.

13. Pharmacotherapy for thyroid storm would *not* include the administration of:
    a. acetaminophen.
    b. iodine.
    c. propylthiouracil.
    d. synthetic levothyroxine.

14. The most common type of goiter is etiologically related to a deficiency of:
    a. thyrotropin.
    b. iodine.
    c. thyroxine.
    d. calcitonin.

15. The nurse knows that the most common and least aggressive type of cancer is:
    a. anaplastic.
    b. follicular adenocarcinoma.
    c. medullary.
    d. papillary adenocarcinoma.

16. A diagnosis of hyperparathyroidism can be established by all of the following signs *except:*
    a. a negative reading on a Sulkowitch test.
    b. a serum calcium level of 12 mg/dL.
    c. an elevated level of parathyroid hormone.
    d. bone demineralization seen on radiographic film.

17. A recommended breakfast for a hyperparathyroid patient would be:
    a. cereal with milk and bananas.
    b. fried eggs and bacon.
    c. orange juice and toast.
    d. pork sausage and cranberry juice.

18. One of the most important and frequently occurring complications of hyperparathyroidism is:
    a. kidney stones.
    b. pancreatitis.
    c. pathologic fractures.
    d. peptic ulcer.

19. The pathophysiology of hypoparathyroidism is associated with all of the following *except:*
    a. a decrease in serum calcium.
    b. an elevation of blood phosphate.
    c. an increase in the renal excretion of phosphate.
    d. a lowered renal excretion of calcium.

20. The goal of medical management for hypoparathyroidism is to:
    a. achieve a serum calcium level of 9 to 10 mg/dL.
    b. eliminate clinical symptoms.
    c. reverse the symptoms of hypocalcemia.
    d. accomplish all of the above.

21. Nursing management for a hypoparathyroid patient would *not* include:
    a. maintaining a quiet, subdued environment.
    b. making certain that calcium gluconate is kept at the bedside.
    c. observing the patient for signs of tetany.
    d. supplementing the diet with milk and milk products.

22. A pheochromocytoma is an adrenal medulla tumor that causes arterial hypertension by increasing the level of circulating:
    a. catecholamines.
    b. enzymes.
    c. hormones.
    d. glucocorticoids.

23. A positive test for overactivity of the adrenal medulla is an epinephrine value of:
    a. 50 pg/mL.
    b. 100 pg/mL.
    c. 100 to 300 pg/mL.
    d. 450 pg/mL.

24. Laboratory findings suggestive of Addison's disease include all of the following *except*:
    a. a relative lymphocytosis.
    b. hyperkalemia and hyponatremia.
    c. hypertension.
    d. hypoglycemia.

25. A positive diagnosis of Cushing's syndrome is associated with:
    a. the disappearance of lymphoid tissue.
    b. a reduction in circulating eosinophils.
    c. an elevated cortisol level.
    d. all of the above.

26. Clinical manifestations of Cushing's syndrome may be modified with a diet that is:
    a. high in protein.
    b. low in carbohydrates.
    c. low in sodium.
    d. all of the above.

27. A patient with aldosteronism would be expected to exhibit all of the following symptoms *except*:
    a. alkalosis.
    b. hypokalemia.
    c. hyponatremia.
    d. an increased pH.

28. The nurse needs to be aware that large-dose corticosteroid therapy is most effective when administered:
    a. at 8:00 AM.
    b. at 8:00 PM.
    c. between 4:00 AM and 5:00 AM.
    d. between 4:00 PM and 6:00 PM.

29. Nursing assessment for a patient who is receiving corticosteroid therapy includes observation for the unacceptable side effect of:
    a. glaucoma.
    b. facial mooning.
    c. potassium loss.
    d. weight gain.

MATCHING

Match the hormonal function column II with its corresponding hormone listed in column I.

Column I

1. _____ Glucagon
2. _____ Aldosterone
3. _____ Oxytocin
4. _____ Somatotropin

5. _____ Vasopressin

6. _____ Calcitonin

7. _____ Prolactin

8. _____ Melatonin

9. _____ Parathormone

10. _____ Insulin

Column II

a. Controls excretion of water by the kidneys

b. Lowers blood sugar

c. Inhibits bone resorption

d. Influences metabolism that is essential for normal growth

e. Supports sexual maturation

f. Promotes the secretion of milk

g. Stimulates the reabsorption of sodium and the elimination of potassium

h. Promotes glycogenolysis

i. Increases the force of uterine contractions during parturition

SHORT ANSWER

Read each statement carefully. Write your response in the space provided.

1. The term used to describe the regulation of hormone concentration in the bloodstream is

_____.

2. Hormones are classified four ways: _____, _____,

_____, and _____.

3. The two major hormones secreted by the posterior lobe of the pituitary gland are

_____, which controls _____, and

_____, which facilitates _____.

4. Oversecretion of adrenocorticotropic hormone (ACTH) or the growth hormone results in

_____ disease.

5. A deficiency of antidiuretic hormone (ADH) or vasopressin can result in the disorder known as

_____, which is characterized by _____ and

_____.

6. The thyroid gland produces three hormones: _____, _____,

and _____.

7. The most common cause of hypothyroidism is _____.

8. Hyperthyroidism is second only to _____ as a common endocrine disorder.

9. The most common type of hyperthyroidism is _____.

10. The two most common medications used to treat hyperthyroidism are _____ and

_____.

11. Name two postoperative conditions that occur when the parathyroid gland is damaged.

_____

_____

12. Tetany is suspected when either of these signs is positive: _____ or

_____.

13. Name the three types of steroid hormones produced by the adrenal cortex:

_____, _____, and _____.

SCRAMBLEGRAM

Unscramble the letters to answer each statement.

1. The master gland of the endocrine system is the _____.

I U I Y T P R T A

2. The pituitary gland is controlled by the _____.

O A T M P U A S H H L Y

3. Another name for the growth hormone is _____.

P O T T I A S N R O O M

4. Excessive secretion of antidiuretic hormone (ADH) results in a syndrome that causes fluid retention, which
is identified by the five letters: _____.

H D A I S

5. The thyroid gland depends on the uptake of _____ to synthesize its hormones.

E O N I D I

6. The term used to describe "bulging eyes" found in patients with hyperthyroidism is

_____.

H M P L O S E A X O H T

7. The term used to describe hyperirritability of the nerves and excessive muscular twitching secondary to
hypocalcemia is _____.

Y T N A E T

II. Critical Thinking Questions and Exercises

DISCUSSION AND ANALYSIS

Discuss the following topics with your classmates.

1. Describe the clinical manifestations, nursing interventions and medical management for diabetes insipidus.
2. Distinguish between four diagnostic thyroid tests: serum thyroid-stimulating hormone, serum free T4, serum T3 and T4, and the T3 resin uptake test.
3. Draft six nursing diagnoses and related goals for a patient with hypothyroidism.
4. Explain how radiation can induce thyroid cancer.
5. Compare and contrast the etiology and clinical manifestations of Addison's disease and Cushing's syndrome.

CLINICAL SITUATIONS

Read the following case studies. Circle the correct answer.

CASE STUDY: Primary Hypothyroidism

Connie has been hospitalized for 1 week for studies to confirm a diagnosis of primary hypothyroidism.

1. Several tests were used in Connie's assessment. All of the following results are consistent with her diagnosis of hypothyroidism *except*:
   a. an increased level of thyrotropin (TSH).
   b. a low uptake of radioactive iodine (^{131}I).
   c. a protein-bound iodine reading of 3 mg/dL.
   d. a T3 uptake value of 45%.

2. Nursing care for Connie includes assessing for clinical manifestations associated with hypothyroidism. A manifestation *not* consistent with her diagnosis is:
   a. a change in her menstrual pattern.
   b. pulse rate of 58 bpm.
   c. temperature of 95.8°F.
   d. weight loss of 10 lb over a 2-week period.

3. The principal objective of medical management is to:
   a. irradiate the gland in an attempt to stimulate hormonal secretion.
   b. replace the missing hormone.
   c. remove the diseased gland.
   d. withhold exogenous iodine to create a negative feedback response, which will force the gland to secrete hormones.

4. Nursing comfort measures for Connie should include:
   a. encouraging frequent periods of rest throughout the day.
   b. offering her additional blankets to help prevent chilling.
   c. using a cleansing lotion instead of soap for her skin.
   d. all of the above.

5. Health teaching for Connie includes making sure that she knows that iodine-based chemotherapy is:
   a. administered intravenously for 1 week so that her symptoms may be rapidly put into remission.
   b. needed for life.
   c. recommended for 1 to 3 months.
   d. used until her symptoms disappear.

CASE STUDY: Hyperparathyroidism

Emily is 65 years old and has been complaining of continued emotional irritability. Her family described her as always being "on edge" and neurotic. After several months of exacerbated symptoms, Emily underwent a complete physical examination and was diagnosed with hyperparathyroidism.

1. Emily's clinical symptoms are all related to an increase in serum:
   a. calcium.
   b. magnesium.
   c. potassium.
   d. sodium.

2. As a nurse, you know that the normal level of the mineral identified in the previous question is:
   a. 8.8 to 10 mg/dL.
   b. 1.3 to 2.1 mEq/L.
   c. 3.5 to 5.0 mEq/L.
   d. 135 to 148 mmol/L.

3. Describe eight symptoms usually seen when hyperparathyroidism involves several body systems.

   _____

   _____

   _____

   _____

   _____

   _____

   _____

   _____

4. One of the most important organ complications of hyperparathyroidism is _____.

5. A musculoskeletal symptom found with hyperparathyroidism is:
   a. deformities due to demineralization.
   b. pain on weight bearing.
   c. pathologic fractures due to osteoclast growth.
   d. all of the above.

6. The recommended treatment for primary hyperparathyroidism is:
   a. pharmacotherapy until the elevated serum levels return to normal.
   b. surgical removal of the abnormal parathyroid tissue.
   c. adrenalectomy.
   d. all of the above treatments.

7. Acute hypercalcemic crises can occur in hyperparathyroidism. The treatment would involve immediate:
   a. administration of diuretic agents to promote renal excretion of calcium.
   b. phosphate therapy to correct hypophosphatemia.
   c. rehydration with large volumes of intravenous fluids.
   d. management with all of the above modalities.

CASE STUDY: Subtotal Thyroidectomy

Darrell, a 37-year-old father of two, has just returned to the clinical area from the recovery room. Darrell has had a subtotal thyroidectomy.

1. Postoperatively, Darrell is assisted from the stretcher to the bed. The most comfortable position for him to assume would be:
   a. high Fowler's with his neck supported by a soft collar.
   b. recumbent with his neck hyperextended and supported by a neck pillow.
   c. recumbent with sandbags preventing his neck from rotating.
   d. semi-Fowler's with his head supported by pillows.

2. Postoperative bleeding when the patient is in the dorsal position would probably be evidenced:
   a. anteriorly.
   b. laterally.
   c. posteriorly.
   d. in any of the above areas.

3. Indicators of internal bleeding include:
   a. a sensation of fullness at the incision site.
   b. hypotension.
   c. tachycardia.
   d. all of the above.

4. The nurse should assess for the common manifestation of recurrent laryngeal nerve damage, which is:
   a. any voice change.
   b. the inability to speak.
   c. pain while speaking.
   d. pain while swallowing.

5. The nurse expects Darrell's postoperative diet to be:
   a. clear liquids, such as tea and carbonated beverages.
   b. high in calories.
   c. low in fat and protein.
   d. low in minerals, especially calcium.

6. The nurse should monitor serum calcium levels for hypocalcemia, which will occur with a serum calcium level of:
   a. 5 mg/dL.
   b. 9 mg/dL.
   c. 13 mg/dL.
   d. 17 mg/dL.

CHAPTER 43

Assessment of Renal and Urinary Tract Function

I. Interpretation, Completion, and Comparison

MULTIPLE CHOICE

Read each question carefully. Circle your answer.

1. An abnormal constituent of urine is:
   a. creatinine.
   b. glucose.
   c. potassium.
   d. urea.

2. The normal quantity of water ingested and excreted in the urine is approximately:
   a. 0.5 L/day.
   b. 1.5 L/day.
   c. 2.5 L/day.
   d. 4.0 L/day.

3. The normal amount of sodium ingested and excreted in the urine is approximately:
   a. 2 to 3 g/day.
   b. 4 to 5 g/day.
   c. 6 to 8 g/day.
   d. 9 to 10 g/day.

4. Increased blood osmolality will result in:
   a. antidiuretic hormone (ADH) stimulation.
   b. an increase in urine volume.
   c. diuresis.
   d. less reabsorption of water.

5. A major sensitive indicator of kidney disease is the:
   a. blood urea nitrogen level.
   b. creatinine clearance level.
   c. serum potassium level.
   d. uric acid level.

6. A major manifestation of uremia is:
   a. a decreased serum phosphorus level.
   b. hyperparathyroidism.
   c. hypocalcemia with bone changes.
   d. increased secretion of parathormone.

7. Significant nursing assessment data relevant to renal function should include information about:
   a. any voiding disorders.
   b. the patient's occupation.
   c. the presence of hypertension or diabetes mellitus.
   d. all of the above.

8. Oliguria is said to be present when urinary output is:
   a. less than 30 mL/hour.
   b. about 100 mL/hour.
   c. between 300 and 500 mL/hour.
   d. between 500 and 1000 mL/hour.

9. A 24-hour urine collection is scheduled to begin at 8:00 AM. The nurse should begin the procedure:
   - a. after discarding the 8:00 AM specimen.
   - b. at 8:00 AM, with or without a specimen.
   - c. 6 hours after the urine is discarded.
   - d. with the first specimen voided after 8:00 AM.

10. The nurse should inform a patient that preparation for intravenous urography includes:
   - a. a liquid restriction for 8 to 10 hours before the test.
   - b. liquids before the test.
   - c. enemas until clear.
   - d. remaining NPO from midnight before the test.

11. Nursing responsibilities after renal angiography include:
   - a. assessment of peripheral pulses.
   - b. color and temperature comparisons between the involved and uninvolved extremities.
   - c. examination of the puncture site for swelling and hematoma formation.
   - d. all of the above.

12. A cystoscope allows visualization of:
   - a. the bladder.
   - b. the ureteral orifices.
   - c. the urethra.
   - d. all of the above areas.

13. Nursing management after a renal brush biopsy includes:
   - a. assessing for the clinical manifestations of hemorrhage.
   - b. encouraging a fluid intake of 3 L every 24 hours.
   - c. obtaining a sample of each voided urine to compare it with a prebiopsy specimen.
   - d. all of the above.

SHORT ANSWER

Read each statement carefully. Write your response in the space provided.

1. The functional unit of each kidney is the ___nephron___, which is located in the ___cortex___ of the kidney.

2. Normal adult bladder capacity is ___300-500___ mL of urine.

3. The regulation of the amount of sodium excreted depends on the hormone ___aldosterone___.

4. The normal urine osmolality ranges between ___300___ and ___900___.

5. When a person is dehydrated, the urine osmolality is ___increased___.

6. Water is reabsorbed, rather than excreted, under the control of the ___ADH___.

7. The major waste product of protein metabolism is ___Urea___.

8. The test that most accurately reflects glomerular filtration and renal excretory function is the ___Creatinine clearance___ test.

II. Critical Thinking Questions and Exercises

IDENTIFYING PATTERNS

Fill in the flow chart of pathophysiologic events that are triggered when the blood pressure decreases and the hormone renin is released from the cells in the kidneys.

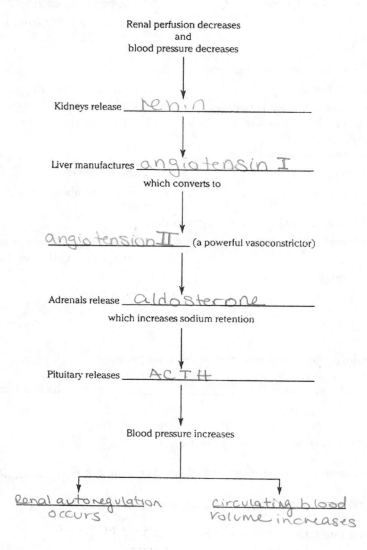

Renal perfusion decreases
and
blood pressure decreases

Kidneys release ___renin___

Liver manufactures ___angiotensin I___
which converts to

___angiotension II___ (a powerful vasoconstrictor)

Adrenals release ___aldosterone___
which increases sodium retention

Pituitary releases ___ACTH___

Blood pressure increases

___Renal autoregulation occurs___   ___Circulating blood volume increases___

CHAPTER 44

Management of Patients With Renal Disorders

I. Interpretation, Completion, and Comparison

MULTIPLE CHOICE

Read each question carefully. Circle your answer.

1. The most accurate indicator of fluid loss or gain in an acutely ill patient is:
   a. blood pressure.
   b. capillary refill.
   c. serum sodium levels.
   d. weight.

2. The nurse notes that a patient who is retaining fluid had a 1-kg weight gain. The nurse knows this is equivalent to about:
   a. 250 mL.
   b. 500 mL.
   c. 750 mL.
   d. 1000 mL.

3. A patient is admitted with electrolyte imbalance. He has carpopedal spasm, electrocardiographic (ECG) changes and a positive Chvostek's sign. The nurse suspects a deficit of:
   a. calcium.
   b. magnesium.
   c. phosphorus.
   d. sodium.

4. Acute glomerulonephritis refers to a group of kidney diseases in which there is:
   a. an inflammatory reaction.
   b. an antigen-antibody reaction to streptococci that results in circulating molecular complexes.
   c. cellular complexes that lodge in the glomeruli and injure the kidney.
   d. a combination of all of the above.

5. In most cases, the major stimulus to acute glomerulonephritis is:
   a. *Escherichia coli.*
   b. group A streptococcal infection of the throat.
   c. *Staphylococcus aureus.*
   d. *Neisseria gonorrhoeae.*

6. Laboratory findings consistent with acute glomerulonephritis include all of the following *except*:
   a. hematuria.
   b. polyuria.
   c. proteinuria.
   d. white cell casts.

7. Chronic glomerulonephritis is manifested by:
   a. anemia secondary to erythropoiesis.
   b. hypercalcemia and decreased serum phosphorus.
   c. hypokalemia and elevated bicarbonate.
   d. metabolic alkalosis.

8. The major manifestation of nephrotic syndrome is:
   a. hematuria.
   b. hyperalbuminemia.
   c. edema.
   d. anemia.

9. A clinical diagnosis of nephrotic syndrome is consistent with an exceedingly high level of:
   a. albumin.
   b. low-density lipoproteins.
   c. protein in the urine.
   d. serum cholesterol.

10. Acute renal failure (ARF) caused by parenchymal damage to the glomeruli or kidney tubules results in all of the following *except:*
    a. decreased glomerular filtration rate (GFR).
    b. an increased urine specific gravity.
    c. an impaired electrolyte balance.
    d. a progressive azotemia.

11. Oliguria is a clinical sign of acute renal failure that refers to a daily urine output of:
    a. 1.5 L.
    b. 1.0 L.
    c. less than 400 mL.
    d. less than 50 mL.

12. A fall in CO_2- combining power and blood pH indicates what state accompanying renal function?
    a. metabolic acidosis
    b. metabolic alkalosis
    c. respiratory acidosis
    d. respiratory alkalosis

13. Hyperkalemia is a serious electrolyte imbalance that occurs in ARF and results from:
    a. protein catabolism.
    b. electrolyte shifts in response to metabolic acidosis.
    c. tissue breakdown.
    d. all of the above.

14. Potassium intake can be restricted by eliminating high-potassium foods such as:
    a. butter.
    b. citrus fruits.
    c. cooked white rice.
    d. salad oils.

15. A patient with ARF and negative nitrogen balance is expected to lose about:
    a. 0.5 kg/day.
    b. 1.0 kg/day.
    c. 1.5 kg/day.
    d. 2.0 kg/day.

16. The leading cause of end-stage renal disease is:
    a. diabetes mellitus.
    b. hypertension.
    c. glomerulonephritis.
    d. toxic agents.

17. A patient with stage 3, chronic renal failure would be expected to have:
    a. a GFR >90 mL/min/1.73 m².
    b. a GFR of 30 to 59 mL/min/1.73 m².
    c. severe decreases in GFR.
    d. kidney failure.

18. In chronic renal failure (end-stage renal disease), decreased glomerular filtration leads to:
    a. increased pH.
    b. decreased creatinine clearance.
    c. increased blood urea nitrogen (BUN).
    d. all of the above.

19. Decreased levels of erythropoietin, a substance normally secreted by the kidneys, leads to what serious complication of chronic renal failure?
    a. anemia
    b. acidosis
    c. hyperkalemia
    d. pericarditis

20. Recent research about the long-term toxicity of aluminum products has led physicians to recommend antacids that lower serum phosphorus, such as:
    a. calcium carbonate.
    b. sodium bicarbonate.
    c. magaldrate.
    d. milk of magnesia.

21. Dietary intervention for renal deterioration includes limiting the intake of:
    a. fluid.
    b. protein.
    c. sodium and potassium.
    d. all of the above.

22. The process that underlies and supports the procedure of hemodialysis is:
    a. diffusion.
    b. osmosis.
    c. ultrafiltration.
    d. all of the above processes.

23. An incomplete protein *not* recommended for the diet of a patient managed by long-term hemodialysis is that found in:
    a. eggs.
    b. fish.
    c. milk.
    d. nuts.

24. With peritoneal dialysis, urea and creatinine pass through the peritoneum by:
    a. active transport.
    b. diffusion and osmosis.
    c. filtration.
    d. ultrafiltration.

25. At the end of five peritoneal exchanges, the patient's fluid loss was 500 mL. This loss is equal to approximately:
    a. 0.5 lb.
    b. 1.0 lb.
    c. 1.5 lb.
    d. 2 lb.

26. The chief danger after renal surgery is:
    a. abdominal distention owing to reflex cessation of intestinal peristalsis.
    b. hypovolemic shock caused by hemorrhage.
    c. paralytic ileus caused by manipulation of the colon during surgery.
    d. pneumonia caused by shallow breathing because of severe incisional pain.

27. Preoperative management for a patient who is to undergo kidney transportation includes:
    a. bringing the metabolic state to as normal a level as possible.
    b. making certain that the patient is free of infection.
    c. suppressing immunologic defense mechanisms.
    d. all of the above.

28. Postoperative management for a recipient of a transplanted kidney includes:
    a. aseptic technique to avoid infection.
    b. hourly urinary output measurements to estimate the degree of kidney function.
    c. protective isolation while immunosuppressive drug therapy is at its maximum dosage.
    d. all of the above.

29. The usual early clinical sign of a renal tumor is:
    a. a palpable mass.
    b. painless hematuria.
    c. localized tenderness.
    d. renal colic.

MATCHING

Match the symptom in column II with its associated fluid or electrolyte imbalance listed in column I.

Column I

1. __A__ Calcium deficit
2. __B__ Calcium excess
3. __C__ Fluid volume deficit
4. __E__ Fluid volume excess
5. __D__ Magnesium deficit
6. __J__ Potassium deficit
7. __H__ Potassium excess
8. __F__ Protein deficit
9. __G__ Sodium deficit
10. __I__ Sodium excess

Column II

a. Carpopedal spasm and tetany
b. Muscle hypotonicity and flank pain
c. Oliguria and weight loss
d. Positive Chvostek's sign
e. Crackles and dyspnea
f. Chronic weight loss and fatigability
g. Fingerprinting on the sternum
h. Irritability and intestinal colic
i. Rough, dry tongue and thirst
j. Soft, flabby muscles and weakness

SHORT ANSWER.

Read each statement carefully. Write your response in the space provided.

1. List the four major clinical manifestations of glomerular injury.

   _____

   _____

   _____

   _____

2. Describe the physical appearance of the urine in the early stage of acute glomerulonephritis:

   _____

   _____

3. Two blood levels that are significantly increased in acute renal failure are _____ and

   _____.

4. Name four physiologic disorders that characterize the nephrotic syndrome.

   _____

   _____

   _____

   _____

5. List three major categories that cause acute renal failure. For each condition, give one to two examples.

    a. _____ Examples: _____

    b. _____ Examples: _____

    c. _____ Examples: _____

6. List at least six clinical manifestations seen in chronic renal failure:

    _____

    _____

7. In ARF, name two clinical signs of hyperkalemia.

    _____

    _____

8. One leading cause of death for patients undergoing chronic hemodialysis is _____.

9. List six potential complications of dialysis treatment.

    _____

    _____

    _____

    _____

    _____

    _____

10. The most common and serious complication of continuous ambulatory peritoneal dialysis (CAPD) is

    _____.

11. Two complications of renal surgery that are believed to be caused by reflex paralysis of intestinal peristalsis and manipulation of the colon or duodenum during surgery are _____ and _____.

II. Critical Thinking Questions and Exercises

DISCUSSION AND ANALYSIS

Discuss the following topics with your classmates.

1. Describe the pathophysiology of acute glomerulonephritis.
2. Explain six measures that a nurse can take to prevent acute renal failure.

3. Describe the signs and symptoms of chronic renal failure, per system (i.e., neurologic, cardiovascular, gastrointestinal, and so on).
4. Compare the indications for acute versus chronic dialysis.
5. Describe the major complications of hemodialysis.
6. Explain the hemodynamics behind and the procedure for peritoneal dialysis.
7. Describe the medical and nursing management for patients who have experienced renal trauma.

APPLYING CONCEPTS

Examine Figure 44-5 in the text and answer the following questions.

1. A needle is inserted into the arterial segment of the fistula to _____.

2. A needle is inserted into the venous segment of the fistula to _____.

3. A new fistula requires _____ weeks to mature. This time is necessary because: _____
   _____

4. Describe the exercise the patient should perform to help increase the vessel size: _____
   _____

5. The most commonly used synthetic graft material is _____. Grafts allow access in as little as _____ days.

CLINICAL SITUATIONS

Read the following case studies. Circle the correct answer.

CASE STUDY: Continuous Ambulatory Peritoneal Dialysis

Edward, a 29-year-old diabetic, chose CAPD as a way of managing his end-stage renal disease.

1. Edward chose CAPD because it helped him:
   a. avoid severe dietary restrictions.
   b. control his blood pressure.
   c. have control over his daily activities.
   d. do all of the above.

2. Using CAPD, Edward needs to dialyze himself:
   a. approximately 4 to 5 times a day with no night changes.
   b. every 3 hours while awake.
   c. every 4 hours around the clock.
   d. once in the morning and once in the evening every day.

3. Edward needs to be aware that toxic wastes are exchanged during the equilibration or dwell time, which usually lasts for:
   a. 10 to 15 minutes.
   b. 30 minutes.
   c. 1 hour.
   d. 2 to 3 hours.

4. Edward needs to be taught how to detect signs of the most serious and most common complication of CAPD, which is:
   a. an abdominal hernia.
   b. anorexia.
   c. edema.
   d. peritonitis.

5. Edward's diet should be modified to be:
   a. high in carbohydrates.
   b. high in fats.
   c. high in protein.
   d. low in bran and fiber.

CASE STUDY: Acute Renal Failure

Fran is hospitalized with a diagnosis of ARF. She had been taking gentamicin sulfate for a pseudomonal infection.

1. The nurse knows that the kidney is susceptible to damage by nephrotoxic antibiotic agents, because it functions as a major excretory pathway and receives what percentage of cardiac output at rest?
   a. 5%
   b. 15%
   c. 25%
   d. 45%

2. The nurse needs to assess for symptoms consistent with pathology secondary to reduced renal blood flow. Symptoms would include:
   a. reduced glomerular filtration.
   b. renal ischemia.
   c. tubular damage.
   d. all of the above.

3. During the oliguric phase of ARF, Fran's protein intake for her 156-lb body weight should be approximately:
   a. 35 g/24 hours.
   b. 70 g/24 hours.
   c. 120 g/24 hours.
   d. 156 g/24 hours.

4. While evaluating laboratory studies, the nurse expects that Fran's oliguric phase will be marked by all of the following *except*:
   a. blood urea nitrogen of 10 mg/dL.
   b. serum creatinine of 0.8 mg/dL.
   c. serum potassium of 6 mEq/L.
   d. urinary volume less than 600 mL/24 hours.

5. After the diuretic phase, the nurse should recommend a:
   a. high-potassium diet.
   b. high-protein diet.
   c. low-carbohydrate diet.
   d. low-fat diet.

6. The nurse expects the period of recovery to follow a period of oliguria and to last approximately:
   a. 2 weeks.
   b. 6 weeks.
   c. 2 months.
   d. 6 to 12 months.

CHAPTER 45

Management of Patients With Urinary Disorders

I. Interpretation, Completion, and Comparison

MULTIPLE CHOICE

Read each question carefully. Circle your answer.

1. An example of an upper urinary tract infection is:
   a. acute pyelonephritis.
   b. cystitis.
   c. prostatitis.
   d. urethritis.

2. A sign of possible urinary tract infection is:
   a. a negative urine culture.
   b. an output of 200 mL to 900 mL with each voiding.
   c. cloudy urine.
   d. urine with a specific gravity of 1.005 to 1.022.

3. The most common site of a lower urinary tract infection (UTI) is the:
   a. bladder.
   b. kidney.
   c. prostate.
   d. urethra.

4. There is an increased risk of UTIs in the presence of:
   a. altered metabolic states.
   b. immunosuppression.
   c. urethral mucosa abrasion.
   d. all of the above.

5. The most common organism responsible for UTIs in women and the elderly is:
   a. *Klebsiella.*
   b. *Escherichia coli.*
   c. *Proteus.*
   d. *Pseudomonas.*

6. A first-line antibacterial agent for UTIs that has been found to be significantly effective is:
   a. Bactrim.
   b. Cipro.
   c. Macrodantin.
   d. Septra.

7. A majority of randomized studies have indicated that daily consumption of what kind of juice decreases the incidence of UTIs?
   a. apple
   b. cranberry
   c. grapefruit
   d. orange

8. Health information for a female patient diagnosed as having cystitis includes all of the following *except:*
   a. cleanse around the perineum and urethral meatus (from front to back) after each bowel movement.
   b. drink liberal amounts of fluid.
   c. shower rather than bathe in a tub.
   d. void no more frequently than every 6 hours to allow urine to dilute the bacteria in the bladder.

9. Complications of chronic pyelonephritis include:
   a. end-stage renal disease.
   b. hypertension.
   c. kidney stone formation.
   d. all of the above.

10. The type of incontinence that results from a sudden increase in intra-abdominal pressure is:
    a. reflex incontinence.
    b. stress incontinence.
    c. overflow incontinence.
    d. urge incontinence.

11. Incontinence or dyssynergia is a voiding dysfunction found in the following neurogenic disorder:
    a. cerebellar ataxia.
    b. diabetes.
    c. multiple sclerosis.
    d. Parkinson's disease.

12. Fluid management as a method of behavioral therapy for incontinence requires a daily liquid intake of:
    a. 0.5 mL.
    b. 1.0 mL.
    c. 1.5 mL.
    d. 2.0 mL.

13. Spastic neurogenic bladder is associated with all of the following *except:*
    a. a loss of conscious sensation and cerebral motor control.
    b. a lower motor neuron lesion.
    c. hypertrophy of the bladder walls.
    d. reduced bladder capacity.

14. The major complication of neurogenic bladder is:
    a. hypertrophy.
    b. infection.
    c. pain.
    d. spasm.

15. The major cause of death for patients with neurologic impairment of the bladder is:
    a. myocardial infection.
    b. pulmonary edema.
    c. septicemia.
    d. renal failure.

16. Nursing measures for the patient with neurogenic bladder include:
    a. encouraging a liberal fluid intake.
    b. keeping the patient as mobile as possible.
    c. offering a diet low in calcium.
    d. all of the above.

17. When managing a closed urinary drainage system, the nurse needs to remember not to:
    a. allow the drainage bag to touch the floor.
    b. disconnect the bag.
    c. raise the drainage bag above the level of the patient's bladder.
    d. do any of the above.

18. A woman is taught to catheterize herself by inserting the catheter into the urethra:
    a. 0.5 to 1 inch.
    b. 2 inches.
    c. 3 inches.
    d. 5 inches.

19. A major clinical manifestation of renal stones is:
    a. dysuria.
    b. hematuria.
    c. infection.
    d. pain.

20. Patients with urolithiasis need to be encouraged to:
    a. increase their fluid intake so that they can excrete 3000 mL to 4000 mL every day, which will help prevent additional stone formation.
    b. participate in strenuous exercises so that the tone of smooth muscle in the urinary tract can be strengthened to help propel calculi.
    c. supplement their diet with calcium needed to replace losses to renal calculi.
    d. limit their voiding to every 6 to 8 hours so that increased volume can increase hydrostatic pressure, which will help push stones along the urinary system.

21. A patient being prescribed a diet moderately reduced in calcium and phosphorus should be taught to avoid:
    a. citrus fruits.
    b. milk.
    c. pasta.
    d. whole grain breads.

22. The most common symptom of cancer of the bladder is:
    a. back pain.
    b. dysuria.
    c. visible, painless hematuria.
    d. infection.

23. The predominant cause of bladder cancer is:
    a. chronic renal failure.
    b. cigarette smoking.
    c. environmental pollution.
    d. metastasis from another primary site.

24. The most effective intravesical agent for recurrent bladder cancer is:
    a. bacille Calmette-Guérin (BCG).
    b. doxorubicin.
    c. etoglucid.
    d. thiotepa.

25. The urinary diversion whereby the patient will void from his rectum for the rest of his life is known as a:
    a. cutaneous ureterostomy.
    b. nephrostomy.
    c. suprapubic cystotomy.
    d. ureterosigmoidostomy.

SHORT ANSWER

Read each statement carefully. Write your response in the space provided.

1. Name common signs and symptoms associated with an uncomplicated lower UTI (cystitis):

    _____

    _____

2. The most common cause of recurrent UTIs in the elderly is _____.

3. Patient's with indwelling catheters are most likely infected by one of the following four organisms:

    _____, _____, _____, and

    _____.

4. List three classifications of medications that cause urinary retention by inhibiting contractility.

_____

_____

_____

5. List four reasons for catheterization.

_____

_____

_____

_____

6. List six pathogens responsible for catheter-associated urinary tract infections.

_____

_____

_____

_____

_____

_____

7. List six signs and/or symptoms associated with catheter-induced urinary tract infections.

_____

_____

_____

_____

_____

_____

8. List three crystalline substances known to form stones in the urinary tract.

_____

_____

_____

II. Critical Thinking Questions and Exercises

RECOGNIZING CONTRADICTIONS

Rewrite each statement correctly. Underline the key concepts.

1. The majority of hospital-acquired urinary tract infections are caused by instrumentation of the urinary tract or catheterization.

_____

2. Urethrovesical reflux refers to the backward flow of urine from the urethra into the bladder.

_____

3. Currently, computerized tomography and ultrasonography are the diagnostic tests of choice.

_____

DISCUSSION AND ANALYSIS

Discuss the following topics with your classmates.

1. Describe six categories of risk factors for UTIs.
2. Discuss the seven factors that contribute to UTIs in the elderly.
3. Compare the clinical symptoms and nursing interventions for acute versus chronic pyelonephritis.
4. Discuss the eight common causes of transient incontinence.
5. Explain general principles/guidelines that a nurse should follow to prevent infections in a catheterized patient.
6. Describe the eight common causes of bladder cancer.

CHAPTER 46

Assessment and Management of Female Physiologic Processes

I. Interpretation, Completion, and Comparison

MULTIPLE CHOICE

Read each question carefully. Circle your answer.

1. The menstrual cycle is dependent on hormone production. The hormone responsible for stimulating progesterone is:

   a. androgens.

   b. estradiol.

   c. the follicle-stimulating hormone.

   d. the luteinizing hormone.

2. A neighbor tells you that she has had vaginal bleeding for the past several days. She is postmenopausal and has not had a menstrual period for the past 4 years. You recommend that she:

   a. see her gynecologist or physician as soon as possible.

   b. mention the bleeding episode to her physician at her next appointment.

   c. disregard this bleeding episode, because it is probably normal.

   d. use a birth control method, because she may be fertile with her next ovulation.

3. An annual pelvic examination should begin at age:

   a. 14 years.

   b. 18 years.

   c. 21 years.

   d. 25 years.

4. During an internal vaginal examination, the nurse practitioner notes a frothy and malodorous discharge. She suspects it is caused by the bacteria:

   a. *Candida.*

   b. *Eschar.*

   c. *Trichomonas.*

   d. *E. coli.*

5. The results of a patient's cytologic test for cancer (Pap test) were interpreted as class II. The nurse explains that a class II finding indicates:

   a. squamous cell abnormalities.

   b. malignancy.

   c. suggestive but not conclusive malignancy.

   d. the absence of atypical or abnormal cells.

6. Newer classifications are being used to describe the findings of the cytologic smear. For example, a high-grade, squamous, intraepithelial lesion corresponds to all of the following *except:*

   a. CIN grade 1.

   b. CIN grade 2.

   c. CIS.

   d. CIN, grade 3.

7. After a cervical cone biopsy, the patient needs to be instructed to:

   a. leave the packing in place for 18 to 24 hours.

   b. report any excessive bleeding.

   c. delay sexual intercourse until healing occurs.

   d. do all of the above.

8. The normal menstrual cycle usually lasts 4 to 5 days with a loss of about how much blood?
   a. 30 mL.
   b. 60 mL.
   c. 90 mL.
   d. 120 mL.

9. To prevent toxic shock syndrome, the nurse advises the 15-year-old girl to change tampons:
   a. every 2 to 3 hours.
   b. every 4 to 6 hours.
   c. every 8 hours.
   d. every 12 hours.

10. A middle-aged woman experiencing dyspareunia can use what medication to diminish the discomfort?
    a. ibuprofen
    b. petroleum jelly
    c. K-Y jelly
    d. aspirin

11. A nutritional recommendation for postmenopausal women would be dietary increase in:
    a. calcium.
    b. iron.
    c. salt.
    d. vitamin K.

12. Premenstrual syndrome (PMS) may be caused by estrogen rising and progesterone decreasing during the phase of the menstrual cycle known as:
    a. follicular.
    b. luteal.
    c. ovulation.
    d. premenstrual.

13. In educating a patient with PMS about changing her dietary practices, the nurse would recommend that she increase her intake of:
    a. magnesium.
    b. vitamin D.
    c. iron.
    d. zinc.

14. Pain at the time of the regular menstrual flow is referred to as:
    a. dysmenorrhea.
    b. amenorrhea.
    c. menorrhagia.
    d. metrorrhagia.

15. In the United States, the percentage of pregnancies that are unplanned is about:
    a. 20%.
    b. 30%.
    c. 50%.
    d. 80%.

16. The most common side effect of the implantable contraceptive, Norplant, is:
    a. breast cancer.
    b. irregular bleeding.
    c. thrombophlebitis.
    d. upper-arm pain at insertion site.

17. Statistically, use of the calendar rhythm method as a means of contraception yields a pregnancy rate of:
    a. less than 10%.
    b. between 10% and 20%.
    c. about 40%.
    d. about 80%.

18. Spontaneous abortion occurs in 10% to 20% of pregnancies. Spontaneous abortion occurs most commonly at:
    a. 4 weeks.
    b. 4 to 6 weeks.
    c. 8 to 12 weeks.
    d. 16 weeks.

19. The highest incidence of ectopic pregnancy occurs in the:
    a. cervix.
    b. interstitial tissue.
    c. fallopian tube.
    d. abdominal area.

20. The incidence of recurrence of an ectopic pregnancy is:
    a. 5%.
    b. 7% to 15%.
    c. 20%.
    d. 25% to 40%.

SHORT ANSWER

Read each statement carefully. Write your response in the space provided.

1. Puberty usually begins at ages _____ to _____ but may occur as early as age _____.

2. The pituitary gland releases two essential hormones: _____ hormone causes the ovaries to secrete estrogen, and _____ stimulates the production of progesterone.

3. Menopause usually begins at age _____ to_____, with a median age of _____. Perimenopause can begin as early as _____.

4. List seven danger signals that any woman should report to a health care professional.

   _____

   _____

   _____

   _____

   _____

   _____

   _____

5. The number of women who experience domestic violence each year is about _____.

6. Approximately _____ percent of women are victims of childhood incest.

7. The most accurate outpatient procedure for evaluating a woman for endometrial cancer is _____.

8. Menopause puts a woman at risk for four serious conditions: _____, _____, _____, and _____.

9. List eight major symptoms a woman with PMS may experience.

   _____

   _____

   _____

   _____

   _____

   _____

   _____

   _____

10. Explain why amenorrhea occurs with anorexia and bulimia: _____

_____

11. Describe the physiologic basis for "the pill" as a contraceptive: _____

_____

12. Identify at least six risk factors that would absolutely contraindicate the use of oral contraceptives.

   _____

   _____

   _____

   _____

   _____

   _____

13. Explain how the injectable contraceptive of Depo-Provera works: _____

_____

14. Explain how the emergency use of estrogen or estrogen and a progestin can prevent pregnancy after an episode of unprotected sexual intercourse (e.g. rape, torn condom):

   _____

   _____

15. Describe in vitro fertilization (IVF): _____

   _____

   _____

MATCHING

Match the term in column II with its corresponding definition listed in column I.

Column I

1. _____ Painful sexual intercourse

2. _____ Bladder protruding into the vagina

3. _____ Beginning of menstruation

4. _____ Description of ovaries and fallopian tubes

5. _____ Painful menstruation

6. _____ Implantation of endometrial tissue in other areas of the pelvis

7. _____ Pain on movement of the cervix

8. _____ Absence of menstrual flow

Column II

a. Adnexa

b. Amenorrhea

c. Chandelier sign

d. Cystocele

e. Dysmenorrhea

f. Dyspareunia

g. Endometriosis

h. Menarche

II. Critical Thinking Questions and Exercises

DISCUSSION AND ANALYSIS

Discuss the following topics with your classmates.

1. Discuss the information that should be obtained during a nursing health assessment, including essential data such as health-related behaviors, annual examinations, and prior immunizations.
2. Describe the practice of female genital mutilation (FGM), common in Africa and the Middle East, and the nurse's role in assessment.
3. Explain the postexposure prophylaxis recommended by the Centers for Disease Control and Prevention (2002) for rape victims, including HIV testing.
4. Outline the health history questions and physical assessment modifications necessary for a woman with a disability.
5. Explain the differences between a hysteroscopy and a hysterosalpingography.
6. Distinguish between the terms menorrhagia and metrorrhagia.

RECOGNIZING CONTRADICTIONS

Rewrite each statement correctly. Underline the key concepts.

1. The Women's Health Initiative (WHI) study (2002) found that hormone replacement therapy, after menopause, greatly reduced the presence of heart disease.

2. Women born to mothers who took diethylstilbestrol (DES) during their pregnancy have a higher than average chance of suffering miscarriage.

3. A cervical cone biopsy may be done without anesthesia because the cervix is less sensitive to pain.

4. Magnetic resonance imaging (MRI) exposes the patient to radiation and is more expensive than other pelvic diagnostic aids.

5. Estrogen prepares the uterus for implantation of the fertilized ovum.

6. Progesterone can cause painful cramps during ovulation because it causes myometrial contractility and arteriolar vasospasm.

7. An abortion drug, methotrexate, can be used during the second trimester.

   _____

8. The leading cause of a pregnancy-related death in the woman's first trimester is hemorrhage after spontaneous abortion.

   _____

EXTRACTING INFERENCES

Refer to the accompanying figure and answer the following questions about ectopic pregnancies.

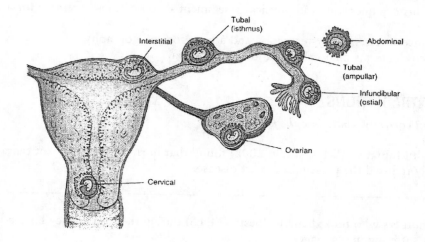

1. Explain what occurs after the ovum is fertilized to cause an ectopic pregnancy: _____

   _____

2. List several possible causes of ectopic implantation: _____

   _____

3. Look at the ovum implanted in the tubal (isthmus) area. What symptoms would you expect the woman to exhibit before tubal rupture occurs?_____

   _____

4. Name three possible surgical options to treat ectopic pregnancies.

   _____

   _____

   _____

5. Postoperative medical management would include assessing the level of beta-HCG to

   _____.

6. Potential maternal complications for ectopic pregnancies are _____ and

   _____.

CLINICAL SITUATIONS

Read the following case study. Circle the correct answer.

Case Study: Toxic Shock Syndrome

Irene, a 23-year-old woman, is admitted to the emergency department in shock with an elevated temperature. She is diagnosed as having toxic shock syndrome (TSS).

1. The nurse knows that TSS is a bacterial infection associated with the use of tampons. The bacterial toxin is believed to be:
   a. *Escherichia coli.*
   b. *Haemophilus influenzae.*
   c. *Staphylococcus aureus.*
   d. *Pseudomonas aeruginosa.*

2. The onset of TSS is characterized by the sudden appearance of:
   a. an elevated fever (up to 102°F).
   b. a red, macular rash.
   c. myalgia and dizziness.
   d. uncontrolled hypotension.

3. Signs associated with TSS include all of the following *except*:
   a. an elevated blood urea nitrogen level.
   b. a decreased bilirubin level.
   c. leukocytosis.
   d. oliguria.

4. Diagnostic evaluation is made from examination of cultures from:
   a. the blood and urine.
   b. the cervix.
   c. the vagina.
   d. all of the above areas.

5. A priority of medical management is:
   a. alleviating respiratory distress.
   b. treating the shock.
   c. controlling the infection.
   d. managing the emotional distress.

CHAPTER 47

Management of Patients With Female Reproductive Disorders

I. Interpretation, Completion, and Comparison

MULTIPLE CHOICE

Read each question carefully. Circle your answer.

1. Conditions that increase a woman's chances of developing candidiasis include:
   a. pregnancy.
   b. diabetes mellitus.
   c. antibiotic therapy.
   d. all of the above.

2. Metronidazole (Flagyl) is the recommended treatment for a vaginal infection caused by:
   a. *Candida albicans.*
   b. *Escherichia coli.*
   c. *Streptococcus.*
   d. *Trichomonas vaginalis.*

3. The nurse knows that a patient diagnosed with bartholinitis would most likely be infected with:
   a. *Candida albicans.*
   b. *Chlamydia.*
   c. *Gardnerella vaginalis.*
   d. *Trichomonas vaginalis.*

4. Nursing interventions for the relief of pain and discomfort for a woman with a vulvovaginal infection include:
   a. warm perineal irrigations.
   b. sitz baths.
   c. cornstarch for chafed inner thighs.
   d. all of the above.

5. The most common sexually transmitted disease among young, sexually active people is:
   a. candidiasis.
   b. human papillomavirus.
   c. endocervicitis.
   d. salpingitis.

6. The bacterium responsible for mucopurulent cervicitis is:
   a. *Chlamydia.*
   b. *Gardnerella.*
   c. *Staphylococcus.*
   d. *Pseudomonas.*

7. The incidence of chlamydia and gonorrhea infections in young females in the United States is:
   a. 5%.
   b. 10%.
   c. 25%.
   d. 40%.

8. The percent of women with gonorrhea who are asymptomatic is:
   a. 20%.
   b. 35%.
   c. 50%.
   d. 80%.

9. The majority of women diagnosed with pelvic inflammatory disease (PID) annually in the United States are:

a. 16 to 24 years of age.

b. 25 to 30 years of age.

c. 35 to 45 years of age.

d. postmenopausal.

10. The leading cause of new HIV infection in women is:

a. heterosexual transmission.

b. homosexual transmission.

c. blood transfusions.

d. intravenous drug use.

11. Women who are HIV positive and are considering getting pregnant need to know that the chance of perinatal transmission is:

a. 10%.

b. 25%.

c. 50%.

d. 100%.

12. Mrs. Jakes has had a pessary inserted for long-term treatment of a prolapsed uterus. As part of your teaching plan, you would advise Mrs. Jakes to:

a. see her gynecologist to remove and clean the pessary at regular intervals.

b. keep the insertion site clean and dry.

c. avoid sexual intercourse.

d. avoid climbing stairs as much as possible.

13. The most common vulvar tumor is known as:

a. Bartholin's cyst.

b. Skene's duct cyst.

c. vulvodynia.

d. vestibular cyst.

14. Ovarian cysts in women older than 50 years of age have the following percent chance of malignancy:

a. 15%.

b. 35%.

c. 50%.

d. 85%.

15. Mrs. Schurman, who has been diagnosed as having endometriosis, asks for an explanation of the disease. The best response for the nurse is to explain that:

a. she has developed an infection in the lining of her uterus.

b. tissue from the lining of the uterus has implanted in areas outside the uterus.

c. the lining of the uterus is thicker than usual, causing heavy bleeding and cramping.

d. the lining of the uterus is too thin because endometrial tissue has implanted outside the uterus.

16. The highest frequency of endometriosis is found in the:

a. cervix.

b. cul-de-sac.

c. ovaries.

d. ureterovesical peritoneum.

17. Mrs. Schurman's treatment involves taking oral danazol (Danocrine), 800 mg/day, for 9 months. Danazol is:

a. a gonadotropin that decreases ovarian and pituitary stimulation.

b. an antigonadotropin that increases pituitary stimulation and decreases ovarian stimulation.

c. a gonadotropin that decreases pituitary stimulation and increases ovarian stimulation.

d. an antigonadotropin that decreases pituitary and ovarian stimulation.

18. Risk factors commonly associated with cancer of the cervix include:

a. chronic cervical infections.

b. exposure to diethylstilbestrol (DES) in utero.

c. multiple sexual partners.

d. all of the above.

19. By incidence, where does cervical cancer rank among the most common female reproductive cancers?
   a. first
   b. second
   c. third
   d. fourth

20. The two chief symptoms of early carcinoma of the cervix are:
   a. leukoplakia and metrorrhagia.
   b. dyspareunia and foul-smelling vaginal discharge.
   c. "strawberry" spots and menorrhagia.
   d. leukorrhea and irregular vaginal bleeding or spotting.

21. Using the International Classification of Carcinoma of the Uterine Cervix, a stage II Pap smear result indicates:
   a. cancer in situ.
   b. vaginal invasion.
   c. pelvic wall invasion.
   d. bladder extension.

22. A postmenopausal woman who has irregular uterine or vaginal bleeding should be encouraged by a nurse to:
   a. stop taking her Premarin (hormonal therapy).
   b. see her gynecologist as soon as possible.
   c. disregard this phenomenon because it is common during this life stage.
   d. mention it to her physician during her next annual examination.

23. Cancer of the uterus is the most common pelvic neoplasm in women; among all cancers for women, it ranks:
   a. first.
   b. second.
   c. third.
   d. fourth.

24. Women who experience postmenopausal bleeding have what chance of developing cancer of the uterus?
   a. 10%
   b. 20%
   c. 35%
   d. 75%

25. The most common symptom of cancer of the vulva is:
   a. a foul-smelling discharge.
   b. bleeding.
   c. pain.
   d. pruritus.

26. The primary treatment for vulvar malignancy is:
   a. chemotherapy creams.
   b. laser vaporization.
   c. radiation.
   d. wide excision.

27. Postoperative nursing care for a simple vulvectomy should include:
   a. cleansing the wound daily.
   b. offering a low-residue diet.
   c. positioning the patient with pillows.
   d. all of the above.

28. As a cause of cancer deaths related to the female reproductive system, ovarian cancer ranks:
   a. first.
   b. second.
   c. third.
   d. fourth.

29. The risk of ovarian cancer peaks when women reach age:
   a. 50 years.
   b. 60 years.
   c. 70 years.
   d. 80 years.

30. The country with the *lowest* incidence of ovarian cancer is:
    a. Japan.
    b. Russia.
    c. Sweden.
    d. United States.

31. A diagnosis of stage III ovarian cancer indicates that growth involves:
    a. only the ovaries.
    b. the ovaries with pelvic extension.
    c. metastases outside the pelvis.
    d. distant metastases.

32. Radiation therapy is the treatment of choice for:
    a. ovarian cancer.
    b. squamous cell carcinoma of the cervix.
    c. uterine carcinoma.
    d. vaginal wall cancer.

SCRAMBLEGRAM

Complete the following scramblegram by circling the word or words that answer each statement below. Terms may be written in any direction.

A	E	E	T	D	A	C	Y	C	L	O	V	I	R
H	L	B	K	E	M	O	M	C	M	U	R	S	C
C	E	D	H	R	A	L	I	T	L	K	L	P	H
V	C	P	A	M	D	E	C	V	Y	L	M	R	A
P	O	A	L	O	N	G	O	S	G	B	E	O	D
B	T	P	U	I	M	D	S	C	A	R	N	L	S
Y	S	S	T	D	Y	L	T	N	L	I	O	A	M
M	Y	M	S	N	M	F	A	B	F	L	R	P	Y
O	C	E	I	R	A	C	T	G	O	T	R	S	T
T	R	A	F	O	S	F	I	Y	E	B	H	E	I
C	E	R	T	S	C	I	N	O	J	K	A	L	R
E	W	D	R	B	D	B	E	P	I	S	G	C	A
R	B	G	B	F	C	R	A	R	M	D	I	B	P
E	R	C	L	M	D	O	I	O	E	S	A	N	I
T	D	S	E	P	T	I	C	S	H	O	C	K	L
S	H	E	R	M	H	D	R	J	R	A	T	H	L
Y	B	A	G	A	C	S	Y	A	T	B	O	L	U
H	B	H	M	D	M	T	P	C	K	T	I	D	N

DEFINITION OF TERMS

1. Intense burning and inflammation of the vulva
2. A preferred treatment for candidiasis
3. The recommended treatment for trichomoniasis
4. The drug of choice for herpes genitalis
5. A potential complication of toxic shock syndrome
6. Downward displacement of the bladder toward the vaginal orifice
7. Test used for diagnosis of cervical cancer
8. Term used to describe the surgical procedure in which the uterus, cervix, and ovaries are removed
9. A term to describe vaginal bleeding
10. Another name for benign tumors of the uterus
11. In utero exposure to this drug increases the incidence of vaginal cancer
12. A risk factor for uterine cancer

13. Exercises that strengthen the pelvic muscles
14. An opening between two hollow organs
15. Displacement of the uterus into the vaginal canal
16. Cysts that arise from parts of the ovum

II. Critical Thinking Questions and Exercises

DISCUSSION AND ANALYSIS

Discuss the following topics with your classmates.

1. Explain why a decrease in estrogen can lead to vaginal infections.
2. Discuss at least ten risk factors for vulvovaginal infections.
3. Describe the pathophysiology and latest treatment (possible vaccine in 2006) for human papillomavirus.
4. Explain the extent of organ involvement with pelvic inflammatory disease.

CLINICAL SITUATIONS

Read the following case studies. Fill in the blanks or circle the correct answer.

CASE STUDY: Bacterial Vaginosis

Maryanne, a 19-year-old college student, has recently noticed increased vaginal discharge that is grey to yellowish white in color.

1. After examination, the nurse prepares a wet mount (vaginal smear). When potassium hydroxide solution is added to the smear, a fishy odor is noted. Maryanne probably has a nonspecific vaginitis known as:

   a. bacterial vaginosis.

   b. candidiasis.

   c. trichomonas vaginalis

   d. atopic vaginitis.

2. A diagnostic sign of bacterial vaginosis is:

   a. a scanty to minimal discharge.

   b. a vaginal pH >4.7.

   c. painful menstruation.

   d. a greenish discharge between periods.

3. Metronidazole (Flagyl) is prescribed to be taken twice a day for 1 week. While taking this medication, Maryanne should be instructed to:

   a. avoid dairy products.

   b. avoid sunlight.

   c. avoid alcohol.

   d. lie down flat for at least 30 minutes after inserting the medication.

4. If Maryanne's vaginal infection recurs, the nurse should recommend that Maryanne:

   a. have her sexual partner tested and treated.

   b. refrain from sexual intercourse.

   c. avoid the use of tampons.

   d. take only showers and no tub baths for awhile.

5. An appropriate nursing diagnosis for Maryanne is:

   a. Altered Comfort: pain and discomfort related to burning or itching from the infectious process.

   b. Self-care Deficit related to inability to perform activities of daily living.

   c. Altered Comfort related to *Gardnerella*-associated vaginitis.

   d. Altered Comfort related to candidiasis.

CASE STUDY: Herpes Genitalis

Paige, a 37-year-old mother of one, has recently been diagnosed with herpes genitalis, a recurrent, life-long viral infection.

1. Herpes genitalis, a sexually transmitted disease, causes blisters on the:
   a. cervix.
   b. external genitalia.
   c. vagina.
   d. all of the above areas.

2. The initial painful infection usually lasts:
   a. 1 week.
   b. 2 weeks.
   c. 4 weeks.
   d. 6 weeks.

3. The herpes virus that is accountable for the majority of genital and perineal lesions is:
   a. Epstein-Barr virus.
   b. cytomegalovirus.
   c. herpes simplex, type 2.
   d. varicella-zoster.

4. At least _____ people, mostly young Caucasian adults, are infected.

5. In order to acquire the infection, one must have had close human contact with one of five sites on the
   body: _____, _____, _____,
   _____, and _____.

6. Because there is no cure for HSV-2 infection, list three antiviral agents that manage symptoms.

   _____

   _____

   _____

7. List four probable nursing diagnoses for Paige.

   _____

   _____

   _____

   _____

CASE STUDY: Pelvic Inflammatory Disease

Donna is a 26-year-old graduate student who has been sexually active with multiple partners for 5 years. Last year she experienced several incidences of cervicitis. She now believes she has PID.

1. Based on your knowledge of PID, you know that the inflammatory condition of the pelvic cavity may involve the following five areas: _____, _____, _____, _____, and _____.

2. Choose six words to describe the characteristics of the infection.

   _____

   _____

   _____

   _____

   _____

   _____

3. Name the two most common causative organisms for PID.

   _____

   _____

4. List five disorders that can result from the PID infection.

   _____

   _____

   _____

   _____

   _____

5. Name four localized symptoms and six generalized symptoms of PID.

LOCALIZED

1. _____

2. _____

3. _____

4. _____

GENERALIZED

1. _____

2. _____

3. _____

4. _____

5. _____

6. _____

CHAPTER 48

Assessment and Management of Patients With Breast Disorders

I. Interpretation, Completion, and Comparison

MULTIPLE CHOICE

Read each question carefully. Circle your answer.

1. The optimal time for breast self-examination is usually at which day after menses begin?
   a. third
   b. fifth
   c. eighth
   d. tenth

2. The average percentage of women who perform breast self-examination is believed to be about:
   a. 15%.
   b. 25%.
   c. 40%.
   d. 80%.

3. Mammography can diagnose breast cancer before it is clinically palpable, meaning that the lump can be detected by x-ray when it is approximately what size?
   a. 1 cm
   b. 1 mm
   c. 2 cm
   d. 1 m

4. As part of health teaching, the nurse needs to alert patients that mammography can yield a false-negative result in how many instances out of 100?
   a. 5 to 10
   b. 10 to 15
   c. 15 to 20
   d. 20 to 25

5. Mammography should be used to annually screen women who are:
   a. younger than 35 years of age.
   b. between the ages of 35 and 40 years.
   c. between 40 and 50 years old.
   d. older than 50 years of age.

6. Characteristics of the lumps present in cystic disease of the breasts include all of the following *except:*
   a. a rapid increase and decrease in size.
   b. increased tenderness before menstruation.
   c. a painless or tender lump.
   d. skin dimpling and nipple retraction.

7. The risk of developing breast cancer is now 1 woman of every:
   a. 8.
   b. 15.
   c. 25.
   d. 40.

8. More than 80% of breast cancers are diagnosed after age:
   a. 40 years.
   b. 50 years.
   c. 65 years.
   d. 75 years.

9. The current 5-year survival rate of breast cancer is:
   a. 60%.
   b. 75%.
   c. 88%.
   d. 98%.

10. Carcinoma in situ, a noninvasive form of cancer, has in incidence rate of:
    a. 5% to 10%.
    b. 15% to 20%.
    c. 25% to 35%.
    d. 50% to 70%.

11. A 1998 clinical study yielded significant reduction in the incidence of breast cancer for those participants who took the chemopreventive agent:
    a. doxorubicin.
    b. methotrexate.
    c. raloxifene.
    d. tamoxifen.

12. The strongest factor (80% correlation) that influences the incidence of breast cancer is:
    a. chemical elements.
    b. environmental pollution.
    c. genetic predisposition.
    d. the number of menstrual cycles.

13. The chance of developing breast cancer doubles if:
    a. the woman had her first child after 30 years of age.
    b. the woman's mother had breast cancer.
    c. the woman was exposed to radiation after puberty.
    d. all of the above are true.

14. The majority of breast cancers occur in the:
    a. upper, inner quadrant.
    b. lower, inner quadrant.
    c. upper, outer quadrant.
    d. lower, outer quadrant.

15. Early clinical manifestations of breast carcinoma include all of the following *except*:
    a. a nontender lump.
    b. asymmetry of the breasts.
    c. nipple retraction.
    d. pain in the breast tissue.

16. A noninvasive breast tumor between 2 cm and 5 cm in size is classified as:
    a. stage I.
    b. stage II.
    c. stage III.
    d. stage IV.

17. Carcinoma of the breast results from cell doubling. A cell that doubles every 60 days for 30 doublings would become palpable (1 cm or larger) after:
    a. 3 years.
    b. 5 years.
    c. 10 years.
    d. 15 years.

18. At diagnosis of breast carcinoma, the risk for presence of metastasis is about:
    a. 25%.
    b. 38%.
    c. 55%.
    d. 73%.

19. The most common site of distant metastasis for breast carcinoma is the:
    a. adrenals.
    b. bone.
    c. lungs.
    d. liver.

20. If the number of positive axillary lymph nodes is between five and six on biopsy, the risk for breast cancer recurrence is:
    a. less than 10%.
    c. 30%.
    b. 15%.
    d. greater than 50%.

21. A patient is scheduled for removal of her left breast and the axillary lymph nodes; the pectoralis minor muscle is to be left in place. This surgical intervention is called:
    a. an extended radical mastectomy.
    c. a quadrantectomy.
    b. a modified radical mastectomy.
    d. a simple mastectomy.

22. The most common hormonal method of intervention is the use of:
    a. Cytadren.
    c. Megace.
    b. diethylstilbestrol.
    d. tamoxifen.

23. A monoclonal antibody that is used for targeted chemotherapy is:
    a. Aranesp.
    c. Herceptin.
    b. Epogen.
    d. Arimidex.

24. Suggested postoperative positioning of the affected arm after surgical intervention (mastectomy) is:
    a. abduction to promote incisional healing.
    c. elevation to promote lymphatic drainage.
    b. adduction to minimize trauma to sensitive tissue.
    d. extension to facilitate isometric exercises.

25. Postmastectomy arm exercises facilitate the development of collateral circulation, which decreases lymphedema. Collateral circulation is usually developed within:
    a. 1 month.
    c. 5 months.
    b. 3 months.
    d. 8 to 10 months.

26. A patient with lymphedema in an arm should be advised to avoid:
    a. blood pressure assessments in that arm.
    c. prolonged exposure of that arm to sunlight.
    b. injections or needles in that arm.
    d. all of the above.

27. The most commonly encountered breast condition in the male is:
    a. breast cancer.
    c. gynecomastia.
    b. mastitis.
    d. cystic breast disease.

MATCHING

Match the term in column II with its corresponding definition listed in column I.

Column I

1. __e___ Overdeveloped breast tissue usually seen in boys

2. __g___ Breast augmentation

3. __A___ Mammography after injection of dye

4. __C___ Breast cancer in the ductal system

5. __b___ Breast pain, usually hormonal in nature

6. __D___ Infection of breast tissue

7. __F___ Partial breast radiation

Column II

a. Galactography

b. Mastalgia

c. Paget's disease

d. Mastitis

e. Gynecomastia

f. Brachytherapy

g. Mammoplasty

II. Critical Thinking Questions and Exercises

CLINICAL SITUATIONS

Read the following case study. Circle the correct answers.

CASE STUDY: Simple Mastectomy

Louise is 53 years old and single. The biopsy findings indicate that she has a malignancy in her breast. She is scheduled for a simple mastectomy.

1. Based on knowledge about the cause of breast cancer, the nurse knows that the highest incidence of this type of cancer is found:
   a. among those who give birth to their first child after 35 years of age.
   b. among those who have had multiple pregnancies.
   c. in the unmarried woman who has not had children.
   d. in the woman who has menopause after 50 years of age.

2. On examination, Louise's tumor is found in the anatomic area where tumors usually develop, the:
   a. medial half of the breast.
   b. nipple area.
   c. posterior segment, inferior to the nipple.
   d. upper, outer quadrant.

3. Louise is advised that if she chooses not to seek treatment, her life expectancy will be:
   a. less than 1 year.
   b. between 2 and 3 years.
   c. about 5 years.
   d. as long as 10 years.

4. The nurse can advise Louise that surgical management for her stage I cancer has a cure rate of:
   a. 30%.
   b. 50%.
   c. 90%.
   d. 100%.

5. Postoperatively, Louise returns to the clinical area and is alert and aware of her surroundings. She experiences moderate pain for the first 72 hours. Postoperative care of the incision includes all of the following *except:*
   a. applying cocoa butter to increase elasticity.
   b. drying the area with slight friction to stimulate the circulation.
   c. gently bathing the area with a nonabrasive soap.
   d. massaging the area.

6. Louise's affected arm should be elevated on a pillow so that her:
   a. entire arm is in a horizontal plane.
   b. forearm is level with her heart.
   c. wrist is higher than her elbow, which should be higher than her shoulder.
   d. wrist is lower than her elbow so that circulation to her hand will not be decreased.

7. The nurse expects that Louise will be allowed out of bed in:

(a.) 1 to 2 days.

b. about 5 days.

c. about 1 week.

d. 1 to 2 weeks.

IDENTIFYING PATTERNS

Five figures of a woman performing breast self-examination follow. Start with the first figure and explain the activity or activities associated with each step.

Step One

1. _____

2. _____

3. _____

Step Two

1. _____

Step Three

1. _____

Step Four

1. _____

2. _____

3. _____

4. _____

5. _____

6. _____

Step Five

1. _____

2. _____

3. _____

CHAPTER 49

Assessment and Management of Problems Related to Male Reproductive Processes

I. Interpretation, Completion, and Comparison

MULTIPLE CHOICE

Read each question carefully. Circle your answer.

1. Health education for a patient with prostatitis includes all of the following *except:*
   a. avoiding drinks that increase prostatic secretions.
   b. forcing fluids to prevent urine from backing up and distending the bladder.
   c. taking several hot sitz baths daily.
   d. using antibiotic therapy for 10 to 14 days.

2. Enlargement of the prostate gland, benign prostatic hyperplasia (BPH), is usually associated with:
   a. dysuria.
   b. dilation of the ureters.
   c. hydronephrosis.
   d. all of the above.

3. The incidence of BPH among men older than 50 years of age is:
   a. 35%.
   b. 50%.
   c. 65%.
   d. 80%.

4. As a cause of death among American men older than 55 years of age, cancer of the prostate ranks:
   a. first.
   b. second.
   c. third.
   d. fourth.

5. The racial group most likely to acquire and die from prostate cancer is:
   a. African Americans.
   b. Caucasians.
   c. Hispanics.
   d. Italians.

6. Prostatic cancer commonly metastasizes to the:
   a. bone.
   b. liver.
   c. lungs.
   d. brain.

7. The 5-year survival rate for prostate cancer is:
   a. 25%.
   b. 50%.
   c. 98%.
   d. 100%.

8. The concentration of prostate-specific antigen (PSA) is proportional to the total prostatic mass. As a diagnostic tool, PSA would indicate all of the following *except:*
   a. local progression of the disease.
   b. patient responsiveness to cancer therapy.
   c. recurrence of prostate cancer.
   d. the presence of malignancy.

9. The closed surgical procedure for a prostatectomy uses which approach?
   a. perineal
   b. retropubic
   c. suprapubic
   d. transurethral

10. The prostatectomy approach that is associated with a high incidence of impotency is:
    a. perineal.
    b. retropubic.
    c. suprapubic.
    d. transurethral.

11. Patients undergoing open surgical removal of the prostate seem to experience a high incidence of:
    a. paralytic ileus.
    b. pneumonia.
    c. impotence.
    d. all of the above.

12. In most instances, patients can be advised that sexual activity may resume, after a prostatectomy, in about:
    a. 4 weeks.
    b. 2 months.
    c. 10 weeks.
    d. 4 months.

13. An expected postoperative outcome of prostatectomy is light pink urine within:
    a. 24 hours.
    b. 48 hours.
    c. 3 days.
    d. 1 week.

14. During the 2 months it takes for the prostatic fossa to heal, the patient is advised not to:
    a. engage in strenuous exercise.
    b. perform the Valsalva maneuver.
    c. take long automobile rides.
    d. do all of the above.

15. In the 15- to 40-year-old age group, testicular cancer has a mortality rate of _____%.
    a. 5
    b. 10
    c. 20
    d. 40

16. Retroperitoneal lymphadenectomy after orchiectomy would probably lead to:
    a. altered libido.
    b. inability to have orgasm.
    c. infertility.
    d. all of the above.

17. One cause of infertility in men is a:
    a. hydrocele.
    b. varicocele.
    c. paraphimosis.
    d. phimosis.

18. Neonatal circumcision is an important protective measure against carcinoma of the:
    a. penis.
    b. testes.
    c. scrotum.
    d. urethra.

19. All of the following are true of priapism *except* that it:
    a. is a urologic emergency.
    b. may result in gangrene.
    c. is painless.
    d. may result in impotence.

SHORT ANSWER

Read each statement carefully. Write your response in the space provided.

1. Two specific tests used to diagnose prostate cancer are _____ and
   _____.

2. List four medications associated with erectile dysfunction.

   _____

   _____

   _____

   _____

3. The most commonly isolated organism that causes prostatitis is _____.

4. List five symptoms associated with prostatitis.

   _____

   _____

   _____

   _____

   _____

5. List five symptoms associated with BPH.

   _____

   _____

   _____

   _____

   _____

6. The most commonly used medication for estrogen therapy in the treatment of prostatic cancer is
   _____; however, newer hormonal therapies, such as _____,
   _____, and _____, suppress testicular androgen.

7. Two chemotherapeutic agents that have been found to prolong survival in patients with prostate cancer
   are _____ and _____.

8. Explain why low-dose heparin is usually given to patients undergoing prostatectomy:

   _____

   _____

9. Describe epididymitis and several of its common causes: _____

   _____

   _____

10. Two tumor markers that may be elevated in testicular cancer are _____ and
    _____.

MATCHING

Match the term in column II with the appropriate description of disorders of the male reproductive system listed in column I.

Column I

1. _____ Collection of fluid in the testes

2. _____ An obstructive complex characterized by increased urinary frequency

3. _____ Constricted foreskin of the penis

4. _____ Failure of the testes to descend into the scrotum

5. _____ Inflammation of the testes

6. _____ Abnormal dilation of the veins in the scrotum

7. _____ Inflammation of the prostrate gland

8. _____ Infection of the epididymis

Column II

a. Cryptorchidism

b. Epididymitis

c. Hydrocele

d. Orchitis

e. Phimosis

f. Prostatism

g. Prostatitis

h. Variocele

II. Critical Thinking Questions and Exercises

DISCUSSION AND ANALYSIS

Discuss the following topics with your classmates.

1. Describe the psychogenic and organic causes of erectile dysfunction.
2. Compare and contrast the actions, side effects, and contraindications of three medications used to treat erectile dysfunction: Viagra, Levitra, and Cialis.
3. Discuss five nursing diagnoses and related goals for a patient with prostate cancer.
4. Describe the physiologic changes in the male reproductive system that occur with age.
5. Compare and contrast the etiology and clinical manifestations of orchitis and epididymitis.

CLINICAL SITUATIONS

Read the following case study. Fill in the blanks or circle the correct answer.

CASE STUDY: Prostatectomy

Tom is a 65-year-old college administrator who is scheduled for a prostatectomy.

1. Preoperatively, two objectives to determine readiness for surgery are _____ and _____.

2. Prostatectomy must be performed before _____.

3. The most commonly performed surgical procedure that is carried out through endoscopy uses which approach?

   a. perineal

   b. retropubic

   c. suprapubic

   d. transurethral

4. List two possible postoperative complications of transurethral resection of the prostate (TURP).

   _____

   _____

5. List four general postoperative complications of a prostatectomy.

   _____

   _____

   _____

   _____

6. Explain why impotence may result from a prostatectomy: _____

   _____

7. List three possible preoperative nursing diagnoses.

   _____

   _____

   _____

8. Identify two nursing activities to help relieve postoperative bladder spasms.

   _____

   _____

9. Explain why the patient is advised not to sit for prolonged periods of time immediately after the operation:

   _____

   _____

10. Describe how you would teach a patient to do perineal exercises: _____

   _____

   _____

CHAPTER 50

Assessment of Immune Function

I. Interpretation, Completion, and Comparison

MULTIPLE CHOICE

Read each question carefully. Circle your answer.

1. A deficient immune system response that is congenital in origin would be classified as what kind of disorder?
   a. autoimmune
   b. gammopathic
   c. primary immune deficiency
   d. hypersensitivity

2. The immune system is essentially composed of:
   a. bone marrow.
   b. lymphoid tissue.
   c. white blood cells.
   d. all of the above components.

3. The primary production site of white blood cells involved in immunity is the:
   a. bone marrow.
   b. adenoids.
   c. thymus gland.
   d. spleen.

4. T lymphocytes, descendants of stem cells, mature in the:
   a. bone marrow.
   b. spleen.
   c. thymus.
   d. lymph nodes.

5. Granulocytes, which fight invasion by releasing histamine, do *not* include:
   a. basophils.
   b. eosinophils.
   c. lymphocytes.
   d. neutrophils.

6. The leukocytes that arrive first at a site where inflammation occurs are:
   a. B lymphocytes.
   b. cytotoxic T cells.
   c. helper T cells.
   d. neutrophils.

7. White blood cells that function as phagocytes are called:
   a. basophils
   b. eosinophils.
   c. monocytes.
   d. lymphocytes.

8. An example of biologic response modifiers that interfere with viruses is:
   a. bradykinin.
   b. eosinophils.
   c. granulocytes.
   d. interferon.

9. The body's first line of defense is the:
   a. antibody response.
   b. cellular immune response.
   c. phagocytic immune response.
   d. white blood cell response.

10. The primary cells responsible for recognition of foreign antigens are:
    a. leukocytes.
    b. lymphocytes.
    c. monocytes.
    d. reticulocytes.

11. Lymphocytes interfere with disease by picking up specific antigens from organisms to alter their function during which stage of an immune response?
    a. effector
    b. proliferation
    c. recognition
    d. response

12. During the proliferation stage:
    a. antibody-producing plasma cells are produced.
    b. lymph nodes enlarge.
    c. lymphocytes rapidly increase.
    d. all of the above occur.

13. Antibodies are believed to be a type of:
    a. carbohydrate.
    b. fat.
    c. protein.
    d. sugar.

14. Cell-mediated immune responses are responsible for all of the following *except*:
    a. anaphylaxis.
    b. graft-versus-host reactions.
    c. transplant rejection.
    d. tumor destruction.

15. It is important to realize that cellular membrane damage results from all of the following *except*:
    a. activation of complement.
    b. antibody-antigen binding.
    c. arrival of killer T cells.
    d. attraction of macrophages.

16. Effector T cells destroy foreign organisms by:
    a. altering the antigen's cell membrane.
    b. causing cellular lysis.
    c. producing lymphokines, which destroy invading organisms.
    d. all of the above mechanisms.

17. Helper T cells accomplish all of the following *except*:
    a. alter the cell membrane by causing cell lysis.
    b. produce lymphokines which activate T cells.
    c. produce cytokines.
    d. activate B cells and macrophages.

18. Complement acts by:
    a. attracting phagocytes to the antigen.
    b. destroying cells through destruction of the antigen's membrane.
    c. rendering the antigen vulnerable to phagocytosis.
    d. a combination of all of the above mechanisms.

19. Interferon is a lymphokine that exerts its effect by:
    a. increasing vascular permeability.
    b. inhibiting the growth of certain antigenic cells.
    c. stopping the spread of viral infections.
    d. suppressing the movement of macrophages.

20. Trace elements, essential for optimum immune function, include all of the following *except:*

   a. cholesterol.
   c. manganese.

   b. copper.
   d. selenium.

MATCHING

Match the immunoglobulin in column II with its associated immunoglobulin (Ig) activity listed in column I. An answer may be used more than once.

Column I

1. _____ Enhances phagocytosis

2. _____ Appears in intravascular serum

3. _____ Helps defend against parasites

4. _____ Activates complement system

5. _____ Protects against respiratory infections

6. _____ Influences B-lymphocyte differentiation

7. _____ Prevents absorption of antigens from food

Column II

a. IgA

b. IgD

c. IgE

d. IgG

e. IgM

Match the immune system effect in column II with its corresponding medication listed in column I. An answer may be used more than once.

Column I

1. _____ Cyclosporine

2. _____ Dactinomycin

3. _____ Indomethacin

4. _____ Methotrexate

5. _____ Mustargen

6. _____ Propylthiouracil

7. _____ Vancomycin

Column II

a. Agranulocytosis, leukopenia

b. Agranulocytosis, neutropenia

c. Leukopenia, aplastic bone marrow

d. Leukopenia, T-cell inhibition

e. Transient leukopenia

II. Critical Thinking Questions and Exercises

DISCUSSION AND ANALYSIS

Discuss the following topics with your classmates.

1. Describe four ways that disorders of the immune system occur.
2. Distinguish between *natural* and *acquired* immunity.
3. Explain what *complement* is and how it is formed.
4. Explain how biologic response modifiers affect the immune response.
5. Explain what research has shown about the role of stem cells.

SCRAMBLEGRAM

Unscramble the letters to answer each statement.

1. A protein substance that responds to a specific antigen: _____

Y N I D T O A B

2. Enzymatic proteins that destroy bacteria: _____

T L P M N C E O E M

3. A substance that stimulates the production of antibodies: _____

G I N T E A N

4. Lymphocytes that directly attack antigens: _____

R P T E L H L E C L E S

5. Cells that engulf and destroy foreign bodies: _____

O G T A E Y P C S H

6. Proteins formed when cells are exposed to foreign agents: _____

F E O T N E S R I R N

CHAPTER 51

Management of Patients With Immunodeficiency

I. Interpretation, Completion, and Comparison

MULTIPLE CHOICE

Read each question carefully. Circle your answer.

1. Immunodeficiency disorders are caused by defects or deficiencies in:
   a. the complement system.
   b. B and T lymphocytes.
   c. phagocytic cells.
   d. all of the above.

2. The cardinal symptoms of immunodeficiency are:
   a. chronic diarrhea.
   b. chronic or recurrent severe infections.
   c. poor response to treatment of infections.
   d. inclusive of all the above.

3. The nitroblue tetrazolium reductase (NTR) test is used to diagnose immunodeficiency disorders related to:
   a. complement.
   b. B lymphocytes.
   c. T lymphocytes.
   d. phagocytic cells.

4. More than 50% of individuals with which disease develop pernicious anemia?
   a. Bruton disease
   b. common variable immunodeficiency (CVID)
   c. DiGeorge syndrome
   d. Nezelof syndrome

5. The most frequent presenting sign in patients with DiGeorge syndrome is:
   a. chronic diarrhea.
   b. hypocalcemia.
   c. neutropenia.
   d. pernicious anemia.

6. The primary cause of death for individuals with ataxia-telangiectasia is:
   a. acute renal failure.
   b. chronic lung disease.
   c. neurologic dysfunction.
   d. overwhelming infection.

7. The most common secondary immunodeficiency disorder is:
   a. AIDS.
   b. DAF.
   c. CVID.
   d. SCID.

8. The recommended dose of intravenous gamma globulin for a 60-kg man, given monthly, is:
   a. 15 g.
   b. 30 g.
   c. 45 g.
   d. 60 g.

9. When gamma globulin is infused intravenously, the rate should not exceed:
   a. 1.5 mL/min.
   b. 3 mL/min.
   c. 6 mL/min.
   d. 10 mL/min.

10. The nurse knows to stop an infusion of gamma globulin if the patient experiences:
   a. flank pain.
   b. shaking chills.
   c. tightness in the chest.
   d. any of the above.

II. Critical Thinking Questions and Exercises

INTERPRETING PATTERNS

For each group of clustered clues, write the corresponding immunodeficiency disorder.

There is an increased incidence of bacterial infections.

Fungal infections from candida organisms develop readily.

The individual is easily infected with herpes simplex.

Chronic eczematoid dermatitis is present.

1. The disorder is: _____
   There is disappearance of germinal centers from lymphatic tissue.
   There is complete lack of antibody production.
   It is associated with the most common immunodeficiency seen in childhood.
   Disease onset occurs most often in the second decade of life.

2. The disorder is: _____
   Lymphopenia is usually present.
   Thymus gland fails to develop.
   Chronic mucocutaneous candidiasis is an associated disorder.

3. The disorder is: _____
   IgA deficiency is present in 40% of individuals.
   T-cell deficiencies become more severe with age.
   Neurologic symptoms usually occur before 5 years of age.

4. The disorder is: _____
   It usually occurs as a result of underlying disease processes.
   It frequently is caused by certain autoimmune disorders.
   It may be caused by certain viruses.

5. The disorder is: _____

EXAMINING ASSOCIATIONS

Read each analogy. Write the best possible response in the space provided.

1. Job's syndrome : phagocytic dysfunction :: Bruton's disease : _____

2. Colony-stimulating factor : HIE syndrome :: Intravenous immunoglobulin : _____

3. CVID : bacterial infections :: Ataxia-telangiectasia : _____

4. Angioneurotic edema : frequent episodes of edema :: Paroxysmal nocturnal hemoglobinuria : _____
   _____

CHAPTER 52

Management of Patients With HIV Infection and AIDS

I. Interpretation, Completion, and Comparison

MULTIPLE CHOICE

Read each question carefully. Circle your answer.

1. The Centers for Disease Control and Prevention (CDC) approved the first antiretroviral drug for AIDS six years after the first cases were reported in:
   a. 1978.
   b. 1982.
   c. 1987.
   d. 1991.

2. According to one early study, the greatest number of reported HIV cases were due to:
   a. male homosexual contact.
   b. male injection drug use.
   c. female homosexual contact.
   d. female injection drug use.

3. The racial/ethnic group that has the highest rate of exposure due to IV injection drug use among men is:
   a. Caucasians.
   b. Hispanics.
   c. African Americans.
   d. Asians.

4. After infection with HIV, the immune system responds by making antibodies against the virus, usually within how many weeks after infection?
   a. 1 to 2
   b. 3 to 6
   c. 3 to 12
   d. 6 to 18

5. Postexposure prophylaxis (PEP) medications should be started within _____ after exposure, but no longer than _____, to offer any benefit, and they must be taken for _____.
   a. 2 hours, 72 hours, and 4 weeks
   b. 4 days, 7 days, and 2 weeks
   c. 1 week, 3 weeks, and 3 months
   d. 1 month, 2 months, and 6 months

6. Up to 85% of individuals infected with HIV develop symptoms of AIDS within how many years after infection?
   a. 3 to 5
   b. 6 to 7
   c. 8 to 10
   d. 12 to 15

7. Abnormal laboratory findings seen with AIDS include:
   a. decreased CD4 and T-cell count.
   b. p24 antigen.
   c. positive enzyme immunoassay (EIA) test.
   d. all of the above.

8. A widely used laboratory test that measures HIV-RNA levels and tracks the body's response to HIV infection is the:

   a. CD4/CD8 ratio.

   b. EIA test.

   c. viral load test.

   d. Western blot.

9. An example of an antiretroviral agent, classified as a fusion inhibitor, that must be injected subcutaneously twice a day is:

   a. Agenerase.

   b. Combivir.

   c. Fuzeon (T20).

   d. Retrovir.

10. One of the most frequent systemic side effects of anti-HIV drugs is:

    a. osteoporosis.

    b. hyperglycemia.

    c. lipodystrophy syndrome.

    d. pancreatitis.

11. The most common infection in persons with AIDS is:

    a. cytomegalovirus.

    b. Legionnaire's disease.

    c. *Mycobacterium tuberculosis.*

    d. *Pneumocystis jiroveci* pneumonia (PCP).

12. The most debilitating gastrointestinal condition found in up to 90% of all AIDS patients is:

    a. anorexia.

    b. chronic diarrhea.

    c. nausea.

    d. vomiting.

13. A diagnosis of "wasting syndrome" can be initially made when involuntary weight loss exceeds what percent of baseline body weight?

    a. 10%

    b. 15%

    c. 20%

    d. 25%

14. The minimum number of daily calories recommended for a 70-kg individual with AIDS-related wasting syndrome is:

    a. 1500.

    b. 2000.

    c. 2800.

    d. 4000.

15. The minimum number of daily *protein* calories for a 70-kg individual with AIDS-related wasting syndrome is:

    a. 20.

    b. 35.

    c. 45.

    d. 60.

16. The most common malignancy seen with HIV infection is:

    a. carcinoma of the skin.

    b. Kaposi's sarcoma.

    c. pancreatic cancer.

    d. stomach cancer.

SHORT ANSWER

Read each statement carefully. Write your response in the space provided.

1. In the United States, three states have reported 43% of cumulative AIDS cases (1999–2003). They are
   _____, _____, and _____.

2. Since 2003, the number of people in the U.S. reported to have AIDS has reached almost
   _____; more than 50% belong to the _____ race, and males
   account for about _____ of these cases.

3. The two major means of HIV transmission are _____ and
_____.

4. List five types of body fluids that can transmit HIV-1.

_____

_____

_____

_____

_____

5. HIV belongs to a group of viruses known as _____.

6. According to the U.S. Department of Health and Human Services Panel on Clinical Practices for HIV
Infection Treatment (2004), there are four criteria that affect treatment decisions:
_____, _____, _____, and
_____.

7. The four goals of treatment are _____, _____,
_____, and _____.

8. All anti-HIV drugs work in one of two ways: _____ or _____.

9. A fungal infection present in almost all patients with AIDS is _____.

10. A recommended chemotherapeutic agent for Kaposi's sarcoma is _____.

MATCHING

Match the AIDS-indicated category in column II with its associated clinical condition listed in column I. An
answer may be used more than once.

Column I

1. _____ Histoplasmosis

2. _____ Hairy leukoplakia

3. _____ Kaposi's sarcoma

4. _____ Acute primary HIV infection

5. _____ *Pneumocystis jiroveci*

6. _____ Bacillary angiomatosis

7. _____ Persistent generalized lymphadenopathy (PGL)

8. _____ Extrapulmonary cryptococcosis

Column II

a. Clinical category A

b. Clinical category B

c. Clinical category C

II. Critical Thinking Questions and Exercises

DISCUSSION AND ANALYSIS

Discuss the following topics with your classmates.

1. Outline and discuss the health teaching points a school nurse would cover to promote safe sexual behaviors in young adults.
2. Give specific examples of how health care providers can maintain "standard precautions" to prevent HIV transmission.
3. Describe the stage of HIV disease known as primary infection.
4. Discuss the current status of research regarding the development of a vaccine for HIV infection.
5. Describe the appearance of the cutaneous lesions seen with Kaposi's sarcoma.
6. Discuss at least eight nursing diagnoses and four collaborative problems for patients with AIDS and HIV infection.

CLINICAL SITUATIONS

Read the following case study. Fill in the blanks or circle the correct answer.

CASE STUDY: Acquired Immunodeficiency Syndrome

Brenden is a 39-year-old homosexual man who has been recently diagnosed with AIDS.

1. On initial assessment, the nurse identifies two major potential risk factors associated with AIDS: _____ and _____.

2. As part of her assessment, the nurse checks Brenden for candidiasis. To do this, she would inspect Brenden's:
   a. heart.
   b. lungs.
   c. oral cavity.
   d. skin.

3. Assessment data indicates dehydration, as evidenced by:
   a. bradycardia.
   b. hypertension.
   c. urine specific gravity greater than 1.025.
   d. urine output greater than 70 mL/hour.

4. The assessment data indicates five possible collaborative problems. List two: _____ and _____.

5. The nurse advises Brenden to avoid certain foods that are bowel irritants to prevent diarrhea. She advises him not to eat:
   a. bland foods.
   b. cooked cereal.
   c. gelatin and pudding.
   d. popcorn.

6. To improve Brenden's nutritional status, the nurse would:
   a. encourage him to rest before eating.
   b. limit fluids 1 hour before meals.
   c. serve five to six small meals per day.
   d. do all of the above.

CHAPTER 53

Assessment and Management of Patients With Allergic Disorders

I. Interpretation, Completion, and Comparison

MULTIPLE CHOICE

Read each question carefully. Circle your answer.

1. The body's first line of defense against potential invaders is the:
   a. gastrointestinal tract.
   b. respiratory tract.
   c. skin.
   d. combination of all the above.

2. An example of an incomplete protein antigen that triggers an allergic response is:
   a. animal dander.
   b. horse serum.
   c. medications.
   d. pollen.

3. The classification of immunoglobulin (Ig) that occupies certain receptors on mast cells and produces an inflammatory response is:
   a. IgA.
   b. IgD.
   c. IgE.
   d. IgG.

4. Histamine acts on major organs by:
   a. contracting bronchial smooth muscle.
   b. dilating small venules.
   c. increasing gastric secretions.
   d. stimulating all of the above mechanisms.

5. A popular medication that has an affinity for histamine-1 (H_1) receptors is:
   a. Benadryl.
   b. Prilosec.
   c. Tagamet.
   d. Zantac.

6. A chemical mediator of hypersensitivity that is released during platelet aggregation and causes bronchial smooth muscle contraction is:
   a. bradykinin.
   b. histamine.
   c. prostaglandin.
   d. serotonin.

7. Hypersensitivity reactions follow reexposure and are classified by type of reaction. An anaphylactic reaction is usually identified as type:
   a. I.
   b. II.
   c. III.
   d. IV.

8. A type II hypersensitivity reaction occurs when a normal constituent is viewed as foreign by the body. An example of a type II reaction is:

   a. bacterial endocarditis.

   b. Rh-hemolytic disease (newborn).

   c. lupus erythematosus

   d. rheumatoid arthritis.

9. Delayed hypersensitivity (type IV) is said to have occurred when the inflammatory response to an allergen peaks within:

   a. 4 to 8 hours.

   b. 24 to 72 hours.

   c. 4 to 6 days.

   d. 1 to 2 weeks.

10. The nurse monitors the patient's eosinophil level. She suspects a definite allergic disorder with an eosinophil value of what percent of the total leukocyte count?

    a. 1% to 3%

    b. 3% to 4%

    c. 5% to 10%

    d. 15% to 40%

11. Atopic disorders that result from an allergic response to an allergen include:

    a. allergic rhinitis.

    b. atopic dermatitis.

    c. bronchial asthma.

    d. all of the above.

12. Pruritus and nasal congestion may be indicators of an impending anaphylactic reaction. These symptoms usually occur within how many hours after exposure?

    a. 2

    b. 6

    c. 12

    d. 24

13. When a patient is experiencing an allergic response, the nurse should initially assess the patient for:

    a. dyspnea, bronchospasm, and/or laryngeal edema.

    b. hypotension and tachycardia.

    c. the presence and location of pruritus.

    d. the severity of cutaneous warmth and flushing.

14. Allergic rhinitis is induced by:

    a. airborne pollens or molds.

    b. ingested foods.

    c. parenteral medications.

    d. topical creams or ointments.

15. Patients who are sensitive to ragweed should be advised that weed pollen begins to appear in:

    a. early spring.

    b. early fall.

    c. summer.

    d. midwinter.

16. A major side effect of antihistamines that requires accurate patient education is:

    a. dryness of the mouth.

    b. anorexia.

    c. palpitations.

    d. sedation.

17. An area of nursing concern when administering a sympathomimetic drug is the drug's ability to:

    a. cause bronchodilation.

    b. constrict integumentary smooth muscle.

    c. dilate the muscular vasculature.

    d. do all of the above.

18. Injected allergens are used for "hyposensitization" and may produce systemic reactions that can be harmful. The medication that should be on hand in case of an adverse reaction is:

    a. Dramamine.

    b. epinephrine.

    c. Phenergan hydrochloride.

    d. Pyribenzamine.

19. For a 132-lb (60-kg) woman who is experiencing anaphylaxis, the nurse should immediately administer intramuscular adrenaline, in a minimum dose of:
    a. 2 mL.
    c. 6 mL.
    b. 4 mL.
    d. 8 mL.

20. The most serious manifestation of hereditary angioedema is:
    a. abdominal pain.
    c. laryngeal edema.
    b. conjunctivitis.
    d. urticaria.

21. One of the most severe food allergies is caused by:
    a. chocolate.
    c. peanuts.
    b. milk.
    d. shrimp.

SHORT ANSWER

Read each statement carefully. Write your response in the space provided.

1. Antibodies react with antigens by _____, _____, and _____.

2. An allergic reaction occurs when: _____

   _____

   _____

3. Prostaglandins are primary chemical mediators that respond to a stimulus by contracting smooth muscle and increasing capillary permeability. This response causes: _____

   _____

4. Type III hypersensitivity reactions involve the binding of antibodies to antigens, as occurs in the following two disorders: _____ and _____.

5. Two examples of a type IV hypersensitivity reaction are _____ and _____.

6. The most common cause of anaphylaxis is _____.

7. People need to be advised that a "rebound" anaphylactic reaction can occur _____ hours after an initial attack, even if epinephrine has been given.

8. The primary treatment available for latex allergy is _____

   _____

II. Critical Thinking Questions and Exercises

DISCUSSION AND ANALYSIS

Discuss the following topics with your classmates.

1. Briefly describe the physiologic response that causes an allergic reaction.
2. Explain the production and function of immunoglobulins.
3. Describe the clinical manifestations that occur with a severe anaphylactic reaction.

4. Distinguish among three types of allergy tests: skin testing, provocative testing, and radioallergosorbent testing.
5. Distinguish between an *atopic* and a *nonatopic* IgE-mediated allergic reaction.
6. Describe the pathophysiology and medical intervention for anaphylaxis.
7. Compare the actions and potential complications of the following: antihistamines, adrenergic agents, mast cell stabilizers, and corticosteroids.
8. Discuss a variety of selected nursing strategies for allergy management.
9. Compare the etiology and clinical manifestations of four types of contact dermatitis.

CLINICAL SITUATIONS

Read the following case study. Fill in the blanks or circle the correct answer.

CASE STUDY: Allergic Rhinitis

Chris is a 26-year-old contractor who specializes in finished basements. Because of his job, he is frequently working in environments where there are substances that stimulate an allergic reaction.

1. Based on assessment data, two likely nursing diagnoses would be _____ and _____.

2. Four probable patient goals would be _____, _____, _____, and _____.

3. The nurse advises Chris that his attacks may be preceded by the symptoms of:
   a. breathing difficulty.
   b. pruritus.
   c. tingling sensations.
   d. all of the above.

4. The nurse also advises him that other symptoms may be more alarming, such as:
   a. hoarseness.
   b. a rash or hives.
   c. wheezing.
   d. all of the above.

5. A teaching plan for Chris would include information about:
   a. reducing exposure to allergens.
   b. desensitization procedures.
   c. correct use of medications.
   d. all of the above.

6. The nurse tells Chris that if the physician recommends a series of inoculations for desensitization, he should expect to receive injections every:
   a. day for 30 days.
   b. week for 1 year.
   c. 2 to 4 weeks.
   d. month for 4 years.

CHAPTER 54

Assessment and Management of Patients With Rheumatic Disorders

I. Interpretation, Completion, and Comparison

MULTIPLE CHOICE

Read each question carefully. Circle your answer.

1. Joint swelling in rheumatic disease may be due to:
   a. bony overgrowth.
   b. fluid accumulation.
   c. hypertrophied synovium.
   d. all of the above.

2. The most common symptom of rheumatic disease that causes a patient to seek medical attention is:
   a. joint swelling.
   b. limited movement.
   c. fatigue.
   d. pain.

3. The nurse knows that a patient who is present with the symptom of "blanching of his fingers on exposure to cold" would be assessed for the rheumatic disease known as:
   a. ankylosing spondylitis.
   b. Raynaud's phenomenon.
   c. Reiter's syndrome.
   d. Sjögren's syndrome.

4. Synovial fluid from an inflamed joint is characteristically:
   a. clear and pale.
   b. milky, cloudy, and dark yellow.
   c. scanty in volume.
   d. straw-colored.

5. A patient is suspected of having myositis. The nurse prepares the patient for what procedure that will confirm the diagnosis?
   a. bone scan
   b. computed tomography (CT)
   c. magnetic resonance imaging (MRI)
   d. muscle biopsy

6. All of the following blood studies are consistent with a positive diagnosis of rheumatoid arthritis *except:*
   a. a positive C-reactive protein (CRP).
   b. a positive antinuclear antibody (ANA).
   c. an RBC count $<4.0 \times 10^6/\mu L$.
   d. a serum complement (C3) level >130 mg/dL.

7. A serum study that is positive for the rheumatoid factor is:
   a. diagnostic for Sjögren's syndrome.
   b. diagnostic for systemic lupus erythematosus (SLE).
   c. specific for rheumatoid arthritis.
   d. suggestive of rheumatoid arthritis.

8. A popular and effective COX-2 inhibitor that increases the patient's risk of stroke is:
   a. Bextra.
   b. Celebrex.
   c. Feldene.
   d. Tolectin.

9. The rheumatoid arthritis reaction produces enzymes that break down:
   a. collagen.
   b. elastin.
   c. hematopoietic tissue.
   d. strong supporting tissue.

10. In rheumatoid arthritis, the autoimmune reaction primarily occurs in the:
    a. joint tendons.
    b. cartilage.
    c. synovial tissue.
    d. interstitial space.

11. In rheumatoid arthritis, the cartilage is replaced with fibrous connective tissue during the stage of synovial joint destruction known as:
    a. cartilage erosion.
    b. increased phagocytic production.
    c. lymphocyte infiltration.
    d. pannus formation.

12. A disease-modifying antirheumatic drug (DMARD) that is successful in the treatment of rheumatoid arthritis yet has retinal eye changes as a side effect is:
    a. Imuran.
    b. Aralen.
    c. Plaquenil.
    d. Solganal.

13. Nonsteroidal anti-inflammatory drugs (NSAIDs) used in rheumatic diseases include all of the following *except*:
    a. Clinoril.
    b. Cytoxan.
    c. Motrin.
    d. Celebrex.

14. When a person with arthritis is temporarily confined to bed, the position recommended to prevent flexion deformities is:
    a. prone.
    b. semi-Fowler's.
    c. side-lying with pillows supporting the shoulders and legs.
    d. supine with pillows under the knees.

15. To immobilize an inflamed wrist, the nurse should splint the joint in a position of:
    a. slight dorsiflexion.
    b. extension.
    c. hyperextension.
    d. internal rotation.

16. A characteristic cutaneous lesion, called the "butterfly rash," appears across the bridge of the nose in 30% to 60% of patients with:
    a. gout.
    b. rheumatoid arthritis.
    c. systemic sclerosis.
    d. SLE.

17. The single, most important type of medication for the treatment of SLE is:
    a. immunosuppressants.
    b. corticosteroids.
    c. NSAIDs.
    d. salicylates.

18. Clinical manifestations of scleroderma include:
    a. decreased ventilation owing to lung scarring.
    b. dysphagia owing to hardening of the esophagus.
    c. dyspnea owing to fibrotic cardiac tissue.
    d. all of the above.

19. The most common type of connective tissue disease in the United States is:
   a. carpal tunnel syndrome.
   b. degenerative joint disease.
   c. fibrositis.
   d. polymyositis.

20. Pathophysiologic changes seen with osteoarthritis include:
   a. joint cartilage degeneration.
   b. the formation of bony spurs at the edges of the joint surfaces.
   c. narrowing of the joint space.
   d. all of the above changes.

21. The nurse knows that a patient diagnosed with a spondyloarthropathy would *not* have:
   a. ankylosing spondylitis.
   b. Raynaud's phenomenon.
   c. reactive arthritis.
   d. psoriatic arthritis.

22. With a diagnosis of gout, a nurse should expect to find:
   a. glucosuria.
   b. hyperuricemia.
   c. hypoproteinuria.
   d. ketonuria.

23. A purine-restricted diet is prescribed for a patient. The nurse should recommend:
   a. dairy products.
   b. organ meats.
   c. raw vegetables.
   d. shellfish.

MATCHING

Match the clinical interpretation/laboratory significance column II with its associated test listed in column I.

Column I

1. _____ Uric acid

2. _____ Complement

3. _____ Rheumatoid factor

4. _____ Hematocrit

5. _____ HLA-B27 antigen

6. _____ Antinuclear antibody (ANA)

Column II

a. A decrease can be seen in chronic inflammation.

b. A positive test is associated with SLE, rheumatoid arthritis, and Raynaud's disease.

c. An increase in this substance is seen with gout.

d. This protein substance is decreased in rheumatoid arthritis and SLE.

e. This is present in 80% of those who have rheumatoid arthritis.

f. This is present in 85% of those with ankylosing spondylitis.

II. Critical Thinking Questions and Exercises

DISCUSSION AND ANALYSIS

Discuss the following topics with your classmates.

1. Explain the theory of *degradation* as it relates to the pathophysiology of rheumatic diseases.
2. Explain the difference between exacerbation and remission.
3. Distinguish between the pathophysiology of inflammatory rheumatic disease and that of degenerative rheumatic disease.
4. Discuss the physiologic rationale supporting the goals and strategies for the treatment of rheumatic diseases.
5. Describe the type of exercises and precautions used to promote mobility for a patient with a rheumatic disease.
6. Compare the process and nursing implications for the following surgical procedures for rheumatoid arthritis: synovectomy, tenorrhaphy, arthrodesis, and arthroplasty.
7. Describe the pathophysiology and clinical manifestations of polymyalgia rheumatica.
8. Describe the pathophysiology and clinical manifestations of degenerative joint disease (osteoarthritis).
9. Explain the pathophysiology and clinical manifestations of gout.
10. Explain the etiology and nursing management for fibromyalgia.

CLINICAL SITUATIONS

Read the following case studies. Fill in the blanks or circle the correct answer.

CASE STUDY: Diffuse Connective Tissue Disease

June, a 33-year-old mother of two, has joint pain and stiffness, decreased mobility, and increased frequency of fatigue. She is depressed.

1. The physician immediately suspects a diagnosis of a diffuse connective tissue disease which the nurse knows manifests primarily in women:

   a. polymyositis.

   b. rheumatoid arthritis.

   c. scleroderma.

   d. systemic lupus erythematosus.

2. On initial examination, the physician notes that Jane's knees are hot, swollen, and painful. The physician orders specific laboratory studies. The test result, which is not significant for a diagnosis of rheumatoid arthritis, is:

   a. a decreased red blood count.

   b. an elevated C4 complement component.

   c. an elevated erythrocyte sedimentation rate.

   d. a positive C-reactive protein.

3. The nurse also assesses the four systemic features usually found with rheumatoid arthritis:

   a. _____

   b. _____

   c. _____

   d. _____

4. Jane is scheduled for an arthrocentesis. The nurse advises her that her knee joint will be anesthetized locally and a fluid specimen will be obtained. There is no special preparation or precautions after the procedure. Jane is told that a positive finding would be joint fluid that:

   a. contains few inflammatory cells.

   b. does not contain leukocytes.

   c. is viscous and tan in color.

   d. will not form a mucin clot.

5. A positive diagnosis of rheumatoid arthritis results in a multidisciplinary approach to treatment. Jane's pharmacotherapy regimen includes several drug classifications. A popular NSAID that may be prescribed is:

   a. Aralen.

   b. Imuran.

   c. Motrin.

   d. Ridaura.

6. If Jane experiences gastric irritation and/or ulceration, the physician may order a new class of NSAIDs called _____.

7. A low-dose corticosteroid regimen is begun for a short period. The nurse advises Jane to be aware of certain drug-induced side effects, such as:

   a. elevated blood pressure.

   b. gastric upset.

   c. weight gain.

   d. all of the above.

CASE STUDY: Systemic Lupus Erythematosus

Brooke is a 41-year-old mother of two teenagers who has had symptoms of joint tenderness for about 10 years. Lately she has noticed significant morning stiffness and a slight rash over the bridge of her nose and cheeks. Her physician suspects a diagnosis of SLE.

1. Before beginning the assessment, the nurse knows that the etiology of SLE is an altered immune regulation that can be caused by disturbances in _____, _____, _____, and _____ factors.

2. The altered immune response can be described as: _____ _____

3. The nurse is aware that the physician will do a complete cardiovascular assessment, checking the patient for _____, _____, and _____.

4. Blood testing will be ordered to determine the presence of _____, _____, _____, _____, and _____.

5. The nurse knows that the physician may order _____ medications for treating Brooke's symptoms, if they are considered mild.

6. As part of health teaching, the nurse reminds Brooke that possible cardiovascular complications require periodic screening for _____ and _____.

IDENTIFYING PATTERNS

Review Fig. 54-1 in the text, which depicts the results of the inflammatory response in the knee joint, as well as Fig. 54-3 in the text, which shows the pathophysiology of rheumatoid arthritis. Outline in detail the series of related steps that lead to the inflammation, beginning with the antigen stimulus that activates monocytes and T lymphocytes, using the following flow chart.

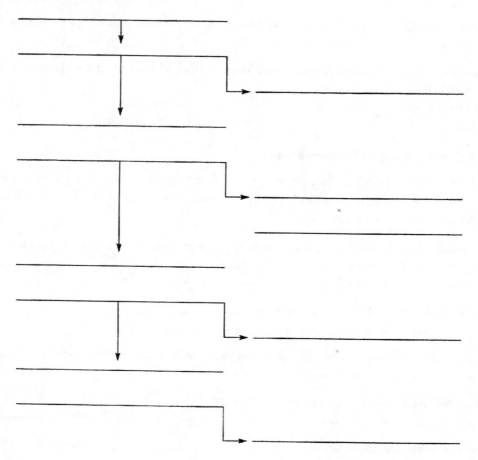

CHAPTER 55

Assessment of Integumentary Function

I. Interpretation, Completion, and Comparison

MULTIPLE CHOICE

Read each question carefully. Circle your answer.

1. For the average adult with a normal body temperature, a nurse needs to know that insensible water loss is approximately:
   a. 250 mL/day.
   b. 600 mL/day.
   c. 800 mL/day.
   d. 1000 mL/day.

2. When a nurse applies a cold towel to a patient's neck to reduce body heat, heat is reduced by:
   a. conduction.
   b. convection.
   c. evaporation.
   d. radiation.

3. Sweating, a process by which the body regulates heat loss, does not occur until the core body temperature exceeds the base level of:
   a. 24°C.
   b. 37°C.
   c. 43°C.
   d. 51°C.

4. In a dark-skinned person, color change that occurs in the presence of shock can be evidenced when the skin appears:
   a. ashen gray and dull.
   b. dusky blue.
   c. reddish pink.
   d. whitish pink.

5. Dark-skinned patients who have cherry-red nail beds, lips, and oral mucosa may be exhibiting signs of:
   a. anemia.
   b. carbon monoxide poisoning.
   c. polycythemia.
   d. shock.

6. A clinical example of a primary skin lesion known as a macule is:
   a. hives.
   b. impetigo.
   c. port-wine stains.
   d. psoriasis.

II. Critical Thinking Questions and Exercises

ANALYZING COMPARISONS

Read each analogy. Write the best response in the space provided.

1. Keratin : skin hardening :: Melanin : _____.
2. Bluish skin color : insufficient oxygenation :: Yellow-green skin : _____.
3. Merkel cells : nervous system :: Langerhans cells : _____.

4. Hirsutism : excessive hair growth :: _____ : hair loss.
5. Vitamin D deficiency : rickets :: Vitamin C deficiency : _____.
6. Palpation : skin turgor :: _____ : vesicle.
7. Acne : a pustule :: Psoriasis : _____.

IDENTIFYING PATTERNS

Consider the cutaneous manifestations listed in each grouping. For each group of clustered clues, write the corresponding systemic disease.

Seen in systemic lupus erythematosus

Characterized by red, spidery lines

Appears in plaques on the nose and ears

Seen on scales on the cheek area

1. _____

Appears as an ulcerated lesion

Is a painless chancre

2. _____

Seen in platelet disorders

Associated with vessel fragility

Characterized by purpura

3. _____

Occurs in infections

Seen with allergic reactions

Characteristic of drug reactions

4. _____

Present as macules, papules, plaques, or nodules

Lesions are visually multiple

Lesions are characteristically blue-red or dark brown

Seen in AIDS

5. _____

For each of the following eight primary or secondary lesions, document two defining characteristics.

1. Cherry angioma

a. _____

b. _____

2. Crust

a. _____

b. _____

3. Cyst

a. _____

b. _____

4. Fissure

a. _____

b. _____

5. Keloid

a. _____

b. _____

6. Telangiectasis

a. _____

b. _____

7. Petechia

a. _____

b. _____

8. Spider angioma

a. _____

b. _____

APPLYING CONCEPTS

For each pathophysiologic change in the skin that occurs with aging, list associated alterations in function.

1. Thinning of the dermis and epidermis at their junction

a. _____

b. _____

c. _____

d. _____

2. Loss of subcutaneous tissue of elastin, fat, and collagen

a. _____

b. _____

c. _____

3. Decreased cellular replacement

    a. _____

    b. _____

4. Decrease in the number and function of sweat and sebaceous glands

    a. _____

5. Reduced hormonal levels of androgens

    a. _____

CHAPTER 56

Management of Patients With Dermatologic Problems

I. Interpretation, Completion, and Comparison

MULTIPLE CHOICE

Read each question carefully. Circle your answer.

1. In the absence of infection or heavy discharge, chronic wounds should remain covered for:
   a. 6 to 12 hours.
   b. 12 to 24 hours.
   c. 24 to 36 hours.
   d. 48 to 72 hours.

2. Moisture-retentive dressings, more effective than wet compresses at removing exudate, should remain in place a minimum of:
   a. 6 hours.
   b. 12 hours.
   c. 18 hours.
   d. 24 hours.

3. A moisture-retentive dressing that promotes débridement and helps form granulation tissue is a:
   a. calcium alginate dressing.
   b. foam dressing.
   c. hydrocolloid dressing.
   d. hydrogel dressing.

4. Occlusive dressings applied to a dermatosis are used to:
   a. enhance the absorption of topical medications.
   b. improve hydration.
   c. increase the local skin temperature.
   d. do all of the above.

5. The nurse caring for a patient with an occlusive dressing knows to assess the skin every 12 hours for the potential complication of:
   a. local atrophy.
   b. striae.
   c. telangiectasia.
   d. all of the above.

6. The patient is advised to apply a suspension-type lotion to a dermatosis site. The nurse advises the patient that the lotion must be applied how often to be effective?
   a. every hour
   b. every 3 hours
   c. every 12 hours
   d. every day at the same time

7. The nurse knows to assess for which local side effect when corticosteroids are used for dermatologic conditions?
   a. skin atrophy
   b. striae
   c. telangiectasia
   d. all of the above

8. An example of a very potent corticosteroid used for treating a dermatologic condition is:
   a. Aclovate.
   b. Aristocort.
   c. Temovate.
   d. Westcort.

9. The most common symptom of pruritus is:
   a. a rash.
   b. itching.
   c. flaking.
   d. pain.

10. A nurse should assess all possible causes of pruritus, including the presence of endocrine disease, such as:
    a. biliary cirrhosis.
    b. hypothyroidism.
    c. lymphoma.
    d. diabetes mellitus.

11. Nurses should advise patients with pruritus to avoid all of the following *except:*
    a. drying soaps.
    b. emollient lubricants.
    c. vigorous towel drying.
    d. warm to hot water.

12. A systemic pharmacologic agent prescribed for nodular cystic acne is:
    a. Accutane.
    b. benzoyl peroxide.
    c. Retin-A.
    d. salicylic acid.

13. Management of follicular disorders includes all of the following *except:*
    a. cleansing of the skin with an antibacterial soap to prevent spillage of bacteria to adjacent tissues.
    b. rupture of the boil or pimple to release the pus.
    c. systemic antibiotic therapy to treat the infection.
    d. warm, moist compresses to increase resolution of the furuncle or carbuncle.

14. Herpes zoster (shingles) is:
    a. a varicella-zoster viral infection related to chickenpox.
    b. an inflammatory condition that produces vesicular eruptions along nerve pathways.
    c. manifested by pain, itching, and tenderness.
    d. characterized by all of the above.

15. The most common fungal infection that frequently affects young adults is:
    a. tinea pedis.
    b. tinea corporis.
    c. tinea cruris.
    d. tinea unguium.

16. Tinea capitis (ringworm of the scalp) can be identified by the presence of:
    a. papules at the edges of inflamed patches.
    b. circular areas of redness.
    c. scaling and spots of baldness.
    d. all of the above.

17. Patient education for the management of pediculosis capitis should include advising the patient to:
    a. comb his or her hair with a fine-toothed comb dipped in vinegar to remove nits.
    b. disinfect all combs and brushes.
    c. wash his or her hair with a shampoo containing lindane (Kwell).
    d. do all of the above.

18. A patient is complaining of severe itching that intensifies at night. The nurse decides to assess the skin using a magnifying glass and penlight to look for the "itch mite." The nurse suspects the skin condition known as:
    a. contact dermatitis.
    b. pediculosis.
    c. scabies.
    d. tinea corporis.

19. Psoriasis is an inflammatory dermatosis that results from:
    a. a superficial infection with *Staphylococcus aureus*.
    b. dermal abrasion.
    c. epidermal proliferation.
    d. excess deposition of subcutaneous fat.

20. The characteristic lesion of psoriasis is a:
    a. raised patch covered with silver scales.
    b. cluster of pustules.
    c. group of raised vesicles.
    d. pattern of bullae that rupture and form a scaly crust.

21. Topical therapy for psoriasis would include all of the following *except*:
    a. Kenalog.
    b. Dovonex.
    c. Tegison.
    d. Valisone.

22. Exfoliate dermatitis is characterized by erythema and scaling and is associated with:
    a. a loss of stratum corneum.
    b. capillary leakage.
    c. hypoproteinemia.
    d. all of the above.

23. Nursing care for a patient with toxic epidermal necrolysis (TEN) should include:
    a. inspection of the oral cavity.
    b. assessment of urinary output.
    c. application of topical skin agents.
    d. all of the above actions.

24. The incidence of skin cancer among fair-skinned Americans is approximately:
    a. 8%.
    b. 12%.
    c. 20%.
    d. 35%.

25. Because sun damage is cumulative, the harmful effects of skin cancer may be severe by age:
    a. 20 years.
    b. 30 years.
    c. 40 years.
    d. 50 years.

26. Basal cell carcinoma tumors appear most frequently on the:
    a. face.
    b. chest.
    c. arms.
    d. hands.

27. Squamous cell metastases have a mortality rate of about:
    a. 25%.
    b. 40%.
    c. 60%.
    d. 75%.

28. The most lethal of all skin cancers is:
    a. basal cell.
    b. squamous cell.
    c. malignant melanoma.
    d. Kaposi's sarcoma.

29. Danger signals of melanoma include changes in a mole's:
    a. color.
    b. shape or outline.
    c. size or surface.
    d. all of the above.

30. The cause of Kaposi's sarcoma is believed to be:
    a. environmental.
    b. genetic.
    c. viral.
    d. a combination of one or all of the above.

31. A living tissue transplant from the same person is known as:

    a. an allograft.

    b. an alloplastic implant.

    c. an autograft.

    d. a xenograft.

32. For a graft to "take,"

    a. the area must be free of infection.

    b. the recipient bed must have an adequate blood supply.

    c. immobilization must be ensured.

    d. all of the above conditions must be present.

SHORT ANSWER

Read each statement carefully. Write your response in the space provided.

1. List four major objectives of therapy for patients with dermatologic problems.

   _____

   _____

   _____

   _____

2. Moisture-retentive dressings are very efficient at removing exudate because they: _____

   _____

3. Cytokines that have potent mitogenic activity work by: _____

   _____

4. A common nursing diagnosis for a patient with dermatosis would be: _____

   _____

5. The most common skin condition in adolescents and young adults between the ages of 12 and 35 years is _____.

6. The most common primary bacterial skin infections are _____ and

   _____.

7. Bullous impetigo, a deep-seated infection characterized by large, fluid-filled blisters, is caused by the bacteria _____.

8. Two major complications of TEN and Stevens-Johnson syndrome (SJS) are _____ and _____; the major cause of death is _____.

9. The most common cancer in the United States is _____. The most common types of this cancer are _____ and _____, and diagnosis is made by _____.

10. A major risk factor for malignant melanoma for young women younger than 30 years of age is use of a tanning bed _____ times per year.

SCRAMBLEGRAM

Complete the scramblegram by circling the word or words that answer each statement. Terms may be written in any direction.

S	C	U	F	A	M	V	I	R	S	O
A	L	A	U	O	X	C	Q	U	C	C
M	I	S	R	L	A	E	P	O	A	H
R	N	I	U	B	R	S	R	T	B	E
E	I	S	N	P	U	A	I	E	I	I
D	M	O	C	S	E	N	A	N	E	L
O	E	R	L	G	E	T	C	S	S	I
Y	N	E	E	A	E	Y	L	L	A	T
P	T	X	E	D	I	L	Y	A	E	I
S	S	C	O	M	E	D	O	N	E	S

DEFINITION OF TERMS

1. Primary lesion of acne
2. Dry, crackling skin at corners of mouth
3. Localized skin infection involving hair follicles
4. Localized skin infection involving only one hair follicle
5. The most common fungal infection of the skin or scalp
6. Bacterial skin infections
7. Lotions with added oil to soften skin
8. Overly dry skin
9. An enzymatic débriding agent
10. A semisolid emulsion that becomes liquid when applied to the skin or scalp
11. A topical corticosteroid with medium to high potency
12. An antiviral agent used to treat herpes zoster
13. An infestation of the skin caused by the itch mite
14. A prescription scabicide
15. A potentially fatal (35% mortality) skin disorder

II. Critical Thinking Questions and Exercises

DISCUSSION AND ANALYSIS

Discuss the following topics with your classmates.

1. Discuss the advantages of moisture-retentive dressings over wet dressings.
2. Explain why a foul odor will be present when autolytic débridement is used.
3. Distinguish between a furuncle and a carbuncle. Mention nursing and medical management.
4. Distinguish between herpes zoster and herpes simplex.
5. Explain the process of photochemotherapy.
6. Discuss the nursing and medical management of patients with TEN and SJS skin disorders.
7. Explain the five risk factors for developing malignant melanoma.

CLINICAL SITUATIONS

Read the following case studies. Fill in the blank spaces or circle the correct answer.

CASE STUDY: Acne Vulgaris

Brian is a 15-year-old boy who has been experiencing facial eruptions of acne for about 1 year. The numerous lesions are inflamed and are present on the face and neck. He has tried many over-the-counter medications and nothing seems to help. His father had a history of severe acne when he was a teenager.

1. Based on knowledge of acne vulgaris, the nurse knows that the skin disorder is characterized by five types of lesions: _____, _____, _____, _____, and _____.

2. The etiology of acne stems from:
   a. genetic factors.
   b. bacterial factors.
   c. hormonal factors.
   d. an interplay of all of the above.

3. Acne, most prevalent at puberty, is the direct result of oversecretion of which glands?
   a. exocrine
   b. lacrimal
   c. sebaceous
   d. mucous

4. Explain the rationale for using benzoyl peroxide: _____
   _____

5. Explain the rationale for using synthetic vitamin A compounds (retinoids): _____
   _____

6. A common antibiotic that is frequently prescribed for treatment of acne is:
   a. terbutaline.
   b. tamoxifen.
   c. tetracycline.
   d. terfenadine.

7. A common oral retinoid that is used for acne is:
   a. Accutane.
   b. Acne-Aid.
   c. Actinex.
   d. Adalat.

8. Based on assessment data, identify two collaborative problems.
   _____
   _____

CASE STUDY: Malignant Melanoma

Steve is a 26-year-old professional baseball player for a Florida farm team. He spent many hours in the sun practicing between 9:00 AM and 4:00 PM. His V-neck uniform left little protection to his chest. Steve had a mole on his chest for 5 years. One day last October he noticed that the margins of the mole were elevated and palpable and the color had become darker. Since his father had malignant melanoma when he was 32 years old, Steve decided to see a physician.

1. Steve knows that malignant melanoma currently comprises 3% of all cancers. Based on statistical predictions, the number of deaths in 10 years will be approximately:
   a. 2%.
   b. 4%.
   c. 6%.
   d. 10%.

2. The peak ages of occurrence are _____ to _____ years.

3. The physician knows that the mortality rate of malignant melanoma is increasing faster than that of any other cancer except for _____.

4. On examination, the physician notes a circular lesion with irregular outer edges and a pinkish hue in the center. The physician suspected the lesion to be:
   a. an acral-lentiginous melanoma.
   b. a lentigo-maligna melanoma.
   c. a nodular melanoma.
   d. a superficial spreading melanoma.

5. The physician confirms the diagnosis by:
   a. complete blood count analysis.
   b. computed tomography.
   c. excisional biopsy.
   d. skin examination.

6. The lesion is greater than 14 mm in thickness and growing vertically. The physician knows that:
   a. dermal invasion is likely.
   b. the prognosis is favorable.
   c. metastasis is probable.
   d. peripheral growth will occur next.

7. The physician considers immunotherapy with a biologic response modifier such as:
   a. interferon alfa.
   b. BCG vaccine.
   c. *Corynebacterium parvum*.
   d. levamisole.

8. The physician advises Steve that with lymph node involvement he only has a _____ percent chance of surviving 5 years.

CHAPTER 57

Management of Patients With Burn Injury

I. Interpretation, Completion, and Comparison

MULTIPLE CHOICE

Read each question carefully. Circle your answer.

1. A full-thickness burn is:
   a. classified by the appearance of blisters.
   b. identified by the destruction of the entire dermis.
   c. not associated with edema formation.
   d. usually very painful because of exposed nerve endings.

2. With partial-thickness (second-degree) burns, skin regeneration begins to take place:
   a. within 7 days.
   b. in 2 to 4 weeks.
   c. after 2 months.
   d. between the third and sixth month.

3. Plasma seeps out into surrounding tissues after a burn. The greatest amount of fluid leaks out in:
   a. the first 2 hours.
   b. 4 to 8 hours.
   c. 12 hours.
   d. 24 to 36 hours.

4. As fluid is reabsorbed after injury, renal function maintains a diuresis for up to:
   a. 3 days.
   b. 1 week.
   c. 2 weeks.
   d. 1 month.

5. Fluid shifts during the first week of the acute phase of a burn injury that cause massive cell destruction result in:
   a. hypernatremia.
   b. hypokalemia.
   c. hyperkalemia.
   d. hypercalcemia.

6. An unexpected laboratory value during the fluid remobilization phase of a major burn is a:
   a. hematocrit of 45%.
   b. a pH of 7.20, with a PaO_2 of 38 mm Hg and a bicarbonate value of 15 mEq/L.
   c. serum potassium of 3.2 mEq/L.
   d. serum sodium of 140 mEq/L.

7. Plasma leakage produces edema, which increases:
   a. circulating blood volume.
   b. the hematocrit level.
   c. systolic blood pressure.
   d. all of the above.

8. The leading cause of death in fire victims is believed to be:
   a. cardiac arrest.
   b. carbon monoxide intoxication.
   c. hypovolemic shock.
   d. septicemia.

9. A serious gastrointestinal disturbance that frequently occurs with a major burn is:
   a. diverticulitis.
   b. hematemesis.
   c. paralytic ileus.
   d. ulcerative colitis.

10. A child tips a pot of boiling water onto his bare legs. The mother should:
    a. avoid touching the burned skin, and take the child to the nearest emergency department.
    b. cover the child's legs with ice cubes secured with a towel.
    c. immerse the child's legs in cool water.
    d. liberally apply butter or shortening to the burned area.

11. A man suffers leg burns from spilled charcoal lighter fluid. His son extinguishes the flames. While waiting for an ambulance, the burn victim should:
    a. have someone assist him into a bath of cool water, where he can wait for emergency personnel.
    b. lie down, have someone cover him with a blanket, and cover his legs with petroleum jelly.
    c. remove his burned pants so that the air can help cool the wound.
    d. sit in a chair, elevate his legs, and have someone cut his pants off around the burned area.

12. As the first priority of care, a patient with a burn injury will initially need:
    a. an airway established.
    b. an indwelling catheter inserted.
    c. fluids replaced.
    d. pain medication administered.

13. Eyes that have been irritated or burned with a chemical should be flushed with cool, clean water:
    a. immediately.
    b. in 5 to 10 minutes.
    c. after an eye examination.
    d. after 24 hours.

14. A nurse knows that a burn injury of 25% of total body surface area is classified as:
    a. minor.
    b. moderate.
    c. major.
    d. severe.

15. Decreased urinary output during the first 48 hours of a major burn is secondary to all of the following *except*:
    a. decreased adrenocortical activity.
    b. hemolysis of red blood cells.
    c. hypovolemia.
    d. sodium retention.

16. Electrolyte changes in the first 48 hours of a major burn include:
    a. base bicarbonate deficit.
    b. hypernatremia.
    c. hypokalemia.
    d. all of the above.

17. The Evans formula for replacing fluid lost during the first 24 to 48 hours recommends the administration of:
    a. colloids.
    b. electrolytes.
    c. glucose.
    d. all of the above.

18. The most recent consensus formula for fluid replacement recommends that a balanced salt solution be administered in the first 24 hours of a burn in the range of 2 mL/kg per percentage of burn. A 176-lb (80-kg) man with a 30% burn should receive how much fluid replacement in the first 8 hours?
    a. 1200 mL
    b. 2400 mL
    c. 3600 mL
    d. 4800 mL

19. A burn patient has been prescribed fluids using the Brooke Army Formula. The nurse knows that D5W (2000 mL) should be administered:
    a. immediately within 12 hours.
    b. slowly over a 36-hour period.
    c. by dividing half in the first 8 hours.
    d. by dividing evenly over 24 hours.

20. Fluid and electrolyte changes in the emergent phase of burn injury include all of the following *except*:
    a. base-bicarbonate deficit.
    b. elevated hematocrit.
    c. potassium deficit.
    d. sodium deficit.

21. During the acute phase of burn injury, the nurse knows to assess for signs of potassium shifting:
    a. within 24 hours.
    b. between 24 and 48 hours.
    c. at the beginning of the third day.
    d. beginning on day 4 or day 5.

22. One parameter of adequate fluid replacement is an hourly urinary output in the range of:
    a. 10 to 30 mL.
    b. 30 to 50 mL.
    c. 80 to 120 mL.
    d. 100 to 200 mL.

23. During the fluid remobilization phase, the nurse knows to expect all of the following *except*:
    a. hemodilution.
    b. increased urinary output.
    c. metabolic alkalosis.
    d. sodium deficit.

24. Fluid remobilization usually begins:
    a. within the first 24 hours, when massive amounts of fluid are being administered intravenously.
    b. after 48 hours, when fluid is being reabsorbed from the interstitial tissue.
    c. after 1 week, when capillary permeability has returned to normal.
    d. after 1 month, when scar tissue covers the wound and prevents evaporative fluid loss.

25. Wound cleansing and débridement usually begin when eschar begins to separate at:
    a. 72 hours.
    b. 1 week.
    c. 1.5 to 2 weeks.
    d. 1 month.

26. Leukopenia within 48 hours is a side effect associated with the topical antibacterial agent:
    a. cerium nitrate solution.
    b. gentamicin sulfate.
    c. sulfadiazine, silver (Silvadene).
    d. mafenide (Sulfamylon).

27. The nurse knows that the topical antibacterial agent that does not penetrate eschar is:
    a. Acticort.
    b. mafenide acetate.
    c. silver nitrate 0.5%.
    d. silver sulfadiazine 1%.

28. The nurse knows to monitor sodium and potassium levels (drug is hypotonic) when a burn patient is being treated with:
    a. Silvadene.
    b. silver nitrate 0.5%.
    c. Sulfamylon.
    d. all of the above.

29. After an occlusive dressing is applied to a burned foot, the foot should be placed in the position of:
    a. adduction.
    b. dorsiflexion.
    c. external rotation.
    d. plantar flexion.

CHAPTER 57 ■ **Management of Patients With Burn Injury** **355**

30. Biologic dressings that use skin from living or recently deceased humans are known as:
    a. autografts.
    b. heterografts.
    c. homografts.
    d. xenografts.

31. An example of a permanent burn wound covering that is used to support an autograft is:
    a. Alloderm.
    b. Aquacel.
    c. Biobrane.
    d. Integra.

32. The nurse knows the physician will most likely prescribe the analgesic of choice for treatment of acute burn pain, which is:
    a. Demerol.
    b. Fentanyl.
    c. morphine sulfate.
    d. OxyContin.

33. The recommended route for administration of low-dose narcotics is:
    a. intramuscular.
    b. intravenous.
    c. oral.
    d. subcutaneous.

34. To meet his early nutritional demands for protein, a 198-lb (90-kg) burned patient will need to ingest a minimum of:
    a. 90 g/day.
    b. 110 g/day.
    c. 180 g/day.
    d. 270 g/day.

35. Early indicators of late-stage septic shock include all of the following *except:*
    a. decreased pulse pressure.
    b. a full, bounding pulse.
    c. pale, cool skin.
    d. renal failure.

SHORT ANSWER

Read each statement carefully. Write your response in the space provided.

1. The two age groups that are at high risk for burn injury are _____ and _____.

2. The majority of burn injuries occur _____ (location).

3. About 1 million persons per year require medical attention for burns. Of these, _____% require acute hospital admission.

4. Burn injuries are classified according to _____ and _____.

5. List two pulmonary complications that occur secondary to inhalation injuries.

   _____

   _____

6. The leading cause of death in thermally injured patients is _____.

7. The first priority of on-the-scene care for a person with a burn injury is to prevent:

   _____

Copyright © 2008 by Lippincott Williams & Wilkins. *Study Guide to Accompany: Brunner and Suddarth's Textbook of Medical-Surgical Nursing,* 11th edition, by Mary Jo Boyer.

8. The analgesic of choice for acute burn pain is: _____

_____

9. List four collaborative problems for a patient during the emergent phase of burn injury.

_____

_____

_____

_____

10. List five bacteria and one fungus that are responsible for infection in a burn wound.

_____

_____

_____

_____

_____

_____

11. List three disorders of wound healing.

_____

_____

_____

II. Critical Thinking Questions and Exercises

DISCUSSION AND ANALYSIS

Discuss the following topics with your classmates.

1. Explain why the survival rate for burn victims has increased significantly over the last 10 years.
2. Explain the pathophysiology of carbon monoxide poisoning.
3. Describe general emergency procedures that a nurse should employ at the burn scene.
4. Describe the nurses' role during the immediate burn injury phase using the ABCs of trauma care.
5. Compare and contrast the extent of burn injury in burns classified as minor, moderate, and major.
6. Discuss general nursing actions for six nursing diagnoses for care of a patient during the emergent phase of burn injury.
7. Discuss why congestive heart failure is a potential complication of an acute burn.

IDENTIFYING PATTERNS

Complete the flow chart illustrating the pathophysiologic sequence of reactions that result from a systemic response to a burn injury.

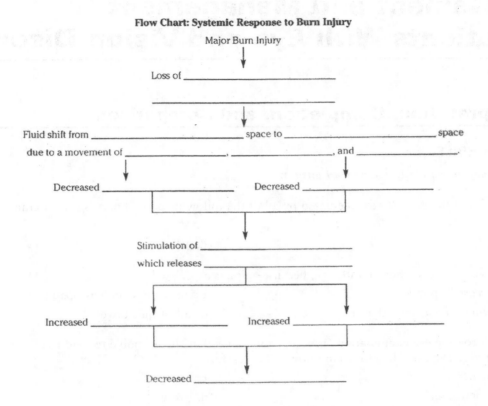

Flow Chart: Systemic Response to Burn Injury

Major Burn Injury

Loss of _____

_____

Fluid shift from _____ space to _____ space due to a movement of _____, _____, and _____.

Decreased _____   Decreased _____

Stimulation of _____

which releases _____

Increased _____   Increased _____

Decreased _____

CLINICAL SITUATIONS

Develop a nursing care plan for each of the two situations described. For each nursing diagnosis, list goals, nursing actions, rationale, and expected outcomes.

1. Aimee, 9 months old, climbed onto a stove where an electric range was on high. Her pajamas caught fire, and she was burned over 60% of her body (excluding her face and neck) with second- and third-degree burns. Her mother managed to extinguish the flames and immerse her in a sink of cool water before emergency help arrived. Aimee was transported to a burn treatment center. There are two other preschool children in her family.
2. Brad, 12 years old, sustained full-thickness burns on his upper chest, face, and neck when he was trying to start a charcoal fire to prepare dinner for his father. His father sprayed him with water from a hose and took him to a hospital emergency department 3 miles away. On arrival Brad was semiconscious and in extreme respiratory distress. He and his divorced father live together.

CHAPTER 58

Assessment and Management of Patients With Eye and Vision Disorders

I. Interpretation, Completion, and Comparison

MULTIPLE CHOICE

Read each question carefully. Circle your answer.

1. The muscles of the eyeball are innervated by all of the following cranial nerves *except* cranial nerve:
   a. III.
   b. IV.
   c. V.
   d. VI.

2. Vision becomes less efficient with age, because aging is associated with:
   a. a decrease in pupil size.
   b. a slowing of accommodation.
   c. an increase in lens opaqueness.
   d. all of the above.

3. During a routine eye examination, a patient complains that she is unable to read road signs at a distance when driving her car. The physician knows to check for:
   a. astigmatism.
   b. anisometropia.
   c. myopia.
   d. presbyopia.

4. Legal blindness refers to visual acuity that is at or worse than:
   a. 20/50.
   b. 20/100.
   c. 20/150.
   d. 20/200.

5. Increased ocular pressure, resulting from optic nerve damage, is indicated by a reading of:
   a. 0 to 5 mm Hg.
   b. 6 to 10 mm Hg.
   c. 11 to 20 mm Hg.
   d. 21 mm Hg or higher.

6. A diagnostic clinical manifestation of glaucoma is:
   a. a significant loss of central vision.
   b. diminished acuity.
   c. pain associated with a purulent discharge.
   d. the presence of halos around lights.

7. When assessing the visual fields in acute glaucoma, the nurse would expect to find a:
   a. clear cornea.
   b. constricted pupil.
   c. marked blurring of vision.
   d. watery ocular discharge.

8. Pharmacotherapy for primary glaucoma that decreases the outflow of aqueous humor would include all of the following *except*:
   a. alpha-adrenergic agonists.
   b. carbonic anhydrase inhibitors.
   c. beta-blockers.
   d. miotics.

9. After cataract surgery, a patient is encouraged to:

   a. maintain bed rest for 1 week.

   b. lie on his or her stomach while sleeping.

   c. avoid bending his or her head below the waist.

   d. lift weights to increase muscle strength.

10. Clinical symptoms of a detached retina include:

    a. a sensation of floating particles.

    b. a definite area of blank vision.

    c. momentary flashes of light.

    d. all of the above.

11. The most common type of retinal detachment is:

    a. exudative.

    b. rhegmatogenous.

    c. traction.

    d. a combination of rhegmatogenous and traction.

12. The most common cause of visual loss in people older than 60 years of age is:

    a. macular degeneration.

    b. ocular trauma.

    c. retinal vascular disease.

    d. uveitis.

13. Chemical burns of the eye are treated with:

    a. local anesthetics and antibacterial drops for 24 to 36 hours.

    b. hot compresses applied at 15-minute intervals.

    c. flushing of the lids, conjunctiva, and cornea.

    d. cleansing of the conjunctiva with a small cotton-tipped applicator.

14. Acute bacterial conjunctivitis is characterized by:

    a. blurred vision.

    b. elevated intraocular pressure.

    c. a mucopurulent ocular discharge.

    d. severe pain.

15. The most common neoplasm of the eyelids is:

    a. basal cell carcinoma.

    b. a chalazion.

    c. xanthelasmas.

    d. squamous cell carcinoma.

16. What type of medication is used in combination with mydriatics to dilate a patient's pupil?

    a. anti-infectives

    b. corticosteroids

    c. cycloplegics

    d. NSAIDs

17. The most common antifungal agent used to treat eye infections is:

    a. acyclovir.

    b. amphotericin.

    c. ganciclovir.

    d. penicillin.

SHORT ANSWER

Read each statement carefully. Write your response in the space provided.

1. A visual acuity examination result of 20/100 is interpreted to mean: _____

   _____

2. List four common causes of visual impairment on blindness in those older than 40 years of age.

   _____

   _____

   _____

   _____

3. The leading cause of irreversible blindness in the world is: _____
_____

4. Two significant changes in the optic nerve in glaucoma are _____ and
_____.

5. The most common laser surgeries for glaucoma are _____ and
_____.

6. According to the World Health Organization, the leading cause of blindness in the world is
_____.

7. List four clinical symptoms indicative of a detached retina.

_____

_____

_____

_____

8. An initial treatment for a splash injury to the eye would be: _____
_____

9. The microorganisms that most commonly cause conjunctivitis are _____,
_____, and _____.

10. A characteristic sign of viral conjunctivitis is _____.

11. One of the most serious ocular consequences of diabetes mellitus is _____.

12. The most common cause of retinal inflammation in patients with AIDS is _____.

Matching

Match the characteristic or function of the eye in column II with its associated structure listed in column I.

Column I

1. _____ Choroid

2. _____ Lens

3. _____ Pupil

4. _____ Retina

5. _____ Vitreous humor

6. _____ Cornea

7. _____ Sclera

8. _____ Iris

9. _____ Uvea

10. _____ Limbus

Column II

a. Maintains the form of the eyeball

b. Area where most of the blood vessels for the eye are located

c. Degree of convexity modified by contraction and relaxation of the ciliary muscles

d. Contractile membrane between the cornea and lens

e. Transparent part of the fibrous coat of the eyeball

f. Accommodates to the intensity of light by dilating or contracting

g. White part of the eye

h. The pigmented, vascular coating of the eye

i. The edge of the cornea where it joins the sclera

j. Contains nerve endings that transmit visual impulses to the brain

CROSSWORD PUZZLE

Complete the crossword puzzle using common ophthalmologic terms.

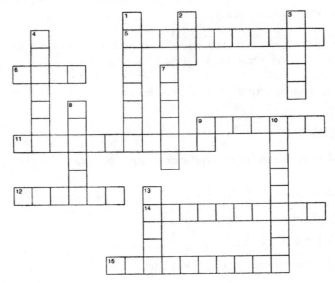

DOWN

1. Excessive production of tears
2. Another term for an external hordeolum
3. The term *oculus dexter* refers to this eye
4. A term used to describe an inflammatory condition of the uveal tract
7. Another term for nearsightedness
8. An inflammatory condition affecting the iris
9. People who are photosensitive function better outdoors during this time of day
10. Inflammation of the cornea
13. A loss of cornea substance or tissue as a result of inflammation

ACROSS

5. Abnormal sensitivity to light
6. The term *oculus sinister* refers to this eye
9. Absence of the lens
11. Uneven curvature of the cornea
12. Drooping of the upper eyelid
14. A tear in the eye tissue
15. A condition in which one eye deviates from the object at which the person is looking

II. Critical Thinking Questions and Exercises

EXTRACTING INFERENCES

Examine Figure 58-1 in the text. List the specific functions for each external structure of the eye.

1. Lacrimal sac, gland, and duct: _____
2. Pupil: _____
3. Iris: _____
4. Limbus: _____
5. Sclera: _____
6. Conjunctiva: _____
7. Outer and inner canthus: _____
8. Upper eyelid: _____
9. Caruncle: _____

DISCUSSION AND ANALYSIS

Discuss the following topics with your classmates.

1. Explain the clinical manifestations of altered vision seen in those with cataracts.
2. Distinguish between two types of refractive surgery: PRK and LASIK.
3. Describe dry eye syndrome.
4. Distinguish among the following surgical procedures: enucleation, evisceration, and exenteration.

INTERPRETING PATTERNS

For each group of clustered clues, identify the specific disorder of the eye.

A chronic inflammation of the eyelid margins

Formation of scales and granulations on the eyelashes

White eyelashes may result from this condition

Staphylococcus aureus may be a primary infecting organism

1. _____
A superficial infection of the glands of the eyelids

Pain and swelling of the eyelids are characteristic signs

Warm, moist compresses on the eyelids facilitate healing

Topical sulfonamides may be prescribed

2. _____
Symptoms include hyperemia and edema of conjunctiva

Etiology may be bacterial, fungal, viral, or allergic

Lay person's term for condition is "pink-eye"

3. _____

Corneal edema is a common sign in this disorder

Ulceration and infection are associated with this disorder

Cycloplegics and mydriatics may be prescribed

Etiology is usually associated with trauma or compromise

Systemic or local defense mechanisms

4. _____

Characterized by an opacification of the lens

Usually associated with the aging process

Vision is clouded because light to the retina is blocked

Associated with compromised night vision

5. _____

CLINICAL SITUATIONS

Read the following case study. Fill in the blank spaces or circle the correct answer.

CASE STUDY: Cataract Surgery

Marcella is a 75-year-old single woman who has had progressive diminished vision and increased difficulty with night driving. Her physician suspects that Marcella has a cataract. He does a complete eye examination and history.

1. As part of an oral history, the physician tries to determine whether Marcella has any of the common factors that contribute to cataract development, such as _____, _____, and _____.

2. Marcella, during her history, told the physician that she was experiencing the three common symptoms found with cataracts: _____, _____, and _____.

3. On ophthalmic examination, the physician noted the major objective finding seen with cataracts: _____.

4. When assessing the need for surgery, the physician determined that Marcella's best corrected vision was worse than the minimal standard of:
   a. 20/15.
   b. 20/25.
   c. 20/35.
   d. 20/50.

5. The physician decided to perform _____, the most preferred technique for cataract surgery.

6. Postoperatively, Marcella knows that she will need to avoid lying on the side of the affected eye for a period of _____.

NURSING CARE PLANS

Develop a nursing care plan for each of the two situations below. For each nursing diagnosis, list goals, nursing actions, rationale, and expected outcomes.

Elise is 65 years old and needs to have cataract surgery on her right eye. Elise lives with her daughter in a three-story house and has rheumatoid arthritis. She needs a cane to walk. Her daughter has a child at home who has Down syndrome and requires constant care. Share your nursing care plan with your instructor for comments.

CHAPTER 59

Assessment and Management of Patients With Hearing and Balance Disorders

I. Interpretation, Completion, and Comparison

MULTIPLE CHOICE

Read each question carefully. Circle your answer.

1. The organ of hearing is known as the:
   a. cochlea.
   b. eardrum.
   c. semicircular canal.
   d. stapes.

2. Mechanical vibrations are transformed into neural activity so that sounds can be differentiated by the:
   a. cochlea.
   b. organ of Corti.
   c. ossicles.
   d. semicircular canals.

3. To straighten the ear canal for examination, the nurse would grasp the auricle and pull it:
   a. backward.
   b. upward.
   c. slightly outward.
   d. in all of these directions.

4. A sensorineural (perceptive) hearing loss results from impairment of the:
   a. eighth cranial nerve.
   b. middle ear.
   c. outer ear.
   d. seventh cranial nerve.

5. The critical level of loudness that most people (without a hearing loss) are comfortable with is a decibel (dB) reading of:
   a. 15 dB.
   b. 30 dB.
   c. 45 dB.
   d. 60 dB.

6. Severe hearing loss is associated with a decibel loss in the range of:
   a. 25 to 40 dB.
   b. 40 to 55 dB.
   c. 70 to 90 dB.
   d. more than 90 dB.

7. A hearing loss that is a manifestation of an emotional disturbance is known as what kind of hearing loss?
   a. conductive
   b. functional
   c. mixed
   d. sensorineural

8. The minimum noise level known to cause noise-induced hearing loss, regardless of duration, is:
   a. 55 to 60 dB.
   b. 65 to 70 dB.
   c. 75 to 80 dB.
   d. 85 to 90 dB.

9. Hearing loss occurs in about what percentage of people between 65 and 75 years of age?
   a. 15%
   b. 30%
   c. 50%
   d. 75%

10. Changes in the ear that occur with aging may include:
    a. atrophy of the tympanic membrane.
    b. increased hardness of the cerumen.
    c. degeneration of cells at the base of the cochlea.
    d. all of the above.

11. The most common fungus associated with ear infections is:
    a. *Staphylococcus albus*.
    b. *Staphylococcus aureus*.
    c. *Aspergillus*.
    d. *Pseudomonas*.

12. Nursing instructions for a patient with external otitis should include the:
    a. application of heat to the auricle.
    b. avoidance of swimming.
    c. ingestion of over-the-counter analgesics such as aspirin.
    d. all of the above.

13. A symptom that is *not* usually found with acute otitis media is:
    a. aural tenderness.
    b. rhinitis.
    c. otalgia.
    d. otorrhea.

14. An incident of otitis media is usually associated with:
    a. ear canal swelling.
    b. discharge.
    c. intense ear pain.
    d. prominent localized tenderness.

15. A myringotomy is performed primarily to:
    a. drain purulent fluid.
    b. identify the infecting organism.
    c. relieve tympanic membrane pressure.
    d. accomplish all of the above.

16. A tympanoplasty, the most common procedure for chronic otitis media, is surgically performed to:
    a. close a perforation.
    b. prevent recurrent infection.
    c. reestablish middle ear function.
    d. accomplish all of the above.

17. Postoperative nursing assessment for a patient who has had a mastoidectomy should include observing for facial paralysis, which might indicate damage to which cranial nerve?
    a. first
    b. fourth
    c. seventh
    d. tenth

18. A facial nerve neuroma is a tumor on which cranial nerve?
    a. third
    b. fifth
    c. seventh
    d. eighth

19. A dietary modification for a patient with Ménière's disease would be:
    a. a decrease in sodium intake to 2000 mg/day.
    b. fluid restriction to 2.0 L/day.
    c. an increase in calcium to 1.0 g/day.
    d. an increase in vitamin C to 1.5 g/day.

20. An acoustic neuroma is a benign tumor of which cranial nerve?
    a. fifth
    b. sixth
    c. seventh
    d. eighth

II. Critical Thinking Questions and Exercises

DISCUSSION AND ANALYSIS

Discuss the following topics with your classmates.

1. Distinguish among three tests used to evaluate gross auditory acuity: the Rhine test, the Weber test, and the whisper test.
2. Distinguish among three types of hearing aids: behind the ear, in the ear, and in the canal.
3. Describe at least six risk factors associated with hearing loss.

EXAMINING ASSOCIATIONS

View the accompanying figure. For each anatomic area labeled, write the associated physiologic function.

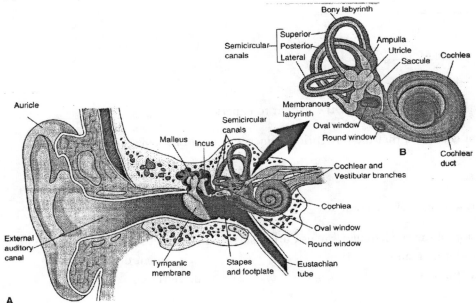

(A) Anatomy of the ear. **(B)** The inner ear.

1. Auricle: _____
2. Malleus: _____
3. Incus: _____
4. Semicircular canals: _____
5. Cochlea: _____
6. Oval window: _____
7. Round window: _____
8. Eustachian tube: _____
9. Stapes: _____
10. Tympanic membrane: _____
11. External auditory canal: _____

CLINICAL SITUATIONS

Read the following case studies. Fill in the blanks or circle the correct answer.

CASE STUDY: Mastoid Surgery

Amber is a 73-year-old grandmother who is scheduled for mastoid surgery to remove a cholesteatoma, a cystlike sac filled with keratin debris, which was large enough to occlude the ear canal.

1. Preoperatively, the physician reviews the results of the audiogram and assesses for the presence of associated ear problems, such as _____, _____, _____, _____, _____, _____, _____, and _____.

2. Identify four major preoperative nursing goals for the patient.

   _____

   _____

   _____

   _____

3. Postoperatively, it is common for the patient to experience _____.

4. The patient is advised that the postauricular incision should be kept dry for:
   a. 7 days.
   b. 2 weeks.
   c. 6 weeks.
   d. 1 month.

5. Two important signs of infection are _____ and _____.

6. Manipulation of the semicircular canals during surgery may result in the symptom of:
   a. sharp, shooting pain.
   b. inner ear fullness.
   c. purulent drainage.
   d. vertigo.

7. The patient is advised that it is normal to hear popping and crackling sounds in the affected ear for about:
   a. 3 days.
   b. 1 week.
   c. 3 to 5 weeks.
   d. 2 to 4 months.

8. The patient is taught to avoid activities that increase intracranial pressure for 2 to 3 weeks after surgery, including _____, _____, and _____.

Case Study: Ménière's Disease

David is a 42-year-old lawyer who travels internationally. He has recently been diagnosed with Ménière's disease.

1. List at least three classic symptoms that are diagnostic for Ménière's disease: _____

   _____

2. The basic pathophysiology causing this classic triad of symptoms is:

   _____

   _____

3. The most common and disrupting clinical symptom of this disease is _____

   _____

4. As part of a diet for Ménière's disease, David should avoid:

   a. bread.

   b. cheese.

   c. eggs.

   d. milk.

5. A popular medication prescribed to suppress the vestibular system is:

   a. Antivert.

   b. Lasix.

   c. Phenergan.

   d. Valium.

6. The most popular surgical procedure used to treat this disease is:

   a. endolymphatic sac decompression.

   b. labyrinthectomy.

   c. middle ear perfusion.

   d. vestibular nerve section.

CHAPTER 60

Assessment of Neurologic Function

I. Interpretation, Completion, and Comparison

MULTIPLE CHOICE

Read each question carefully. Circle your answer.

1. A neurotransmitter that helps control mood and sleep is:
   a. acetylcholine.
   b. dopamine.
   c. enkephalin.
   d. serotonin.

2. Parkinson's disease is caused by an imbalance in the neurotransmitter known as:
   a. acetylcholine.
   b. dopamine.
   c. GABA.
   d. endorphin.

3. A person's personality and judgment are controlled by that area of the brain known as the:
   a. frontal lobe.
   b. occipital lobe.
   c. parietal lobe.
   d. temporal lobe.

4. The lobe of the cerebral cortex that is responsible for visual interpretation is the:
   a. frontal lobe.
   b. occipital lobe.
   c. parietal lobe.
   d. temporal lobe.

5. Voluntary muscle control is governed by a vertical band of "motor cortex" located in the:
   a. frontal lobe.
   b. occipital lobe.
   c. parietal lobe.
   d. temporal lobe.

6. The sleep regulator and the site of the hunger center is known as the:
   a. hypothalamus.
   b. medulla oblongata.
   c. pituitary gland.
   d. thalamus.

7. The overall supervision of the autonomic nervous system is the function of the:
   a. cerebellum.
   b. hypothalamus.
   c. pons.
   d. temporal lobe of the cerebral cortex.

8. The "master gland" is also known as the:
   a. adrenal gland.
   b. thyroid gland.
   c. pineal gland.
   d. pituitary gland.

9. The major receiving and communication center for afferent sensory nerves is the:
   a. medulla oblongata.
   b. pineal body.
   c. pituitary gland.
   d. thalamus.

10. The normal adult produces about 150 mL of cerebrospinal fluid daily from the:
    a. ventricles.
    b. dura mater.
    c. circle of Willis.
    d. corpus callosum.

11. The spinal cord tapers off to a fibrous band of tissue at the level of the:
    a. coccygeal nerve.
    b. first lumbar vertebra.
    c. lateral ventricle.
    d. medulla oblongata.

12. The preganglionic fibers of the sympathetic neurons are located in those segments of the spinal cord identified as:
    a. C1 to T1.
    b. C3 to L1.
    c. C8 to L3.
    d. T1 to S5.

13. Parasympathetic impulses are mediated by the secretion of:
    a. acetylcholine.
    b. epinephrine.
    c. norepinephrine.
    d. all of the above.

14. Motor axons form pyramidal tracts that cross to the opposite side. This crossed pyramidal tract occurs in the brain in the area of the:
    a. frontal cerebrum.
    b. lateral portion of the cerebellum.
    c. medulla oblongata.
    d. pons.

15. The brain center responsible for balancing and coordination is the:
    a. cerebellum.
    b. second lumbar vertebra.
    c. first sacral nerve.
    d. sacrum.

16. The Romberg test is used to assess:
    a. balance and coordination.
    b. muscle strength.
    c. biceps reflex.
    d. muscle tone.

17. The Babinski response is used to assess:
    a. muscle strength.
    b. coordination.
    c. central nervous system disease.
    d. optical nerve damage.

18. To reduce leakage of cerebrospinal fluid after myelography with an oil-based medium, the patient must lie for 12 to 24 hours in what position?
    a. high Fowler's position
    b. with the head of the bed elevated 30 to 45 degrees
    c. prone
    d. recumbent

19. Patient preparation for electroencephalography includes omitting, for 24 hours before the test, all of the following *except:*
    a. coffee and tea.
    b. solid foods.
    c. stimulants.
    d. tranquilizers.

20. For a lumbar puncture, the nurse should assist the patient to flex his or her head and thighs while lying on the side so that the needle can be inserted between the:

a. fourth and fifth cervical vertebrae.

b. fifth and sixth thoracic vertebrae.

c. third and fourth lumbar vertebrae.

d. first and second sacral vertebrae.

21. After a lumbar puncture, the nurse knows to assess for the most common (30% occurrence) complication:

a. epidural abscess.

b. epidural hematoma.

c. throbbing headache.

d. meningitis.

MATCHING

Match the nervous system response in column II with the neurotransmitter listed in column I.

Column I

1. _____ Gamma-aminobutyric acid

2. _____ Enkephalin

3. _____ Norepinephrine

4. _____ Dopamine

5. _____ Acetylcholine

6. _____ Serotonin

Column II

a. Primarily excitatory; can produce vagal stimulation of heart

b. Inhibits pain pathways and can control sleep

c. Affects behavior, attention, and fine movement

d. Excitatory response, mostly affecting moods

e. Muscle and nerve inhibitory transmissions

f. Excitatory; inhibits pain transmission

II. Critical Thinking Questions and Exercises

EXAMINING ASSOCIATIONS

Write the effects produced by the parasympathetic and sympathetic nervous systems on each organ or tissue. Use the terms provided, and document in the space below. An example is provided.

Autonomic Nervous System

TERMS TO BE USED

Acceleration
Inhibition
Constriction
Increased motility
Dilation
Secretion

ORGAN OR TISSUE

a. Bronchi
b. Cerebral vessels
c. Coronary vessels
d. Heart
e. Iris of the eye
f. Salivary glands
g. Smooth muscle of bladder wall
h. Smooth muscle of large intestine
i. Smooth muscle of small intestine

PARASYMPATHETIC EFFECT

Constriction _____

_____

_____

_____

_____

_____

_____

_____

SYMPATHETIC EFFECT

Dilation _____

_____

_____

_____

_____

_____

_____

_____

Cranial Nerves

Next to each cranial nerve listed by number, write the name of the nerve in column I and a major associated function in column II. An example is provided.

CRANIAL NERVE	COLUMN I	COLUMN II
I	Olfactory	Smell
II		
III		
IV		
V		
VI		
VII		
VIII		
IX		
X		
XI		
XII		

APPLYING CONCEPTS

View the diagram of the brain below and list the major functions of each identified area.

Medial view of the brain.

THALAMUS

1. _____
2. _____

HYPOTHALAMUS

1. _____
2. _____
3. _____
4. _____
5. _____
6. _____
7. _____
8. _____

PITUITARY

1. _____
2. _____

CHAPTER 61

Management of Patients With Neurologic Dysfunction

I. Interpretation, Completion, and Comparison

MULTIPLE CHOICE

Read each question carefully. Circle your answer.

1. Unconsciousness may have what type of origin?

   a. neurologic

   b. metabolic

   c. toxicologic

   d. multisystem involvement

2. The first priority of treatment for a patient with altered level of consciousness is:

   a. assessment of pupillary light reflexes.

   b. determination of the cause.

   c. positioning to prevent complications.

   d. maintenance of a patent airway.

3. A nurse assesses the patient's level of consciousness using the Glasgow Coma Scale. Which score indicates severe impairment of neurologic function?

   a. 3

   b. 6

   c. 9

   d. 12

4. The most severe neurologic impairments are evidenced by the abnormal body posturing defined as:

   a. decerebrate.

   b. decorticate.

   c. flaccid.

   d. rigid.

5. The normal range of intracranial pressure (ICP) is:

   a. 5 to 8 mm Hg.

   b. 10 to 20 mm Hg.

   c. 20 to 30 mm Hg.

   d. 25 to 40 mm Hg.

6. Intracranial pressure can be increased by a:

   a. decrease in venous outflow.

   b. dilation of the cerebral blood vessels.

   c. rise in $PaCO_2$.

   d. change in all of the above.

7. Initial compensatory vital sign changes with increased ICP include all of the following *except*:

   a. a slow, bounding pulse.

   b. an increased systemic blood pressure.

   c. a decreased temperature.

   d. respiratory rate irregularities.

8. A patient is admitted to the hospital with an ICP reading of 20 mm Hg and an arterial pressure of 90 mm Hg. The nurse knows that the cerebral perfusion pressure would be calculated at:

   a. 50 mm Hg.

   b. 60 mm Hg.

   c. 70 mm Hg.

   d. 80 mm Hg.

9. Irreversible neurologic dysfunction occurs when the cerebral perfusion pressure (CPP) is:
   a. less than 50 mm Hg.
   b. 60 to 80 mm Hg.
   c. 75 to 95 mm Hg.
   d. greater than 100 mm Hg.

10. A nurse knows that a patient experiencing Cushing's triad would *not* exhibit:
    a. bradycardia.
    b. bradypnea.
    c. hypertension.
    d. tachycardia.

11. The earliest sign of serious impairment of brain circulation related to increasing ICP is:
    a. a bounding pulse.
    b. bradycardia.
    c. hypertension.
    d. lethargy and stupor.

12. As ICP rises, the nurse knows that she may be asked to give a commonly used osmotic diuretic:
    a. glycerin.
    b. isosorbide.
    c. mannitol.
    d. urea.

13. An indicator of compromised respiratory status significant enough to require mechanical ventilation for an average-weight adult patient with a neurologic dysfunction would be:
    a. an expiratory reserve volume of 1300 mL.
    b. an inspiratory capacity of 3000 mL.
    c. a residual volume of 1400 mL.
    d. a vital capacity of 1000 mL.

14. Nursing care activities for a patient with increased ICP would *not* include:
    a. assisting the patient with isometric exercises.
    b. avoiding activities that interfere with venous drainage of blood from the head.
    c. use of a cervical collar.
    d. teaching the patient to exhale when being turned (to avoid the Valsalva maneuver).

15. A nurse assessing urinary output as an indicator of diabetes insipidus knows that an hourly output of what volume over 2 hours may be a positive indicator?
    a. 50 to 100 mL/hour
    b. 100 to 150 mL/hour
    c. 150 to 200 mL/hour
    d. more than 200 mL/hour

16. Neurologic and neurosurgical approaches to pain relief would include:
    a. stimulation procedures.
    b. administration of intraspinal opiates.
    c. interruption of nerve tracts that conduct pain.
    d. all of the above mechanisms.

17. Postcraniotomy cerebral edema is at a maximum how long after brain surgery?
    a. 6 hours
    b. 12 to 20 hours
    c. 24 to 72 hours
    d. 3 to 5 days

18. The majority of cases of epilepsy occur in those:
    a. younger than 20 years of age.
    b. 25 to 35 years of age.
    c. approximately 45 years of age.
    d. older than 60 years of age.

19. Long-term use of anti-seizure medication in women leads to an increased incidence of:
    a. anemia.
    b. osteoarthritis.
    c. osteoporosis.
    d. obesity.

20. Nursing care for a patient who is experiencing a convulsive seizure includes all of the following *except:*
    a. loosening constrictive clothing.
    b. opening the patient's jaw and inserting a mouth gag.
    c. positioning the patient on his or her side with head flexed forward.
    d. providing for privacy.

21. A seizure characterized by loss of consciousness and tonic spasms of the trunk and extremities, rapidly followed by repetitive generalized clonic jerking, is classified as a:
    a. focal seizure.
    b. generalized seizure.
    c. Jacksonian seizure.
    d. partial seizure.

22. A nutritional approach for seizure management includes a diet that is:
    a. low in fat.
    b. restricts protein to 10% of daily caloric intake.
    c. high in protein and low in carbohydrate.
    d. at least 50% carbohydrate.

23. Headaches classified as primary would include all of the following *except:*
    a. aneurysm.
    b. cluster.
    c. migraine.
    d. tension.

24. A most widely used drug for the treatment of a migraine headache is:
    a. Amerge.
    b. Imitrex.
    c. Maxalt.
    d. Zomig.

SHORT ANSWER

Read each statement carefully. Write your response in the space provided.

1. Potential collaborative problems for a patient with an altered level of consciousness would include _____, _____, _____, _____, and _____.

2. List three major potential complications in a patient with a depressed level of consciousness.

   _____

   _____

   _____

3. The earliest sign of increased ICP is _____.

4. List three primary complications of increased ICP.

   _____

   _____

   _____

5. List six treatment goals for the prompt management of increased ICP.

   _____

   _____

   _____

   _____

   _____

   _____

6. Name four ICP monitoring devices that a nurse may be asked to manage.

   _____

   _____

   _____

   _____

7. The primary, lethal complication of ICP is _____.

8. Name three complications of intracranial surgery.

   _____

   _____

   _____

9. The leading cause of seizures in the elderly is _____.

10. A major potential complication of epilepsy is _____.

11. List six "triggers" known to cause migraine headaches.

    _____

    _____

    _____

    _____

    _____

    _____

MATCHING

Match the neurologic dysfunction in column II with its associated nursing intervention listed in column I. An answer may be used more than once.

Column I

1. _____ Assist with daily active or passive range of motion

2. _____ Elevate the head of the bed 30 degrees

3. _____ Institute a bowel-training program

4. _____ Maintain dorsiflexion to affected area

5. _____ Place the patient in a lateral position

Column II

a. Footdrop

b. Incontinence

c. Impaired cough reflex

d. Keratitis

e. Paralyzed diaphragm

f. Paralyzed extremity

II. Critical Thinking Questions and Exercises

DISCUSSION AND ANALYSIS

Discuss the following topics with your classmates.

1. Describe several nursing interventions for maintaining the airway for a patient with an altered level of consciousness.
2. Discuss 6 of 12 major goals for a patient with an altered level of consciousness.
3. Explain two new trends in neurologic monitoring: microdialysis and cerebral oxygenation monitoring.
4. Distinguish between the early and late signs of ICP that a nurse would be responsible for assessing.
5. Explain the rationale for reducing body temperature in patients with cerebral disorders.
6. Describe the nursing management of a patient during a seizure.

INTERPRETING PATTERNS

Read each analogy. Write the best response in the space provided.

1. Craniotomy : surgery involving entry into the cranial vault :: Craniectomy :

   _____

2. Cushing's response : increased arterial pressure in response to increased intracranial pressure :: Cushing's triad : _____

3. Decerebration : extreme extension of the upper and lower extremities :: _____ : abnormal flexion of the upper extremities

4. A primary headache : controllable localized pain :: Migraine headache :

   _____

5. Ataxic breathing : random sequences of deep and shallow breaths :: Cheyne-Stokes breathing :

   _____

CLINICAL SITUATIONS

Develop a nursing care plan for the situation described. For each nursing diagnosis, list goals, nursing actions, rationale, and expected outcomes.

Miss Potter, a 32-year-old, single circus performer has been unconscious since she was admitted to the hospital 1 week ago after falling from a high wire. Her family must leave the area to travel with the circus and is expected to return in 2 months.

Nursing Diagnoses:

Goals	Nursing Actions	Rationale	Expected Outcomes

APPLYING CONCEPTS

Look at Table 61-1, Nursing Assessment for the Unconscious Patient, in the text. List the clinical assessment technique in column I and the clinical significance in column II for the eyes and the foot. An example is provided.

Eyes

COLUMN I	COLUMN II
Fixed, dilated pupils (example)	Injury at midbrain (example)

Foot

COLUMN I	COLUMN II

CHAPTER 62

Management of Patients With Cerebrovascular Disorders

I. Interpretation, Completion, and Comparison

MULTIPLE CHOICE

Read each question carefully. Circle your answer.

1. As a cause of death in the United States, stroke currently ranks:
   a. second.
   b. third.
   c. fourth.
   d. fifth.

2. The most common cause of cerebrovascular disease is:
   a. arteriosclerosis.
   b. embolism.
   c. hypertensive changes.
   d. vasospasm.

3. The etiology of an ischemic stroke would include:
   a. cardiogenic embolus.
   b. cerebral aneurysm.
   c. arteriovenous malformation.
   d. intracerebral hemorrhage.

4. The majority of ischemic strokes have what type of origin?
   a. cardiogenic embolic
   b. cryptogenic
   c. large artery thrombotic
   d. small artery thrombotic

5. The nurse knows that symptoms associated with a transient ischemic attack (TIA), which is frequently a precursor of stroke, usually subside in:
   a. 1 hour.
   b. 3 to 6 hours.
   c. 12 hours.
   d. 24 to 36 hours.

6. Approximately what percentage of patients who experience a TIA will have a stroke within 3 years?
   a. 5%
   b. 20%
   c. 40%
   d. 80%

7. The degree of neurologic damage that occurs with an ischemic stroke depends on the:
   a. location of the lesion.
   b. size of the area of inadequate perfusion.
   c. amount of collateral blood flow.
   d. combination of the above factors.

8. A stroke victim is experiencing memory loss and impaired learning capacity. The nurse knows that brain damage has most likely occurred in which lobe?
   a. frontal
   b. occipital
   c. parietal
   d. temporal

9. The initial mortality rate for a stroke can be as high as:
   a. 10%.
   b. 20%.
   c. 30%.
   d. 50%.

10. The most common motor dysfunction of a stroke is:
    a. ataxia.
    b. diplopia.
    c. dysphagia.
    d. hemiplegia.

11. The initial diagnostic test for a stroke, usually performed in the emergency department, is a:
    a. 12-lead electrocardiogram.
    b. carotid ultrasound study.
    c. noncontrast computed tomogram.
    d. transcranial Doppler flow study.

12. To be effective, thrombolytic therapy with recombinant tissue plasminogen activator (t-PA) must be given to a stroke patient within a timeframe of how many hours after onset of the stroke?
    a. 3
    b. 6 to 12
    c. 18
    d. 24 to 48

13. An emergency room nurse understands that a 110-lb patient with recent stroke will receive at least the minimum dose of recombinant t-PA. The patient will receive a minimum dose of:
    a. 50 mg.
    b. 60 mg.
    c. 85 mg.
    d. 100 mg.

14. The most common side-effect of t-PA is:
    a. an allergic reaction.
    b. bleeding.
    c. severe vomiting.
    d. a second stroke in 6 to 12 hours.

15. Eighty percent of hemorrhagic strokes are primarily caused by:
    a. an embolus.
    b. a cerebral thrombus.
    c. a brain tumor.
    d. uncontrolled hypertension.

16. A classic diagnostic symptom of hemorrhagic stroke is the patient's complaint of:
    a. numbness of an arm or leg.
    b. double vision.
    c. severe headache.
    d. dizziness and tinnitus.

17. Most patients with hemorrhagic stroke are placed in bed in which position?
    a. high Fowler's
    b. prone
    c. supine
    d. semi-Fowler's (head of bed at 15 to 30 degrees)

SHORT ANSWER

Read each statement carefully. Write your response in the space provided.

1. The primary cerebrovascular disorder in the United States is _____, which was recently given the term _____ to emphasize the urgency of its occurrence.

2. Four nonmodifiable risk factors for stroke are _____, _____, _____, and _____.

3. Four classifications of stroke based on time course are _____, _____, _____, and _____.

4. Define the term *bruit:* _____

_____

5. The main surgical procedure for managing TIAs is: _____

_____

6. Three possible collaborative problems for a patient recovering from an ischemic stroke are

_____, _____, and _____.

7. Four primary complications of carotid endarterectomy are _____,

_____, _____, and _____.

8. Hemorrhagic strokes are caused by bleeding into _____,

_____, or _____.

9. Almost 50% of the mortality and morbidity associated with hemorrhagic stroke is due to

_____.

10. Immediate complications of a hemorrhagic stroke are _____ and

_____.

MATCHING

Match the each of the clinical manifestations of specific neurologic deficits in column II with its associated cause listed in column I.

Column I

1. _____ Ataxia
2. _____ Receptive aphasia
3. _____ Dysphagia
4. _____ Homonymous hemianopsia
5. _____ Loss of peripheral vision
6. _____ Expressive aphasia
7. _____ Diplopia
8. _____ Paresthesia

Column II

a. Difficulty judging distances
b. Unaware of the borders of objects
c. Double vision
d. Staggering, unsteady gait
e. Difficulty in swallowing
f. Difficulty with proprioception
g. Unable to form words that are understandable
h. Unable to comprehend the spoken word

II. Critical Thinking Questions and Exercises

DISCUSSION AND ANALYSIS

Discuss the following topics with your classmates.

1. Explain the pathophysiology of a brain attack.
2. Describe clinical manifestations of a stroke that a nurse should interpret. Organize those symptoms according to a classification of deficits: visual field, motor, sensory, verbal, cognitive, and emotional.
3. Describe the focus of nursing interventions when helping a patient recover from an ischemic stroke.

CLINICAL SITUATIONS

Develop a nursing care plan for the situation described. For each nursing diagnosis, list goals, nursing actions, rationale, and expected outcomes.

Mrs. Coe recently sustained an ischemic stroke. She is 41 years old and lives with her husband and three sons. In your nursing care plan, emphasize the rehabilitative phase, which should have begun with her diagnosis, and stress the retraining of her flaccid right upper and lower extremities. She also needs to be taught how to sit, stand, and walk with balance and how to use a wheelchair.

Nursing Diagnoses:

Goals	Nursing Actions	Rationale	Expected Outcomes

CHAPTER 63

Management of Patients With Neurologic Trauma

I. Interpretation, Completion, and Comparison

MULTIPLE CHOICE

Read each question carefully. Circle your answer.

1. All of the following statements about the occurrence of head injuries are correct *except:*
   a. The majority of all victims are younger than 25 years of age.
   b. An estimated 50,000 persons die annually from these injuries.
   c. Motor vehicle crashes are the primary cause.
   d. The majority of injuries occur in females.

2. A cerebral hemorrhage located within the brain is classified as:
   a. an epidural hematoma.
   b. an extradural hematoma.
   c. an intracerebral hematoma.
   d. a subdural hematoma.

3. The Glasgow Coma Scale is used to determine the level of consciousness. A score considered indicative of coma is:
   a. 1.
   b. 3.
   c. 15.
   d. 0.

4. Assessing the level of consciousness is an important nursing measure after injury. Signs of increasing intracranial pressure (ICP) include:
   a. bradycardia.
   b. increased systolic blood pressure.
   c. widening pulse pressure.
   d. all of the above.

5. Comatose patients are mechanically ventilated to control ICP. Hypocapnia is a goal that can be achieved with a $PaCO_2$ in the range of:
   a. 10 to 25 mm Hg.
   b. 25 to 30 mm Hg.
   c. 30 to 35 mm Hg.
   d. 35 to 40 mm Hg.

6. A cause of elevated body temperature in a head-injured patient is:
   a. cerebral irritation from hemorrhage.
   b. damage to the hypothalamus.
   c. infection.
   d. all of the above.

7. To prevent decreased cerebral perfusion after brain injury, the nurse knows that cerebral perfusion pressure must be at a minimum reading of:
   a. 15 mm Hg.
   b. 30 mm Hg.
   c. 50 mm Hg.
   d. 70 mm Hg.

8. A common cause of increased ICP is cerebral edema and swelling that peaks how long after the injury?

   a. 12 hours

   b. 12 to 24 hours

   c. 2 to 3 days

   d. 7 days

9. Posttraumatic seizures that are classified as *late* occur how long after the injury?

   a. more than 48 hours

   b. more than 72 hours

   c. more than 4 to 6 days

   d. more than 7 days

10. More than 50% of patients with new spinal cord injury are:

    a. 30 years of age or younger.

    b. 30 to 40 years of age.

    c. 40 to 50 years of age.

    d. 50 years of age or older.

11. In the United States, the number of new spinal cord injuries each year averages approximately:

    a. 5000 cases.

    b. 13,000 cases.

    c. 20,000 cases.

    d. 25,000 cases.

12. The primary cause of spinal cord injuries (35%) is:

    a. gunshot wounds.

    b. industrial accidents.

    c. sports activities.

    d. motor vehicle crashes.

13. Spinal cord injury can be classified according to the area of spinal cord damage. Motor deficits in the upper rather than the lower extremities, usually caused by edema in the cervical area, is classified as:

    a. anterior cord syndrome.

    b. Brown-Sequard syndrome.

    c. central cord syndrome.

    d. peripheral syndrome.

14. Respiratory difficulty and paralysis of all four extremities occur with spinal cord injury located:

    a. above C4.

    b. at C6.

    c. at C7.

    d. around C8.

15. High doses of which drug have been found to reduce swelling and disability if given within 8 hours after injury?

    a. mannitol

    b. methylprednisolone

    c. naloxone

    d. Neomycin

16. Loss of autonomic nervous system function below the level of the lesion causes what kind of shock?

    a. cardiac

    b. hypovolemic

    c. septic

    d. neurogenic

17. Recovery of vital organ functions resulting from spinal shock can take up to:

    a. 4 months.

    b. 12 months.

    c. 2 years.

    d. 4 years.

18. Orthostatic hypotension is a common problem for spinal cord injuries at the level of:

    a. C4.

    b. T7.

    c. L4.

    d. S1.

19. A common complication of immobility in a spinal cord injury is:

    a. pressure ulcers.

    b. deep vein thrombosis.

    c. urinary tract infections.

    d. pneumonia.

SHORT ANSWER

Read each statement carefully. Write your response in the space provided.

1. A characteristic sign of a basal skull fracture is: _____

    _____

2. A brain injury can cause serious brain damage because: _____

    _____

3. Five symptoms of postconcussion syndrome are _____,

    _____, _____, _____, and

    _____.

4. After concussion, a patient needs to know to seek medical attention if any of the following six symptoms occur:

    _____

    _____

    _____

    _____

    _____

    _____

5. The most serious brain injury that can develop within the cranial vault is a: _____

    _____

6. Identify four signs of a rapidly expanding, acute subdural hematoma that would require immediate surgical intervention.

    _____

    _____

    _____

    _____

7. The three cardinal signs of brain death are _____, _____,

    and _____.

8. List five collaborative problems that a nurse should assess for a patient with a brain injury.

    _____

    _____

    _____

    _____

    _____

9. Name the three criteria used to assess level of consciousness using the Glasgow Coma Scale.

   _____

   _____

   _____

10. Complications after traumatic head injuries can be classified according to _____,

    _____, and _____.

11. The five vertebrae most commonly involved in spinal cord injuries are the: _____,

    _____, _____, _____, and

    _____.

12. List four common manifestations of pulmonary embolism.

    _____

    _____

    _____

    _____

13. Three potential complications that may develop in spinal cord injury are _____,

    _____, and _____.

14. Patients with tetraplegia and paraplegia are at increased risk for infection and sepsis from three common

    sources: _____, _____, and _____.

II. Critical Thinking Questions and Exercises

DISCUSSION AND ANALYSIS

Discuss the following topics with your classmates.

1. Discuss the annual frequency of head injuries in the United States.
2. Describe the clinical manifestations of traumatic brain injury.
3. Distinguish between a cerebral *concussion* and a cerebral *contusion*.
4. Explain why the most important consideration in any head injury is whether the brain is injured.
5. Explain what the Uniform Determination of Brain Death Act regulates.
6. Discuss the nursing measures that should be used to control ICP in severely brain-injured patients.
7. Describe the pathophysiology and nursing interventions for autonomic dysreflexia.

CLINICAL SITUATIONS

Develop a nursing care plan for each of the two situations described. For each nursing diagnosis, list goals, nursing actions, rationale, and expected outcomes.

CASE STUDY: Cervical Spine Injury

Katie is an 11-year-old who suffered a cervical spine injury after diving into a swimming pool. Katie is in traction applied by Crutchfield tongs and is on a Stryker frame. She is the oldest of three children and has never been hospitalized before. Develop a nursing care plan for Katie, and share it with your instructor for comments.

Nursing Diagnoses:

Goals	Nursing Actions	Rationale	Expected Outcomes

CASE STUDY: Paraplegia

Matthew, a 29-year-old Navy pilot, was recently injured in a training maneuver. Matthew is a paraplegic. He has been hospitalized for 1 week. He was recently married, and his wife is expecting their first child in 2 months. Emphasize the following areas in your nursing care plan: psychological support, weight-bearing activities, muscle exercises, mobilization, and sexual needs. Share your work with your clinical instructor.

Management of Patients With Neurologic Infections, Autoimmune Disorders, and Neuropathies

I. Interpretation, Completion, and Comparison

MULTIPLE CHOICE

Read each question carefully. Circle your answer.

1. Identify the bacteria *not* associated with the cause of septic meningitis:
   a. *C. neoformans*
   b. *H. influenzae*
   c. *N. meningitidis*
   d. *S. pneumoniae*

2. The most severe form of meningitis is considered to be:
   a. bacterial.
   b. aseptic.
   c. septic.
   d. viral.

3. Bacterial meningitis alters intracranial physiology, causing:
   a. cerebral edema.
   b. increased permeability of the blood–brain barrier.
   c. raised intracranial pressure.
   d. all of the above changes.

4. A brain abscess is a collection of infectious material within the substance of the brain that is caused by:
   a. direct invasion of the brain.
   b. spread of infection from nearby sites.
   c. spread of infection by other organs.
   d. all of the above mechanisms.

5. During assessment, the nurse knows that the most frequently reported disabling symptom found in multiple sclerosis is:
   a. depression.
   b. double vision.
   c. fatigue.
   d. pain.

6. A positive diagnosis of myasthenia gravis can be reached using the following test:
   a. anticholinesterase levels
   b. magnetic resonance imaging
   c. computed tomography (CT) scan
   d. electromyography

7. A surgical intervention that can cause substantial remission of myasthenia gravis is:
   a. esophagostomy.
   b. myomectomy.
   c. thymectomy.
   d. splenectomy.

8. The initial neurologic symptom of Guillain-Barré syndrome is:
   a. absent tendon reflexes.
   b. dysrhythmias.
   c. paresthesia of the legs.
   d. transient hypertension.

9. Tic douloureux is characterized by paroxysms of pain and burning sensations. It is a disorder of which cranial nerve?
   a. third
   b. fifth
   c. seventh
   d. eighth

10. Bell's palsy is characterized by weakness or paralysis of the facial muscles. It is a disorder of which cranial nerve?
    a. third
    b. fifth
    c. seventh
    d. eighth

11. Tinnitus and vertigo are clinical manifestations of damage to which cranial nerve?
    a. fourth
    b. sixth
    c. eighth
    d. tenth

SHORT ANSWER

Read each statement carefully. Write your response in the space provided.

1. Name the five infectious disorders of the nervous system.

   _____

   _____

   _____

   _____

   _____

2. List six signs of bacterial meningitis that a nurse should assess.

   _____

   _____

   _____

   _____

   _____

   _____

3. The most common cause of acute encephalitis in the United States is _____. The medication of choice for this disorder is _____.

4. The diagnosis of Creutzfeldt-Jakob disease can now be supported by the presence of _____ in the cerebrospinal fluid.

5. The primary pathology of multiple sclerosis is damage to the _____.

6. List the three forms of multiple sclerosis based on the frequency and progression of symptoms.

   _____

   _____

   _____

7. Myasthenia gravis is considered an autoimmune disease in which antibodies are directed against

   _____.

8. The most common causes of peripheral neuropathy are _____,

   _____, and _____.

MATCHING

Match the cranial nerve column II with its associated clinical disorder listed in column I. An answer may be used more than once.

Column I

1. _____ Optic neuritis

2. _____ Pituitary tumor

3. _____ Brainstem ischemia

4. _____ Trigeminal neuralgia

5. _____ Bell's palsy

6. _____ Herpes zoster

7. _____ Ménière's syndrome

8. _____ Guillain-Barré syndrome

9. _____ Vagal body tumors

10. _____ Sinus tract tumor

Column II

a. I

b. II

c. IV

d. V

e. VI

f. VII

g. VIII

h. X

II. Critical Thinking Questions and Exercises

DISCUSSION AND ANALYSIS

Discuss the following topics with your classmates.

1. Explain how a nurse would assess for the Kernig sign and the Brudzinski sign in determining a diagnosis of bacterial meningitis.
2. Explain what *demyelination* refers to in reference to multiple sclerosis.
3. Discuss the various disease-modifying medications used to treat multiple sclerosis.
4. Explain the etiology and clinical manifestations of myasthenic crises.

CLINICAL SITUATIONS

Read the following case study. Circle the correct answer.

Case Study: Multiple Sclerosis

Toni, a 32-year-old mother of two, has had multiple sclerosis for 5 years. She is currently enrolled in a school of nursing. Her husband is supportive and helps with the care of their preschool sons. Toni has been admitted to the clinical area for diagnostic studies related to symptoms of visual disturbances.

1. The nurse is aware that multiple sclerosis is a progressive disease of the central nervous system characterized by:

   a. axon degeneration.

   b. demyelination of the brain and the spinal cord.   d. all of the above.

   c. sclerosed patches of neural tissue.

2. During the physical assessment, the nurse recalls that the areas most frequently affected by multiple sclerosis are:
   a. the lateral, third, and fourth ventricles.   c. the pons, medulla, and cerebellar peduncles.
   b. the optic nerve and chiasm.   d. all of the above areas.

3. During the nursing interview, Toni minimizes her visual problems, talks about remaining in school to attempt advanced degrees, requests information about full-time jobs in nursing, and mentions her desire to have several more children. The nurse recognizes Toni's emotional responses as being:
   a. an example of inappropriate euphoria characteristic of the disease process.   c. indicative of the remission phase of her chronic illness.
   b. a reflection of coping mechanisms used to deal with the exacerbation of her illness.   d. realistic for her current level of physical functioning.

4. Toni's disease process involves the sacral plexus. Assessment should include:
   a. bladder problems or urinary tract infections.   c. sexual activity.
   b. bowel management.   d. all of the above.

CHAPTER 65

Management of Patients With Oncologic or Degenerative Neurologic Disorders

I. Interpretation, Completion, and Comparison

MULTIPLE CHOICE

Read each question carefully. Circle your answer.

1. The highest incidence of brain tumors occurs during which decade of life?
   a. earlier than the third
   b. in the third
   c. in the fourth
   d. between the fifth and seventh

2. The most frequently seen brain neoplasm is:
   a. an acoustic neuroma.
   b. an angioma.
   c. a glioma.
   d. a meningioma.

3. A patient is diagnosed with an intracerebral tumor. The nurse knows that the diagnosis may include all of the following *except:*
   a. astrocytoma.
   b. ependymoma.
   c. medulloblastoma.
   d. meningioma.

4. The most common benign encapsulated brain tumor (representing 20% of primary brain tumors) is:
   a. angioma.
   b. glioblastoma multiforme.
   c. meningioma.
   d. neuroma.

5. A nurse knows that a patient exhibiting seizure-like movements localized to one side of the body most likely has:
   a. a cerebellar tumor.
   b. a frontal lobe tumor.
   c. a motor cortex tumor.
   d. an occipital lobe tumor.

6. All of the following tumor types are commonly seen in the elderly *except:*
   a. anaplastic astrocytoma.
   b. cerebral metastasis from other sites.
   c. glioblastoma multiforme.
   d. medulloblastoma.

7. The majority of brain tumors are treated by:
   a. neurosurgery.
   b. chemotherapy.
   c. radioisotope implants.
   d. all of the above mechanisms.

8. Metastatic brain lesions occur in what percentage of patients with cancer?
   a. 10%
   b. 25%
   c. 40%
   d. 50% to 70%

9. The median survival time for patients with brain lesion metastasis, when no surgery is performed and radiation therapy is used, is:
   a. 3 to 6 months.
   b. 9 to 12 months.
   c. 18 months.
   d. 24 months.

10. Parkinsonian symptoms usually appear during which decade of life?
    a. fourth
    b. fifth
    c. sixth
    d. seventh

11. The clinical manifestations of Parkinson's disease (bradykinesia, rigidity, and tremors) are directly related to a decreased level of:
    a. acetylcholine.
    b. dopamine.
    c. serotonin.
    d. phenylalanine.

12. An example of an anticholinergic agent effective in controlling the tremor of parkinsonism is:
    a. Requip.
    b. cycrimine.
    c. Symmetrel.
    d. Permax.

13. Clinical manifestations of Huntington's disease include:
    a. abnormal involuntary movements (chorea).
    b. emotional disturbances.
    c. intellectual decline.
    d. all of the above.

14. The average time from onset to death for patients diagnosed with amyotrophic lateral sclerosis (ALS) is:
    a. 3 years.
    b. 5 to 8 years.
    c. 10 years.
    d. 15 to 20 years.

15. The majority of lumbar disc herniations occur at the level of:
    a. L1–L2.
    b. L3–L4.
    c. L4–L5.
    d. S1–S2.

SHORT ANSWER

Read each statement carefully. Write your response in the space provided.

1. The majority of metastatic lesions to the brain occur from six areas:

   _____

   _____

   _____

   _____

   _____

   _____

2. Name the three most common systemic signs of increased intracranial pressure.

   _____

   _____

   _____

3. List three common focal or localized symptoms of a brain tumor:

   _____

   _____

   _____

4. A spinal cord tumor located within the spinal cord is classified as _____.

5. List five degenerative disorders of the central and peripheral nervous system.

   _____

   _____

   _____

   _____

   _____

6. Identify the four cardinal signs of Parkinson's disease.

   _____

   _____

   _____

   _____

7. List the five chief symptoms of amyotrophic lateral sclerosis.

   _____

   _____

   _____

   _____

   _____

8. Identify the common characteristics of muscular dystrophies: _____,

   _____, and _____.

9. Cervical disk herniation usually occurs at the _____ interspaces.

10. Identify two major collaborative problems for patients with a cervical discectomy.

    _____

    _____

MATCHING

Match the neurologic disorder in column II with its associated clinical manifestation listed in column I.

Column I

1. _____ Impaired ability to execute voluntary movements
2. _____ Rapid, jerky, purposeless movements of extremities or facial muscles
3. _____ A sensation of "pins and needles"
4. _____ Restlessness and agitation
5. _____ Disease of the spinal nerve root
6. _____ Minute and illegible handwriting
7. _____ Very slow voluntary movements and speech
8. _____ Abnormal voice quality caused by incoordination of speech muscles

Column II
a. Akathisia
b. Bradykinesia
c. Chorea
d. Dyskinesia
e. Dysphonia
f. Micrographia
g. Paresthesia
h. Radiculopathy

II. Critical Thinking Questions and Exercises

DISCUSSION AND ANALYSIS

Discuss the following topics with your classmates.

1. Discuss a variety of physiologic changes that result from the infiltration of tissue subsequent to the growth of a brain tumor.
2. Describe the various classifications of brain tumors based on their pathophysiology.
3. Discuss the primary nursing diagnoses and interventions for a patient with cerebral metastases or an incurable brain tumor.
4. Describe the benefits and limitations of thalamotomy and pallidotomy in the treatment of Parkinson's disease.
5. Explain the basic pathophysiology and clinical manifestations of Huntington's disease.
6. Describe the six types of surgical procedures used to treat degenerative disk disease.

CLINICAL SITUATIONS

Read the following case study. Circle the correct answer.

CASE STUDY: Parkinson's Disease

Charles is a 76-year-old retired professional golfer. He has recently been diagnosed as having Parkinson's disease.

1. The nurse knows that Parkinson's disease, a progressive neurologic disorder, is characterized by:
   a. bradykinesia.
   b. muscle rigidity.
   c. tremor.
   d. all of the above.

2. The nurse assesses for the characteristic movement of Parkinson's disease, which is:
   a. an exaggerated muscle flaccidity that leads to frequent falls.
   b. a hyperextension of the back and neck that alters normal movements.
   c. a pronation–supination of the hand and forearm that interferes with normal hand activities.
   d. a combination of all of the above.

3. Charles is started on chemotherapy which is aimed at restoring dopaminergic activities. An example of such a drug is:
   a. Artane.
   b. Benadryl.
   c. Elavil.
   d. Dopar.

4. Nutritional considerations as part of the nursing care plan would include all of the following *except*:
   a. the diet should be semisolid to facilitate the passage of food.
   b. calcium should be avoided.
   c. the patient should be sitting in an upright position during feeding.
   d. thick fluids should be encouraged to provide additional calories.

CASE STUDY: Huntington's Disease

Develop a nursing care plan for the situation described. For each nursing diagnosis, list goals, nursing actions, rationale, and expected outcomes.

Mike is a 49-year-old television producer who has been diagnosed as having Huntington's disease. He lives alone in a penthouse apartment and is extremely busy and successful in his business. He has no living relatives. He is experiencing uncontrollable movements and difficulties feeding himself. He recently started chemotherapy with haloperidol (Haldol). Develop a nursing care plan for Mike and share it with your instructor for comments. Your care plan should include the following nursing diagnosis: Potential for accidental injury related to abnormal involuntary movements.

Nursing Diagnoses:

Goals	Nursing Actions	Rationale	Expected Outcomes

EXTRACTING INFERENCES

Look at Figure 65-1 in the text. For each brain tumor site, describe the expected clinical symptoms, nursing assessments, and medical/surgical interventions.

CHAPTER 66

Assessment of Musculoskeletal Function

I. Interpretation, Completion, and Comparison

MULTIPLE CHOICE

Read each question carefully. Circle your answer.

1. The vertebrae can be classified as a type of:
   a. flat bone.
   b. irregular bone.
   c. long bone.
   d. short bone.

2. The sternum, a bone that is a site for hematopoiesis, is classified as a:
   a. flat bone.
   b. irregular bone.
   c. long bone.
   d. short bone.

3. The basic cells responsible only for the formation of bone matrix are:
   a. osteoblasts.
   b. osteoclasts.
   c. osteocytes.
   d. all of the above.

4. About 3 weeks after fracture, an internal bridge of fibrous material, cartilage, and immature bone joins bone fragments so that ossification can occur. The building of a "fracture bridge" occurs during the stage of bone healing known as:
   a. inflammation.
   b. cellular proliferation.
   c. callus formation.
   d. ossification.

5. The hip and shoulder are examples of diarthroses that are classified as:
   a. ball-and-socket joints.
   b. hinge joints.
   c. pivot joints.
   d. saddle joints.

6. The primary energy source for muscle cells is:
   a. adenosine triphosphate (ATP).
   b. creatine phosphate.
   c. glucose.
   d. glycogen.

7. Isometric contraction of the vastus lateralis is part of the exercises known as:
   a. biceps-tightening exercises.
   b. triceps-resisting exercises.
   c. gluteal-setting exercises.
   d. quadriceps exercises.

8. Patient education for musculoskeletal conditions for the aging is based on the understanding that there is a gradual loss of bone after a peak of bone mass at age:
   a. 20 years.
   b. 35 years.
   c. 40 years.
   d. 50 years.

9. By age 75 years, the average woman is susceptible to bone fractures and has lost about what percentage of cancellous bone?

   a. 15%

   b. 40%

   c. 60%

   d. 75%

10. The removal of synovial fluid from a joint is called:

    a. arthrectomy.

    b. arthrocentesis.

    c. arthrography.

    d. arthroscopy.

MATCHING

Match the range-of-motion term in column II with its associated description listed in column I.

Column I

1. _____ Pulling down toward the midline of the body

2. _____ The act of turning the foot inward

3. _____ The opposite movement of flexion

4. _____ Turning around on an axis

5. _____ Turning the palms down

6. _____ Pulling the jaw forward

7. _____ Moving away from the midline

8. _____ Conelike circular movement

9. _____ Turning the palm up

10. _____ Turning the foot outward

Column II

a. Supination

b. Extension

c. Circumduction

d. Abduction

e. Protraction

f. Eversion

g. Pronation

h. Adduction

i. Inversion

j. Rotation

SHORT ANSWER

Read each statement carefully. Write your response in the space provided.

1. The leading cause of disability in the United States is _____.

2. The most common musculoskeletal condition that necessitates hospitalization in those older than 65 years of age is _____.

3. The approximate percentage of total body calcium present in the bones is _____.

4. In the human body, there are _____ bones.

5. Approximately _____ mg of calcium daily is essential to maintain adult bone mass.

6. Red bone marrow is located in the shaft of four long and flat bones: _____, _____, _____, and _____.

7. The major hormonal regulators of calcium homeostasis are _____ and _____.

8. Ossification for major adult long bone fractures can take up to _____.

9. The term used to describe the grating, crackling sound heard over irregular joint surfaces such as the knee is _____.

SCRAMBLEGRAM

Unscramble the letters to answer each statement.

1. The fibrous membrane that covers the bone: _____

E O P T R M E S U I

2. These connect muscles to muscles: _____

A N S I G M L T E

3. The contractile unit of skeletal muscle: _____

O E S E A R M R C

4. These attach muscles to bone: _____

N T S O E D N

5. Loss of bone mass common in postmenopausal women: _____

I S S T P O O R E O O S

6. A lateral curving deviation of the spine: _____

L S O S O S I I C

7. Excessive fluid within a joint capsule: _____

N E O F I F S U

8. Aspiration of a joint to obtain synovial fluid: _____

S A I R E T T H N R E O C

II. Critical Thinking Questions and Exercises

DISCUSSION AND ANALYSIS

Discuss the following topics with your classmates.

1. List several general functions of the musculoskeletal system.
2. Compare and contrast the function of osteoblasts, osteocytes, and osteoclasts. Include a description of the Haversian system.
3. Describe the process of osteogenesis.
4. Explain how vitamin D regulates the balance between bone formation and bone resorption.
5. Explain the role of the sex hormones testosterone and estrogen on bone remodeling.
6. Describe the process of fracture healing, mentioning the six stages of progression.

7. Contrast the difference between *isotonic* and *isometric* contractions.
8. Describe the age-related changes of the musculoskeletal system specific to bones, muscles, joints, and ligaments.
9. Distinguish between three common deformities of the spine: kyphosis, lordosis, and scoliosis.
10. Compare and contrast the purpose of three diagnostic procedures commonly prescribed for musculoskeletal conditions: computed tomography, magnetic resonance imaging, and arthrography.

EXTRACTING INFERENCES

Look at Figure 66-2 in the text and describe the physiologic function of the following structures.

1. Synovial cavity

_____

2. Bursa

_____

3. Patella

_____

4. Fat pad

_____

5. Articular cartilage

_____

6. Medial meniscus

_____

7. Intrapatellar bursa

_____

CHAPTER 67

Musculoskeletal Care Modalities

I. Interpretation, Completion, and Comparison

MULTIPLE CHOICE

Read each question carefully. Circle your answer.

1. Choose the *incorrect* statement about the traditional plaster cast. After a plaster cast has been set, it:
   a. will take 1 to 3 days to dry.
   b. may be dented with pressure from the fingers of the hands when being moved.
   c. should be covered with a blanket to promote quick drying.
   d. will not have maximum strength until it is dry.

2. A patient with an arm cast complains of pain. The nurse should do all of the following *except:*
   a. assess the fingers for color and temperature.
   b. administer a prescribed analgesic to promote comfort and allay anxiety.
   c. suspect that the patient may have a pressure sore.
   d. determine the exact site of the pain.

3. The nurse who assesses bone fracture pain expects the patient to describe the pain as:
   a. a dull, deep, boring ache.
   b. sharp and piercing.
   c. similar to "muscle cramps."
   d. sore and aching.

4. The nurse suspects "compartment syndrome" for a casted extremity. She would assess for characteristic symptoms such as:
   a. decreased sensory function.
   b. excruciating pain.
   c. loss of motion.
   d. all of the above.

5. The nurse knows to assess the patient in an arm cast for possible pressure ulcers in the following area:
   a. lateral malleolus.
   b. olecranon.
   c. radial styloid.
   d. ulna styloid.

6. After removal of a cast, the patient needs to be instructed to do all of the following *except:*
   a. apply an emollient lotion to soften the skin.
   b. control swelling with elastic bandages, as directed.
   c. gradually resume activities and exercise.
   d. use friction to remove dead surface skin by rubbing the area with a towel.

7. A common pressure problem area for a long leg cast is the:
   a. dorsalis pedis.
   b. peroneal nerve.
   c. popliteal artery.
   d. posterior tibialis.

8. The nurse assesses for peroneal nerve injury by checking the patient's casted leg for the primary symptom of:
   a. burning.
   b. numbness.
   c. tingling.
   d. all of the above indicators.

9. The nurse is very concerned about the potential debilitating complication of peroneal nerve injury, which is:
   a. permanent paresthesia.
   b. footdrop.
   c. deep vein thrombosis.
   d. infection.

10. Choose the *incorrect* statement about turning a patient in a hip spica cast.
    a. A minimum of three persons are needed so that the cast can be adequately supported by their palms.
    b. Points over body pressure areas need to be supported to prevent the cast from cracking.
    c. The abduction bar should be used to ensure that the lower extremity can be moved as a unit.
    d. The patient should be encouraged to use the trapeze or side rail during repositioning.

11. Skin traction is usually limited to a weight between:
    a. 1 and 3 lb.
    b. 4 and 8 lb.
    c. 10 and 12 lb.
    d. 13 and 15 lb.

12. A patient in pelvic traction needs his or her circulatory status assessed. The nurse should check for a positive (+) Homans' sign by asking the patient to:
    a. extend both hands while the nurse compares the volume of both radial pulses.
    b. extend each leg and dorsiflex each foot to determine if pain or tenderness is present in the lower leg.
    c. plantar flex both feet while the nurse performs the blanch test on all of the patient's toes.
    d. squeeze the nurse's hands with his or her hands to evaluate any difference in strength.

13. Nursing assessment of a patient in traction should include:
    a. lung sounds and bowel sounds.
    b. circulation, sensation, and motion of the extremities in traction.
    c. the patient's level of anxiety and apprehension.
    d. all of the above interventions.

14. The nurse expects that up to how much weight can be used for a patient in skeletal traction?
    a. 10 lb
    b. 25 lb
    c. 40 lb
    d. 60 lb

15. When a patient is in continuous skeletal leg traction, it is important for the nurse to remember to do all of the following *except:*
    a. encourage the patient to use the trapeze bar.
    b. maintain adequate countertraction.
    c. remove the weights when pulling the patient up in bed to prevent unnecessary pulling on the fracture site.
    d. use a fracture bedpan to prevent soiling and to maintain patient comfort.

16. Patients with a hip and knee replacement begin ambulation with a walker or crutches how long after surgery?
    a. 24 hours
    b. 72 hours
    c. 1 week
    d. 2 to 3 weeks

17. An artificial joint for total hip replacement involves an implant that consists of:
    a. an acetabular socket.
    b. a femoral shaft.
    c. a spherical ball.
    d. all of the above.

18. The recommended leg position to prevent prosthesis dislocation after a total hip replacement is:
    a. abduction.
    b. adduction.
    c. flexion.
    d. internal rotation.

19. Postoperatively a patient with a total hip replacement is allowed to turn:
    a. 45 degrees onto his or her unoperated side if the affected hip is kept abducted.
    b. from the prone to the supine position only, and the patient must keep the affected hip extended and abducted.
    c. to any comfortable position as long as the affected leg is extended.
    d. to the operative side if his or her affected hip remains extended.

20. The nurse caring for a postoperative hip-replacement patient knows that the patient should not cross his or her legs, at any time, for how long after the surgery?
    a. 2 months.
    b. 3 months.
    c. 4 months.
    d. 6 months.

21. One of the most dangerous of all postoperative complications is:
    a. atelectasis.
    b. hypovolemia.
    c. pulmonary embolism.
    d. urinary tract infection.

22. After a total hip replacement, stair climbing is kept to a minimum for the first:
    a. 3 months.
    b. 4 months
    c. 6 months.
    d. 8 months.

23. The patient with a total hip replacement is usually able to resume daily activities after:
    a. 3 months.
    b. 6 months.
    c. 9 months.
    d. 1 year.

24. Preoperative nursing measures that are appropriate for an orthopedic patient should include:
    a. encouraging fluids to prevent a urinary tract infection.
    b. teaching isometric exercises and encouraging active range of motion.
    c. discouraging smoking to improve respiratory function.
    d. all of the above interventions.

25. Postoperative nursing concerns when caring for an orthopedic patient should include:
    a. determining that the patient's pain is controlled by administering prescribed analgesics.
    b. observing for signs of shock, such as hypotension and tachycardia.
    c. preventing infection by using aseptic technique when giving wound care.
    d. all of the above interventions.

SHORT ANSWER

Read each statement carefully. Write your response in the space provided.

1. List four purposes for applying a cast.

   _____

   _____

   _____

   _____

2. The advantages of a fiberglass cast compared to a plaster cast are: _____

_____

3. Unrelieved pain for a patient in a cast must be immediately reported to avoid four possible and serious potential problems: _____, _____, _____, and _____.

4. Name several indicators of neurovascular status that the nurse should assess to determine circulatory status for a casted extremity: _____

_____

5. List the five "P's" that should be assessed as part of the neurovascular check.

   _____

   _____

   _____

   _____

   _____

6. List several danger signs of possible circulatory constriction for a casted extremity:

   _____

   _____

7. List three major complications of a casted extremity.

   _____

   _____

   _____

8. Name four purposes for traction application.

   _____

   _____

   _____

   _____

9. The most effective cleansing solution for care of a pin site is _____.

10. A nursing goal for a patient with skeletal traction is to avoid infection and the development of _____ at the site of pin insertion.

11. List seven potential complications that may develop when a patient is in skeletal traction.

   _____

   _____

   _____

   _____

   _____

   _____

   _____

12. The nurse knows to assess a patient for deep vein thrombosis (DVT) by assessing the lower extremities for _____, _____, _____, and _____.

13. The incidence of DVT after hip replacement can be as high as _____ percent, with occurrence expected _____ to _____ days after surgery. Those who experience DVT have a _____ percent chance of developing a pulmonary embolism, with a _____ percent chance of fatality.

14. Name four possible complications of a total knee replacement.

    _____

    _____

    _____

    _____

II. Critical Thinking Questions and Exercises

DISCUSSION AND ANALYSIS

Discuss the following topics with your classmates.

1. Discuss three potential collaborative problems for a patient with a cast.
2. Discuss the major nursing goals for a patient with a cast.
3. Describe the complication of compartment syndrome, and its recommended treatment.
4. Describe the serious complication known as Volkmann's contracture.
5. Describe the psychological behavior and the physiologic symptoms seen in patients with cast syndrome.
6. Discuss the major nursing goals for a patient in traction.
7. Describe the 11 types of frequently seen orthopedic surgeries.
8. Describe the seven methods for preventing hip prosthesis dislocation that a nurse would teach a patient.
9. Outline in detail the patient education guidelines for home care after hip replacement.
10. Discuss the nursing assessments for five nursing diagnoses for the preoperative and postoperative care of a patient undergoing orthopedic surgery.

CLINICAL SITUATIONS

Read the following case studies. Fill in the blanks or circle the correct answer.

CASE STUDY: Buck's Traction

Bernadette is a 32-year-old bank secretary who was admitted to the hospital for unilateral Buck's extension traction to the left leg after a hip injury. Bernadette is the single parent of three children younger than 12 years of age.

1. Based on her knowledge of running traction, the nurse knows to expect that:
   a. the patient's leg will be flat on the bed to allow for a straight pulling force.
   b. the patient's leg will be flexed at the knee to allow for mobility without disruption of the pulling force.
   c. the traction will be applied directly to the bony skeleton to maintain a constant pulling force.
   d. the traction will allow the patient's leg to be suspended off the bed so that no further damage can occur to the hip.

2. The nurse knows that countertraction must be considered whenever traction is applied. Countertraction for Buck's traction is provided by _____ and _____.

3. In preparing the patient's skin for Buck's traction application, the nurse knows that it is necessary to
_____ and _____.

4. The nurse makes certain that the weights applied will not exceed:
   a. 2 lb.   c. 6 lb.
   b. 4 lb.   d. 8 lb.

5. The nurse consistently assesses neurovascular status when traction is in place. List seven indicators that the nurse would evaluate.

   _____

   _____

   _____

   _____

   _____

   _____

   _____

6. On assessment, the nurse notes a positive Homans' sign. Explain what this means:

   _____

   _____

CASE STUDY: Total Hip Replacement

Tom is a 62-year-old athletic coach at a high school. Sports activities, especially baseball, have been the focus of his energies since he was in high school and college. Because of prior hip joint injuries and degenerative joint disease, he is scheduled for a total hip replacement.

1. Preoperatively, the nurse assesses the status of the cardiovascular system based on the knowledge that

   mortality for patients older than 60 years of age is directly related to the complications of

   _____ and _____.

2. As part of preoperative teaching, the nurse makes the patient aware of four major potential complications

   of hip replacement: _____, _____,

   _____, and _____.

3. Based on the knowledge that limited hip flexion decreases hip prosthesis dislocation, the nurse knows to:
   a. keep the patient flat in bed with the leg extended.
   b. gatch the knees to decrease the effect of pulling force on the hip.
   c. raise the head of the bed between 30 and 45 degrees.
   d. maintain the patient in semi-Fowler's position.

4. The nurse teaches Tom how to minimize hip extension during transfers and while sitting. The nurse should encourage him to:
   a. rotate the hip inward slightly during sitting to prevent pressure on the external border of the hip.
   b. hyperextend the leg during transfers so the hip socket will not "pop out."
   c. maintain adduction and flexion when moving around to minimize strain at the surgical site.
   d. always pivot on the unoperated leg to protect the operated leg from unnecessary work.

5. A dislocated prosthesis is evidenced by any of the following five indicators: _____,
_____, _____, _____, and
_____.

6. In assessing postoperative wound drainage, the nurse knows that Tom's drainage of how much in the first 24 hours is within normal range?
   a. 150 mL
   b. 350 mL
   c. 600 mL
   d. 1000 mL

7. The nurse is careful to assess for evidence of DVT (3% mortality), which occurs in approximately what percent of patients?
   a. 20% to 30%
   b. 45% to 70%
   c. 75% to 85%
   d. more than 85%

CHAPTER 68

Management of Patients With Musculoskeletal Disorders

I. Interpretation, Completion, and Comparison

MULTIPLE CHOICE

Read each question carefully. Circle your answer.

1. The intervertebral disks that are subject to the greatest mechanical stress and greatest degenerative changes are:
   a. C3, C4, and L2.
   b. L1, L2, and L4.
   c. L2, L3, and L5.
   d. L4, L5, and S1.

2. Back pain is classified as "chronic" when the pain lasts without improvement for longer than:
   a. 4 weeks.
   b. 3 months.
   c. 6 months.
   d. 1 year.

3. The best position to ease low back pain is:
   a. high Fowler's to allow for maximum hip flexion.
   b. supine with the knees slightly flexed and the head of the bed elevated 30 degrees.
   c. prone with a pillow under the shoulders.
   d. supine with the bed flat and a firm mattress in place.

4. When lifting objects, patients with low back pain should be encouraged to maximize the use of the:
   a. gastrocnemius.
   b. latissimus dorsi.
   c. quadriceps.
   d. rectus abdominis.

5. The nurse should encourage a patient with low back pain to do all of the following *except*:
   a. lie prone with legs slightly elevated.
   b. strengthen abdominal muscles.
   c. avoid prolonged sitting or walking.
   d. maintain appropriate weight.

6. Carpal tunnel syndrome is a neuropathy characterized by:
   a. bursitis and tendonitis.
   b. flexion contracture of the fourth and fifth fingers.
   c. median nerve compression at the wrist.
   d. pannus formation in the shoulder.

7. The term for onychocryptosis, a common foot condition, is:
   a. callus.
   b. bunion.
   c. flatfoot.
   d. ingrown toenail.

8. An overgrowth of the horny layer of epidermis on the foot is called a:
   a. bunion.
   b. clawfoot.
   c. corn.
   d. hammer toe.

9. The average 75-year-old woman with osteoporosis has lost about how much of her cortical bone?
   a. 5%
   b. 10%
   c. 25%
   d. 40%

10. The estimated intake of calcium to prevent bone loss for a postmenopausal woman is _____ mg/day. The actual intake is about _____ mg/day.
    a. 600, 200
    b. 900, 300
    c. 1200, 400
    d. 1500, 600

11. Bone formation is enhanced by:
    a. calcium intake.
    b. muscular activity.
    c. weight bearing.
    d. all of the above.

12. The most common symptoms of osteomalacia are:
    a. bone fractures and kyphosis.
    b. bone pain and tenderness.
    c. muscle weakness and spasms.
    d. softened and compressed vertebrae.

13. Most cases of osteomyelitis are caused by:
    a. *Proteus.*
    b. *Pseudomonas.*
    c. *Salmonella.*
    d. *Staphylococcus aureus.*

14. Signs and symptoms of osteomyelitis may include all of the following *except*:
    a. pain, erythema, and fever.
    b. leukopenia, swelling, and purulent drainage.
    c. elevated erythrocyte sedimentation rate and increased white blood cell count.
    d. positive wound cultures and localized discomfort.

15. The specific treatment for chronic osteomyelitis would probably be:
    a. antibiotic therapy.
    b. drainage of localized foci of infection.
    c. immobilization.
    d. surgical removal of the sequestrum.

16. The most common benign bone tumor is:
    a. an enchondroma.
    b. a giant cell tumor.
    c. an osteochondroma.
    d. an osteoid osteoma.

17. The multiple myeloma tumor has its origin and principal location in the:
    a. bone marrow.
    b. liver.
    c. lymph nodes.
    d. spleen.

18. Appropriate nursing actions when caring for a patient with a primary malignant bone tumor would include all of the following *except*:
    a. allowing the patient to independently plan his or her daily routine.
    b. estimating the size and location of the mass daily by vigorously palpating the affected area.
    c. assuring the patient receiving chemotherapy that alopecia, if it occurs, is temporary.
    d. encouraging range-of-motion exercises to prevent atrophy of unaffected muscles.

SHORT ANSWER

Read each statement carefully. Write your response in the space provided.

1. Identify at least five causes of acute low back pain.

   _____

   _____

   _____

   _____

   _____

2. List four nursing diagnoses for a patient undergoing foot surgery.

   _____

   _____

   _____

   _____

3. Two significant characteristics of osteoporosis are _____ and

   _____.

4. The onset of osteoporosis begins in the _____ decade of life, when bone mass peaks and then begins to decline.

5. Explain the effects of the following on the development of age-related osteoporosis:

   a. Calcitonin: _____

   b. Estrogen: _____

   c. Parathyroid hormone: _____

6. Using a bone mineral density (BMD) score, *osteoporosis* is present if the score is _____ standard deviations (SD) below the young adult mean score; *osteopenia* is diagnosed if the score is _____ SDs below the mean.

7. The primary deficit in osteomalacia is _____.

8. Three medications used to treat Paget's disease are _____,

   _____, and _____.

II. Critical Thinking Questions and Exercises

DISCUSSION AND ANALYSIS

Discuss the following topics with your classmates.

1. Distinguish between the two inflammatory conditions, bursitis and tendonitis.
2. Explain the pathophysiology of carpal tunnel syndrome and Dupuytren's disease.
3. Discuss the etiology and medical treatment for the nine common foot problems listed in the chapter (eg, plantar fascitis, corn, hammer toe).
4. Describe the pathophysiology of Paget's disease.

APPLYING CONCEPTS

Review the pictures of common foot deformities found in Figure 68–6 of the text and complete the exercises.

1. Identify each foot ailment and list the associated clinical manifestations.
2. For each ailment, list associated nursing diagnoses.
3. From each diagnosis, draft a nursing plan of care.
4. Broadly explain the medical/surgical management for each ailment.

CLINICAL SITUATIONS

Read the following case study. Fill in the blanks or circle the correct answer.

CASE STUDY: Osteoporosis

Emily is a 49-year-old administrative assistant at a community college who has just been diagnosed with osteoporosis. The physician has asked you to answer some of Emily's questions and to explain the physician's directions for Emily's level of activity and her nutritional needs.

1. Emily asks the nurse to explain why she is losing her bone mass. The nurse's explanation is based on the

   physiologic rationale that bone mass loss occurs when: _____

   _____

2. What two reasons could the nurse use to explain why women develop osteoporosis more frequently than men? _____

   _____

3. The nurse advises Emily that about what percent of Caucasian women older than 50 years of age have some degree of osteoporosis?
   a. 10%   c. 50%
   b. 25%   d. 80%

4. The nurse advises Emily that the development of osteoporosis is significantly dependent on:
   a. decreased estrogen, which inhibits bone breakdown.
   b. increased calcitonin, which enhances bone resorption.
   c. increased vitamin D use, which interferes with calcium use.
   d. increased parathyroid hormone, which decreases with aging.

5. Part of Emily's teaching plan includes nutritional information about dietary calcium and vitamin D. The nurse advises Emily that she needs how much calcium each day?
   a. 500 mg   c. 1200 mg
   b. 1000 mg   d. 1500 mg

6. Emily is told that her x-ray results indicated bone radiolucency. The nurse knows that Emily has probably already exhibited about what percentage of demineralization?
   a. 5%   c. 20%
   b. 10%   d. 30%

CHAPTER 69

Management of Patients With Musculoskeletal Trauma

I. Interpretation, Completion, and Comparison

MULTIPLE CHOICE

Read each question carefully. Circle your answer.

1. A muscle tear that is microscopic and due to overuse is called a:
   a. contusion.
   b. dislocation.
   c. sprain.
   ✳d. strain.

2. The acute inflammatory stage of a strain or sprain usually lasts:
   a. less than 24 hours.
   b. between 24 and 48 hours.
   c. about 72 hours.
   d. at least 1 week.

3. After arthroscopic surgery for a rotator cuff tear, a patient can usually resume full activity in:
   a. 3 to 4 weeks.
   b. 8 weeks.
   c. 3 to 4 months.
   ✳d. 6 to 12 months.

4. A patient who has a meniscectomy by arthroscopic surgery needs to know that normal athletic activities can usually be resumed after:
   a. 2 weeks.
   ✳b. 3 weeks.
   c. 2 months.
   d. 6 months.

5. An open fracture with extensive soft tissue damage is classified as a what grade of fracture?
   a. I
   b. II
   c. III
   d. IV

6. Emergency management of a fracture should include:
   a. covering the area with a clean dressing, if the fracture is open.
   b. immobilizing the affected site.
   c. splinting the injured limb.
   d. all of the above nursing interventions.

7. The most serious complication of an open fracture is:
   ✳ a. infection.
   b. muscle atrophy caused by loss of supporting bone structure.
   c. necrosis of adjacent soft tissue caused by blood loss.
   d. nerve damage.

8. Shock, as an immediate complication of fractures, is usually classified as:

   a. cardiogenic.

   b. hypovolemic.

   c. neurogenic.

   d. septicemic.

9. As a complication of fractures, fat emboli:

   a. represent the major cause of death in fracture patients.

   b. result in symptoms of decreased mental alertness.

   c. may compromise the patient's respiratory status, necessitating ventilator support.

   d. are characterized by all of the above.

10. After a fracture, the onset of symptoms for fat embolism syndrome occurs:

   a. within 1 to 3 days.

   b. 1 to 2 weeks after the fracture is set.

   c. about 4 weeks after the bone fragments solidify.

   d. immediately after the fracture heals, when activity begins.

11. The femur fracture that commonly leads to avascular necrosis or nonunion because of an abundant supply of blood vessels in the area is a fracture of the:

   a. condylar area.

   b. neck.

   c. shaft.

   d. trochanteric region.

12. Patients who experience a fracture of the humeral neck are advised that healing will take an average of _____ weeks, with restricted vigorous activity for an additional _____ weeks.

   a. 6, 2

   b. 10, 4

   c. 10, 6

   d. 16, 2

13. After an arm fracture, pendulum exercises are begun:

   a. as soon as tolerated.

   b. in 2 to 3 weeks, when callus ossification prevents easy movements of bony fragments.

   c. in about 4 to 5 weeks, after new bone is well established.

   d. in 2 to 3 months, after normal activities are resumed.

14. The most serious complication of a supracondylar fracture of the humerus is:

   a. hemarthrosis.

   b. paresthesia.

   c. malunion.

   d. Volkmann's ischemic contracture.

15. The two most serious complications of pelvic fractures are:

   a. paresthesias and ischemia.

   b. hemorrhage and shock.

   c. paralytic ileus and a lacerated urethra.

   d. thrombophlebitis and infection.

16. Nursing assessment for a pelvic fracture includes:

   a. checking the urine for hematuria.

   b. palpating peripheral pulses in both lower extremities.

   c. testing the stool for occult blood.

   d. all of the above.

17. An acetabular fracture of the femur involves the:

   a. neck of the femur.

   b. shaft of the femur.

   c. supracondylar area of the femur.

   d. trochanteric region of the femur.

18. The most common complication of a hip fracture in the elderly is:
    a. avascular necrosis.
    b. infection.
    c. nonunion.
    d. pneumonia.

19. An immediate nursing concern for a patient who has suffered a femoral shaft fracture is assessment for:
    a. hypovolemic shock.
    b. infection.
    c. knee and hip dislocation.
    d. pain resulting from muscle spasm.

20. The longest immobilization time necessary for fracture union occurs with a fracture of the:
    a. intratrochanteric area of the femur.
    b. midshaft of the humerus.
    c. pelvis.
    d. tibial shaft.

21. The major indicator of lower extremity amputation is:
    a. congenital deformity.
    b. malignant tumor.
    c. peripheral vascular disease.
    d. trauma.

22. A nurse can foster a positive self-image in a patient who has had an amputation by all of the following *except*:
    a. encouraging the patient to care for the residual limb.
    b. allowing the expression of grief.
    c. introducing the patient to local amputee support groups.
    d. encouraging family and friends to refrain from visiting temporarily because this may increase the patient's embarrassment.

MATCHING

Match the type of fracture in column II with its descriptive terminology listed in column I.

PART I

Column I
1. _____ A break occurs across the entire section of the bone.
2. _____ A fragment of the bone is pulled off by a ligament or tendon.
3. _____ Bone is splintered into several fragments.
4. _____ One side of a bone is broken and the other side is bent.

Column II
a. Avulsion
b. Comminuted
c. Complete
d. Epiphyseal
e. Greenstick

PART II

Column I
1. _____ A fracture occurs at an angle across the bone.
2. _____ Fragments are driven inward.
3. _____ The fractured bone is compressed by another bone.
4. _____ The fracture extends through the skin.

Column II
a. Compressed
b. Depressed
c. Oblique
d. Open
e. Pathologic

SHORT ANSWER

Read each statement carefully. Write your response in the space provided.

1. Joint dislocations can lead to avascular necrosis if it is not treated. Avascular necrosis is:

   _____

   _____

2. Crepitus, a grating sensation felt when the hands are placed over an extremity, is caused by:

   _____

   _____

3. Patients with open fractures risk three major complications: _____,

   _____, and _____.

4. List three early complications of fractures and three delayed complications:

   Early: _____

   _____

   Delayed: _____

   _____

5. Treatment of early shock in fractures consists of four activities: _____,

   _____, _____, and _____.

6. List three early and serious complications associated with bed rest and reduced skeletal muscle contractions for a patient with an open fracture.

   _____

   _____

   _____

7. The most common fracture of the distal radius is _____.

8. The most common complication of hip fractures in the elderly is _____.

9. Common pulmonary complications, post hip fracture, for the elderly include _____ and _____.

II. Critical Thinking Questions and Exercises

EXAMINING ASSOCIATIONS

Read each analogy. Fill in the space provided with the best response. Explain the correlation.

1. A strain : a microscopic muscle tear :: A sprain : _____

2. A dislocation : lack of contact between the articular surfaces of bones ::
   _____ : partial dislocation of associated joint structures

3. Closed reduction : the alignment of bone fragments into opposition :: Open reduction :
   _____

4. Delayed union : delayed healing due to infection or poor nutrition :: Nonunion :
   _____

5. Autograft : donor to donor tissue :: _____ : tissue from donor or other

6. Intracapsular fracture : neck of the femur :: Extracapsular fracture : _____

DISCUSSION AND ANALYSIS

Discuss the following topics with your classmates.

1. Compare the nursing assessment and medical management for strains and sprains of first degree, second degree, and third degree.
2. Describe immediate nursing and medical management for an open fracture.
3. Distinguish between open and closed reduction as a management technique for fractures.
4. Discuss in detail those factors that enhance and inhibit fracture healing.
5. Explain the clinical manifestations and underlying pathophysiology of fat embolism.
6. Explain the etiology, clinical manifestations, and medical management for compartment syndrome.
7. Distinguish between the clinical manifestations and medical management of intravascular and extravascular fractures.

EXTRACTING INFERENCES

Examine Figure 69-2 in the text and answer the following questions.

1. The foot is firmly planted and the knee is struck laterally, as in basketball or soccer. This hit can result in a
   torn _____. The patient will immediately experience _____,
   _____, _____, and the inability to walk without assistance.
   Bleeding into the joint, _____, may occur.

2. The foot is firmly planted and the knee is hyperextended as in football. A "pop" sound is heard.
   This indicates a possible tear to the _____. Surgical reconstruction can be scheduled
   after _____. Rehabilitation takes _____ to
   _____ months.

3. Patients who report that their knees "give way" or "lock" after twisting or repetitive squatting are most likely experiencing a _____. Diagnosis is confirmed by _____. The most common postoperative complication is _____. Normal activities can be resumed in _____ (weeks/months).

CLINICAL SITUATIONS

Read the following case study. Circle the correct answers.

CASE STUDY: Above-the-Knee Amputation

William, a 70-year-old Catholic priest, lives in a center city rectory. He is scheduled to have an above-the-knee amputation of his left leg because of peripheral vascular disease.

1. Preoperatively the nurse knows that the circulatory status of the affected limb should be evaluated by assessing for:
   a. color and temperature.
   b. palpable pulses.
   c. positioning responses.
   d. all of the above.

2. The level of William's amputation was determined after assessing:
   a. the circulatory status of the affected limb.
   b. the type of prosthesis to be used.
   c. William's ability to understand and use the prosthetic device.
   d. all of the above.

3. Preoperatively, the nurse needs to assist William in exercising the muscles needed for crutch walking. The major muscle to be strengthened is the:
   a. pectoralis major.
   b. gastrocnemius.
   c. quadriceps femoris.
   d. triceps brachii.

4. Postoperatively, William experiences phantom limb sensations. The most appropriate nursing response is to:
   a. agree with his statements, recognizing that he is expressing a psychological need.
   b. consistently stress the absence of the lower leg.
   c. disagree with him and reorient him to reality.
   d. keep him as active as possible and encourage self-expression.

5. William's amputation is treated with a soft compression dressing. Nursing care would include all of the following *except:*
   a. keeping the residual limb slightly elevated on a pillow to decrease edema.
   b. monitoring vital signs to detect any indication of bleeding.
   c. placing the residual limb in an extended position, with brief periods of elevation.
   d. keeping a tourniquet nearby in case of hemorrhage.

6. Preprosthetic nursing care should attempt to avoid any problem that can delay prosthetic fitting, such as:
   a. abduction deformities of the hip.
   b. flexion deformities.
   c. nonshrinkage of the residual limb.
   d. all of the above.

7. The nurse who is preparing to apply a bandage to William's residual limb knows that she should:

   a. anchor the bandage on the posterior surface of the residual limb.

   b. begin the vertical turns on the anterior surface of the residual limb.

   c. maintain the residual limb in a position of flexion while bandaging.

   d. use circular turns that run in a horizontal plane from the proximal to the distal segment.

8. The nurse teaches William to massage his residual limb to:

   a. decrease local tenderness.

   b. improve vascularity.

   c. mobilize the scar.

   d. accomplish all of the above.

CHAPTER 70

Management of Patients With Infectious Diseases

I. Interpretation, Completion, and Comparison

MULTIPLE CHOICE

Read each question carefully. Circle your answer.

1. It is recommended that the measles, mumps, and rubella (MMR) vaccine should be initially given to children at age:
   a. 2 months.
   b. 6 months.
   c. 12 to 15 months.
   d. 18 to 24 months.

2. Chickenpox and herpes zoster (also known as shingles), are both caused by the same viral agent:
   a. *Clostridium difficile*.
   b. *Shigella*.
   c. *Plasmodium vivax*.
   d. Varicella zoster.

3. Each year nosocomial infections affect about how many patients?
   a. 250,000
   b. 500,000
   c. 1 million
   d. 2 million

4. The single most important means of preventing the spread of infection is:
   a. antibiotic therapy.
   b. gowning and gloving.
   c. handwashing.
   d. isolation measures.

5. The bacterium with significant nosocomial potential that is gram-positive, spore-forming, and highly resistant to antimicrobial therapy is:
   a. *Clostridium difficile*.
   b. methicillin-resistant *Staphylococcus aureus* (MRSA).
   c. *Staphylococcus aureus*.
   d. vancomycin-resistant enterococcus (VRE).

6. MRSA is a common nosocomial infection. The most frequently occurring pathogen identified with this disorder is:
   a. *Escherichia coli*.
   b. *Proteus*.
   c. *Pseudomonas aeruginosa*.
   d. *Staphylococcus aureus*.

7. A gram-positive organism that is less virulent than a gram-negative organism is:
   a. *Escherichia coli*.
   b. *Pseudomonas aeruginosa*.
   c. *Proteus*.
   d. *Staphylococcus aureus*.

8. Choose the *incorrect* statement about West Nile virus infection.

   a. It was first seen in the United States in 1999.

   b. It is caused by an infected mosquito.

   c. It is treated successfully by intravenous antibiotics if diagnosed within 72 hours after onset of symptoms.

   d. Its symptoms are similar to those of meningitis.

9. A person diagnosed with Legionnaire's disease would have a primary infection in his or her:

   a. bloodstream.

   b. central nervous system.

   c. gastrointestinal tract.

   d. lungs.

10. The antibiotic of choice for Legionnaire's disease is:

    a. Biaxin.

    b. Ilotycin.

    c. Levaquin.

    d. Zithromax.

11. The most common viral cause of diarrhea in children is:

    a. *Campylobacter.*

    b. *Shigella.*

    c. rotavirus.

    d. *Salmonella.*

12. A common bacterial cause of diarrhea that has been linked to the ingestion of undercooked beef is:

    a. *Escherichia coli.*

    b. *Campylobacter.*

    c. *Salmonella.*

    d. *Shigella.*

13. The rehydration goal for a 70-kg patient who has moderate dehydration would be how many milliliters over 4 hours?

    a. 3000

    b. 5000

    c. 7000

    d. 9000

14. Acquired immunodeficiency syndrome (AIDS) is a:

    a. condition of unknown cause.

    b. disorder of immunoregulation.

    c. syndrome associated with high mortality.

    d. condition consistent with all of the above.

15. The transmission route for human immunodeficiency virus (HIV) is through:

    a. contaminated blood.

    b. semen and vaginal secretions.

    c. maternal-fetal blood.

    d. all of the above.

16. Latent syphilitic lesions may still be treated with penicillin G benzathine for up to:

    a. 2 to 3 months.

    b. 3 to 6 months.

    c. 6 to 9 months.

    d. 1 year.

17. A chancre initially appears 2 to 3 weeks after inoculation with the spirochete, *Treponema pallidum*, in the sexually transmitted disease known as:

    a. chlamydia.

    b. gonorrhea.

    c. HIV/AIDS.

    d. syphilis.

18. Gonorrhea is a sexually transmitted infection that involves the mucosal surface of the:

    a. genitourinary tract.

    b. pharynx.

    c. rectum.

    d. all of the above.

19. The primary site for gonorrhea in women is the:
    a. urethra.
    b. kidney.

    c. vagina.
    d. uterine cervix.

20. The most deadly microorganism used as a biowarfare agent, which has a mortality rate of 90%, is:
    a. anthrax.
    b. Ebola virus.

    c. plague.
    d. smallpox.

SHORT ANSWER

Read each statement carefully. Write your response in the space provided.

1. Define the term *colonization:* _____
   _____

2. Define the term *infection:* _____
   _____

3. List the three components of a microbiology report, the primary source of information about most bacterial infections.
   _____
   _____
   _____

4. The two primary agencies involved in setting guidelines about infection prevention are the
   _____ and the _____.

5. List three specific organisms that are consistently associated with infection potential.
   _____
   _____
   _____

6. List at least six infectious diseases that have been controlled by successful vaccine programs.
   _____
   _____
   _____
   _____
   _____
   _____

7. It is recommended that immunosuppressed adults be vaccinated for _____,
   _____, and _____.

8. According to the Centers for Disease Control and Prevention (CDC), there are five emerging infectious diseases that have increased in the past two decades:

   _____

   _____

   _____

   _____

   _____

9. The most common infectious diseases in the United States are _____, infecting approximately _____ million Americans.

10. The most well known viral hemorrhagic fever viruses are _____ and

    _____.

MATCHING

Match the disease or condition in column II with its associated causative organism listed in column I.

Column I

1. _____ Varicella zoster

2. _____ *Neisseria gonorrhoeae*

3. _____ Hepatitis B virus

4. _____ *Staphylococcus aureus*

5. _____ Epstein-Barr virus

6. _____ *Salmonella* species

7. _____ *Streptococcus pneumoniae*

8. _____ *Microsporum* species

Column II

a. Chickenpox

b. Bloodborne hepatitis

c. Diarrheal disease

d. Gonorrhea

e. Impetigo

f. Mononucleosis

g. Pneumococcal pneumonia

h. Ringworm

II. Critical Thinking Questions and Exercises

EXAMINING ASSOCIATIONS

Examine the accompanying figure. For each of the six links in the infection cycle, describe specific nursing interventions that can be used to break transmission. The first entry is filled in as an example.

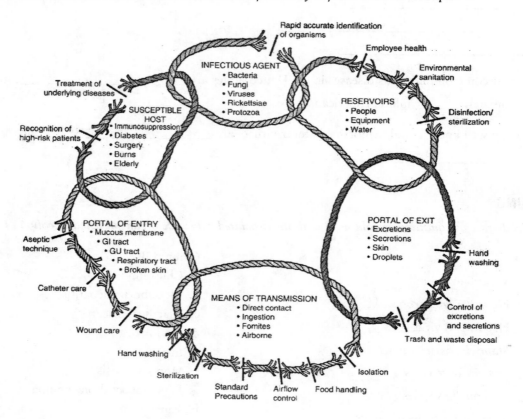

1. Infectious Agent

    a. Educate patient about immunization (example)

    b. _____

    c. _____

2. Reservoirs

    a. _____

    b. _____

    c. _____

3. Portal of Exit

    a. _____

    b. _____

    c. _____

4. Means of Transmission

   a. _____

   b. _____

   c. _____

5. Portal of Entry

   a. _____

   b. _____

   c. _____

6. Susceptible Host

   a. _____

   b. _____

   c. _____

DISCUSSION AND ANALYSIS

Discuss the following topics with your classmates.

1. Distinguish between the terms *infection* and *infectious disease.*
2. Distinguish between *standard* and *transmission-based* isolation precautions.
3. Review the CDC's standard recommended vaccination schedule and discuss the ages for initial and catch-up vaccinations.
4. Based on assessment data, describe eight potential complications for a patient with an infectious disease.
5. Compare and contrast diarrheal diseases caused by *Salmonella* and *Shigella* infections.

CHAPTER 71

Emergency Nursing

I. Interpretation, Completion, and Comparison

MULTIPLE CHOICE

Read each question carefully. Circle your answer.

1. A triage nurse in the emergency department determines that a patient with dyspnea and dehydration is not in a life-threatening situation. The triage category that the nurse would choose is:
   a. delayed.
   b. emergent.
   c. immediate.
   d. urgent.

2. A nurse at the scene of an industrial explosion uses "field triage" to categorize victims for treatment. A patient in need of emergent care would be tagged using the color:
   a. blue.
   b. green.
   c. red.
   d. yellow.

3. In the United States, the elderly, who are major consumers of emergency health care, account for about how many visits to the emergency room annually?
   a. 20 million
   b. 50 million
   c. 100 million
   d. 150 million

4. John, 16 years old, is brought to the emergency department after a vehicular accident. He is pronounced dead on arrival (DOA). When his parents arrive at the hospital, the nurse should:
   a. ask them to sit in the waiting room until she can spend time alone with them.
   b. speak to both parents together and encourage them to support each other and express their emotions freely.
   c. speak to one parent at a time in a private setting so that each can ventilate feelings of loss without upsetting the other.
   d. ask the emergency physician to medicate the parents so that they can handle their son's unexpected death quietly and without hysteria.

5. The first priority in treating any patient in the emergency department is:
   a. controlling hemorrhage.
   b. establishing an airway.
   c. obtaining consent for treatment.
   d. restoring cardiac output.

6. An oropharyngeal airway should be inserted:
   a. at an angle of 90 degrees.
   b. upside down and then rotated 180 degrees.
   c. with the concave portion touching the posterior pharynx.
   d. with the convex portion facing upward.

7. Clinical indicators for emergency endotracheal intubation include:
   a. airway obstruction.
   b. respiratory arrest.
   c. respiratory insufficiency.
   d. all of the above.

8. The initial nursing measure for the control of hemorrhage caused by trauma is to:
   a. apply a tourniquet.
   b. apply firm pressure over the involved area or artery.
   c. elevate the injured part.
   d. immobilize the area to control blood loss.

9. Indicators of hypovolemic shock associated with internal bleeding include all of the following *except:*
   a. bradycardia.
   b. cool, moist skin.
   c. hypotension.
   d. thirst.

10. The most common cause of shock in emergency situations is:
    a. cardiac failure.
    b. decreased arterial resistance.
    c. hypovolemia.
    d. septicemia.

11. The leading cause of death in children and adults younger than 44 years of age is:
    a. cancer.
    b. drowning.
    c. pneumonia.
    d. trauma.

12. Nursing measures for a penetrating abdominal injury (gunshot and stab wound) would include:
    a. assessing for manifestations of hemorrhage.
    b. covering any protruding viscera with sterile dressings soaked in normal saline solution.
    c. looking for any associated chest injuries.
    d. all of the above actions.

13. A patient has experienced blunt abdominal trauma from a motor vehicle crash. The nurse assesses the patient with the knowledge that the most frequently injured solid abdominal organ is the:
    a. duodenum.
    b. large bowel.
    c. liver.
    d. spleen.

14. Nursing management for a crushing lower extremity wound includes:
    a. applying a clean dressing to protect the wound.
    b. elevating the site to limit the accumulation of fluid in the interstitial spaces.
    c. splinting the wound in a position of rest to prevent motion.
    d. all of the above measures.

15. Identify the sequence of medical or nursing management for a patient who experiences multiple injuries.
    a. Assess for head injuries, control hemorrhage, establish an airway, prevent hypovolemic shock.
    b. Control hemorrhage, prevent hypovolemic shock, establish an airway, assess for head injuries.
    c. Establish an airway, control hemorrhage, prevent hypovolemic shock, assess for head injuries.
    d. Prevent hypovolemic shock, assess for head injuries, establish an airway, control hemorrhage.

16. Nursing measures for an extremity fracture would include:
    a. assessing for manifestations of shock.
    b. immobilizing the fracture site.
    c. palpating peripheral pulses.
    d. all of the above actions.

17. Progressive deterioration of body systems occurs when hypothermia lowers the body temperature to:
    a. 98°F.
    b. 97°F.
    c. 96°F.
    d. 95°F.

18. Approximately how many women experience domestic violence every year in the United States?

   a. 2 million

   b. 3 million

   c. 4 million

   d. 5 million

19. Rose, a 19-year-old student, has been sexually assaulted. When assisting with the physical examination, the nurse should do all of the following *except:*

   a. have the patient shower or wash the perineal area before the examination.

   b. assess and document any bruises and lacerations.

   c. record a history of the event, using the patient's own words.

   d. label all torn or bloody clothes and place each item in a separate brown bag so that any evidence can be given to the police.

SHORT ANSWER

Read each statement carefully. Write your response in the space provided.

1. Emergency room personnel are at increased risk for exposure to communicable disease through blood or body fluids because of the number of people infected with _____ and _____.

2. A patient with a foreign body airway obstruction demonstrates the inability to _____, _____, or _____.

3. Describe the appearance of a wound classified as a hematoma: _____

   _____

   _____

4. The most frequently injured solid organ from intra-abdominal injuries is the _____.

5. The second most common cause of unintentional death in children younger than 14 years of age is _____.

6. The most common victims of snake bites are those between the ages of _____ and _____ years.

7. An easy and immediate treatment for an ingested poison that is not caustic is _____, which immediately induces vomiting.

8. Name two agents of major concern that could be released as part of biological warfare.

   _____

   _____

II. Critical Thinking Questions and Exercises

DISCUSSION AND ANALYSIS

Discuss the following topics with your classmates.

1. Describe the criteria distinguishing the five levels of the triage system: resuscitation, emergent, urgent, nonurgent, and minor.
2. Explain the five major reasons for endotracheal intubation.
3. Describe the emergency room nursing management of a patient in hypovolemic shock.

4. Explain why lactated Ringer's solution is initially useful as fluid replacement for a patient experiencing hypovolemic shock.
5. Describe the nursing and medical intervention for a patient with heat stroke.
6. Explain the immediate nursing and medical interventions for someone who has swallowed a corrosive poison.
7. Explain the immediate intervention for a victim of carbon monoxide poisoning.
8. Describe the immediate nursing and medical management for a patient experiencing delirium tremors.
9. Describe the clinical symptoms of posttraumatic stress disorder.

APPLYING CONCEPTS

For each of the following situations, identify a nursing action with supporting rationale for managing a foreign body obstruction.

CONDITION	ACTION	RATIONALE
Heimlich maneuver for standing or sitting conscious patient	_____	_____
Heimlich maneuver with patient lying unconscious	_____	_____
Finger sweep	_____	_____
Chest thrusts with conscious patient standing or sitting		

CLINICAL SITUATIONS

For each of the following situations, supply nursing diagnoses, nursing actions, and supporting rationale for each intervention.

1. Consider a patient who has experienced blunt abdominal trauma. List your results in order of the priority of the nursing intervention.
2. List the emergency nursing measures you would carry out if you were present when someone experienced an anaphylactic reaction to a bee sting.
3. Ann is admitted to the emergency department because she ingested approximately 30 diet capsules 1 hour before admission. The nurse is to assist with gastric lavage.

Read each statement carefully. Write your response in the space provided.

4. List specific nursing interventions that can be used for drug abuse with each of the following drugs. It is assumed that the patient is presenting to the emergency department for treatment.

   a. Cocaine: _____
   b. Dexedrine: _____
   c. Valium: _____
   d. Aspirin: _____

5. List nursing actions for psychiatric emergencies in dealing with the following patients.

   a. An overactive patient: _____

   b. A violent patient: _____

   c. A depressed patient: _____

   d. A suicidal patient: _____

CHAPTER 72

Terrorism, Mass Casualty, and Disaster Nursing

I. Interpretation, Completion, and Comparison

MULTIPLE CHOICE

Read each question carefully. Circle your answer.

1. Disasters are assigned designations based on the anticipated level of response needed. A disaster that requires statewide and federal assistance would be classified as:
   a. level I.
   b. level II.
   c. level III.
   d. level IV.

2. The National Medical Response Team for Weapons of Mass Destruction is a subdivision of the:
   a. Department of Health and Human Services.
   b. Department of Justice.
   c. Federal Emergency Management Agency.
   d. National Disaster Medical System.

3. The NATO triage system uses color-coded tagging to identify severity of injuries. A patient with survivable but life-threatening injuries (eg, incomplete amputation) would be color-tagged with:
   a. black.
   b. green.
   c. red.
   d. yellow.

4. A triaged patient with a significant injury that can wait several hours for treatment would be assigned:
   a. priority 1.
   b. priority 2.
   c. priority 3.
   d. priority 4.

5. A triaged patient with psychological disturbances would be color-tagged with:
   a. black.
   b. green.
   c. red.
   d. yellow.

6. Those patients in a disaster who are unlikely to survive are triaged as:
   a. priority 1.
   b. priority 2.
   c. priority 3.
   d. priority 4.

7. The Environmental Protection Agency has identified four categories of personal protection equipment for health care workers in response to biological, chemical, or radiation exposure. The highest level of respiratory protection that includes a self-contained breathing apparatus and a chemical resistant suit is:
   a. level A.
   b. level B.
   c. level C.
   d. level D.

8. In natural disasters, what percent of trapped victims survive up to 6 hours?
   a. 80%   c. <50%
   b. 60%   d. >80%

9. The most severe form of anthrax exposure is through:
   a. skin contact.   c. ingestion.
   b. inhalation.   d. open wounds or sores.

10. An example of a chemical agent that acts by inhibiting cholinesterase is a:
    a. nerve agent.   c. corrosive acid.
    b. blood agent.   d. vesicant.

11. The type of chemical agents that do not act within seconds (latency period) are:
    a. cyanide-based.   c. nerve agents.
    b. sulfur mustards.   d. vesicants.

12. An example of the most toxic chemical agent in existence is:
    a. chlorine.   c. mustard nitrogen.
    b. cyanide.   d. sarin.

13. A common chemical agent that causes harm by separating the alveoli from the capillary bed is:
    a. chlorine.   c. phosgene.
    b. cyanide.   d. sarin.

14. There are five phases of radiation exposure related to the dose, duration, and degree of radiation penetration. The phase characterized by decreasing amounts of leukocytes and lymphocytes is the:
    a. prodromal phase.   c. illness phase.
    b. latent phase.   d. recovery phase.

SHORT ANSWER

Read each statement carefully. Write your response in the space provided.

1. An example of a biological weapon of mass destruction is _____; an example of a chemical weapon of mass destruction is _____.

2. Three federal agencies that provide disaster assistance are _____, _____, and _____.

3. Only four states in the country have locations for Disaster Medical Assistance Teams. These states are _____, _____, _____, and _____.

4. Describe the Incident Command System: _____

   _____

5. Identify five factors that influence an individual's response to disaster: _____,

   _____, _____, _____, and

   _____.

6. Distinguish between the terms *defusing* and *debriefing* as they relate to the Critical Incident Stress

   Management process: _____

   _____

7. Two biologic agents most likely to be used during a terrorist attack are _____ and

   _____.

8. Exposure to anthrax, without clinical signs and symptoms of the disease, requires a 60-day treatment

   with one of two antibiotics: _____ or _____. The mortality

   rate associated with respiratory distress is _____ percent.

9. Smallpox has a case-fatality rate of _____ percent.

10. Explain how pulmonary chemical agents (eg, phosgene) act: _____

    _____

    _____

II. Critical Thinking Questions and Exercises

DISCUSSION AND ANALYSIS

Discuss the following topics with your classmates.

1. Compare and contrast the three disaster levels.
2. Discuss the 13 components of an emergency operations plan.
3. Explain why patients who are most critically ill, with a high mortality rate, would be assigned a low triage priority in a disaster situation.
4. Discuss some of the cultural variables that health care providers need to consider in any disaster situation in which a large number patients of diverse religious and ethnic groups need to be treated.
5. Describe common behavioral responses seen in victims of mass disaster.
6. Select one of three ethical theories (utilitarianism, beneficence, justice) and apply its constructs to solving ethical conflicts in a disaster situation.
7. Describe the clinical manifestations seen with smallpox.
8. Describe the clinical manifestations of nerve gas exposure.
9. Distinguish among the three types of radiation-induced injury.
10. Describe the phases of acute radiation syndrome.

Answer Key

Chapter 1

I. Interpretation, Completion, and Comparison

MULTIPLE CHOICE

1. d   6. a
2. a   7. c
3. d   8. d
4. b   9. d
5. c   10. d

SHORT ANSWER

1. Refer to chapter heading, "The Health Care Industry and the Nursing Profession: Nursing Defined."
2. Current major health care concerns are emerging infectious diseases, trauma, obesity, and bioterrorism.
3. Human responses requiring nursing intervention should include self-image changes, impaired ventilation, and anxiety and fear. Answer may also include pain and discomfort, grief, and impaired functioning in areas such as rest and sleep.
4. Four major concepts are the capacity to perform to the best of one's ability, the flexibility of adjusting and adapting to various situations, a reported feeling of well-being, and a feeling of "harmony"—that everything is together.
5. In Maslow's hierarchy of needs, needs are ranked as follows (refer to Fig. 1-1):
   Physiologic: Food
   Safety and security: Financial security
   Belongingness and affection: Companionship
   Esteem and self-respect: Recognition by society
   Self-actualization: Achieved potential in an area
   Self-fulfillment: Creativity (painting)
   Knowledge and understanding: Information and explanation
   Aesthetics: Attractive environment
6. Stress, improper diet, lack of exercise, smoking, drugs, high-risk behaviors (including risky sexual practices), and poor hygiene are all lifestyle behaviors known to have a negative effect on health.
7. Tuberculosis, acquired immunodeficiency syndrome (AIDS), and sexually transmitted diseases.
8. Clinical pathways are tools for tracking a patient's progress toward positive outcomes within a specific period of time. Pathways include tests, treatments, activities, medications, consultations, and education within a set time period from admission to discharge.
9. Care mapping is more beneficial than a clinical pathway when a patient's complex condition defies prediction and a specific timeframe for achieving outcomes is excluded.
10. Managed care is characterized by prenegotiated payment rates, mandatory precertification, utilization review, limited choice of provider, and fixed-price reimbursement.
11. Managed care has contributed to declining in-patient hospital days, shorter lengths of hospital stay, increased acuity of patients, and expansion of ambulatory care.
12. Case management is a system where one person or team coordinates the care for the patient and family. The goals include quality care, appropriate and timely care delivery, and cost reduction.
13. Three roles for nurses are practitioner, researcher, and leader.

II. Critical Thinking Questions and Exercises

DISCUSSION AND ANALYSIS

1. Three factors that should be part of the discussion are the decline in the number of nurses entering the profession compared with 10 to 20 years ago, the approaching retirement of many currently practicing nurses, and the increased complexity of patient care that is forcing nurses to leave the profession prematurely for another job that is less demanding.
2. Discussion and analysis should include the definition of primary nursing, the scope of practice responsibility, and the challenges facing practice (e.g., increasing patient acuity, cost and staffing concerns).
3. The primary differences between community-based and community-oriented/public health nursing are the emphasis on primary, secondary, and tertiary care and prevention; the settings; and the focus of care.
4. The advanced practice nurse is able to perform functions that were previously restricted to the practice of medicine. Such functions include the performance of selected invasive procedures and the prescription of medications and treatments. The scope of practice is stipulated by individual state nurse practice acts.

SUPPORTING ARGUMENTS

Share your data and discuss your response with your instructor and classmates. There are no specific right or wrong answers. The validity of your response is determined by your ability to consciously support your argument. Refer to chapter heading, "Health Care in Transition."

RECOGNIZING CONTRADICTIONS

1. The majority of health problems today are chronic in nature.
2. A person with chronic illness can attain a high level of wellness if he or she is successful in meeting his or her health potential within the limits of the chronic illness.
3. The World Health Organization's definition of health is restrictive, not allowing for any variation in degrees of health or illness.
4. By 2030, it is predicted that the elderly in the United States will constitute 20% of the total population; racial and ethnic minorities will constitute 40% of the population.
5. The prospective payment system legislation created a level of payment that reimburses hospitals at a fixed rate and restricts patient length of stay to a predetermined number of days based on each diagnosis.
6. The main focus of continuous quality improvement (CQI) is on the processes that affect quality and patient outcomes.
7. Health care costs averaged about 15% to 22% of the GDP in 2000.
8. Home health care nursing is a major component of community-based nursing.

EXAMINING ASSOCIATIONS

1. The description should explain how a patient's medical condition is so severe that the individual can only focus on maintaining his or her basic physiologic needs. The patient is unable, either physically, mentally, or emotionally, to address the need for safety and security.
2. The collaborative model of clinical decision making is usually found in a decentralized organizational structure in which shared participation, responsibility, and accountability are promoted.

CLINICAL SITUATIONS

FLOW CHART: SMOKING

Refer to chapter heading, "Clinical Pathways and Care Mapping," and your current knowledge about anatomy and physiology.

Smoking

Respiratory Changes
- ↓ ciliary action
- ↑ mucous production
- ↑ airway resistance

Cardiovascular change
- ↑ CO levels
- ↑ arterial vasoconstriction
- ↑ blood pressure

Illnesses
- Coronary artery disease
- Emphysema
- Lung cancer

FLOW CHART: RADIAL PULSE ASSESSMENT

Refer to your knowledge of fundamental skills.

2. Radial Pulse Assessment

1.0 Patient ID	**2.0** Explain Procedure	**3.0** Identify Site	**4.0** Palpate Pulse	**5.0** Document Results
1.1 ID Patient 1.2 Ask patient's name 1.3 Check patient's name on bed	2.1 Give instruction at level of patient's learning.	3.1 Extend patient's forearm 3.2 Locate pulse on inner thumb-side of wrist	4.1 Place pads of index and middle fingers over radial artery. 4.2 Palpate for rate, rhythm, amplitude, and symmetry. 4.3 Count rate for 60 seconds if irregular, 30 seconds × 2, if regular. 4.4 Reassess for any abnormalities	5.1 Note rate and character of pulse 5.2 Record on graphic sheet on patient's chart 5.3 Report appropriate information

FLOW CHART: CQI CAUSE-AND-EFFECT DIAGRAM—DELAYED MEDICATION

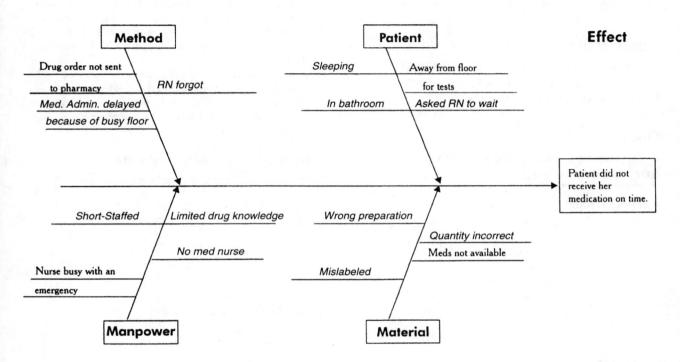

CQI Cause and Effect Diagram: Delayed Medication
Possible Causes

Method — Drug order not sent to pharmacy; RN forgot; Med. Admin. delayed because of busy floor

Patient — Sleeping; Away from floor for tests; In bathroom; Asked RN to wait

Effect — Patient did not receive her medication on time.

Manpower — Short-Staffed; Limited drug knowledge; No med nurse; Nurse busy with an emergency

Material — Wrong preparation; Quantity incorrect; Meds not available; Mislabeled

Chapter 2

I. Interpretation, Completion, and Comparison

MULTIPLE CHOICE

1. d
2. d
3. c
4. d

5. c
6. c
7. b

SHORT ANSWER

1. Hypertension, diabetes, and obesity.
2. Federal legislation, tighter insurance regulations, decreasing hospital revenues, and alternative health care delivery systems.
3. Nurses will need to be expert, independent decision makers who are self-directed, flexible, adaptable, and competent in critical thinking, physical assessment, health education, and basic nursing care.
4. Community-based nursing practice focuses on promoting and maintaining the health of individuals and families, preventing and minimizing the progression of disease, and improving the quality of life.
5. Self-care, preventive care, continuity of care, and collaboration.
6. Skilled nursing services may include intravenous therapy, injections, parenteral nutrition, venipuncture, catheter insertion, pressure ulcer and wound care, and ostomy care.
7. Call the patient to obtain permission for a visit, schedule the visit, and verify the address.
8. During the initial home visit, the patient is evaluated and a plan of care is established.
9. Ambulatory health care can be provided in medical clinics, ambulatory care units, urgent care centers, cardiac rehabilitation programs, mental health and student health facilities, community outreach programs, and nurse-managed centers.
10. Trauma, tuberculosis, anemia, lice, scabies, hypothermia, skin disorders, dental problems, sexually transmitted diseases, and mental illness.

II. Critical Thinking Questions and Exercises

DISCUSSION AND ANALYSIS

1. Refer to the book, *Community and Public Health Nursing,* by M. Stanhope and J. Lancaster, 2004, St. Louis, Mosby.
2. Primary prevention focuses on health promotion and disease prevention (e.g., diabetic counseling).

Secondary prevention focuses on health maintenance, early detection, and prompt intervention
(e.g., health care screening). Tertiary prevention
focuses on minimizing deterioration and improving
the quality of life (e.g., health care screening, rehabilitation).
3. Refer to chapter heading, "The Growing Need for
Community-Based Health Care."

CLINICAL SITUATION

CASE STUDY: ASSESSING THE NEED FOR A HOME VISIT

Refer to chapter heading, "Home Health Visits" and
Chart 2-2 to complete the case study.

Chapter 3

I. Interpretation, Completion, and Comparison

MULTIPLE CHOICE

1. b	7. d	13. c
2. c	8. d	14. a
3. b	9. c	15. a
4. d	10. b	16. d
5. a	11. d	17. b
6. a	12. d	

SHORT ANSWER

1. Answer may include active thinker, fair, independent
and open-minded, persistent, empathic, honest, organ-
ized and systematic, proactive, flexible, realistic, hum-
ble, logical, curious, and insightful. Critical thinkers are
good communicators and are committed to excellence.
2. Analysis, evaluation, explanation, inference, interpretation, and self-regulation.
3. Critical thinking is influenced by the culture, attitude,
and experiences of the individual, who sees the situation through the lens of his or her experiences.
4. Moral distress occurs when one is aware of the correct course of action but institutional constraints
stand in the way of pursuing the correct action.
5. Nursing practice encompasses the protection, promotion, and optimization of health and abilities, prevention of illness and injury, alleviation of suffering
through the diagnosis and treatment of human
response, and advocacy in the care of individuals,
families, communities, and populations.
6. Two types of "advanced directive" are a living will
and a durable power of attorney.
7. An "advanced directive" provides health care practitioners with information about the patient's wishes for
health care before his or her illness or hospitalization.
8. Suggested statements include "Please tell me what
brought you to the hospital," "Please tell me what
you think your needs are," and "Please tell me about
your past history."

9. A nursing diagnosis identifies actual or potential
health problems that guide nurses in the development
of a plan of care, and it is amenable to resolution by
nursing actions. Collaborative problems are potential
problems or complications that are medical in origin
and require collaborative interventions with the physician and the health care team. The nursing diagnosis
and collaborative problems are the patient's nursing
problems. A medical diagnosis identifies diseases, conditions, or pathology that can be medically managed.
Refer to Figure 3-2.
10. Expected outcomes of nursing intervention should be
stated in behavioral terms and should be realistic as
well as measurable. Expected behavioral outcomes
serve as the basis for evaluating the effectiveness of
nursing intervention.

NURSING OR COLLABORATIVE PROBLEMS

Refer to Figures 3-1 and 3-2 and Charts 3-6 and 3-7.

1. N	6. N
2. N	7. C
3. C	8. C
4. C	9. N
5. N	10. C

MATCHING (CRITICAL THINKING)

Refer to Chart 3-1.

1. e	5. a
2. g	6. c
3. f	7. b
4. d	

MATCHING (ETHICAL PRINCIPLES)

Refer to Chart 3-2.

1. d	4. f
2. e	5. a
3. b	6. c

II. Critical Thinking Questions and Exercises

DISCUSSION AND ANALYSIS

Refer to chapter heading, "Using the Nursing Process:
Planning," for questions 1 to 3 and Chart 3-9.

RECOGNIZING CONTRADICTIONS

1. Nursing ethics is a distinct form of applied ethics
because nursing is its own separate profession.
2. A moral dilemma occurs when a clear conflict
between one or more principles exist.
3. Moral distress exists when a nurse is prevented from
doing what he or she believes is correct.

4. A request for withdrawal of food and hydration necessitates an evaluation of harm and may not be routinely supported even for competent patients.

5. Living wills are not always honored because they refer to terminal illnesses and patients frequently change their perspective as they become sicker.

SUPPORTING ARGUMENTS

Answers are individualized; there are no right or wrong responses. Refer to chapter heading, "Ethical Nursing Care," for questions 1 to 3.

CLINICAL SITUATIONS

Outcomes per Nursing Diagnosis (refer to NOC, Chart 3-8).

1. Patient will be able to walk from his room to the nursing station every morning with respiratory rate within normal limits.

2. Patient will move from bed to chair on second postoperative day with legs abducted.

3. Patient will achieve a balance between fluid intake and output with a weight gain no greater than 1 lb/week.

4. Patient will eat 1800 cal/day to maintain a desired weight of 135 lb.

5. Patient will sleep 6 to 8 hours, without interruption, every evening.

CASE STUDY: ETHICAL ANALYSIS

Assessment

Your answer should include the conflict between the nurse's professional obligation to provide treatment to all and the unpleasant outcome of choosing "the lesser of two evils."

Planning

You should be able to analyze the medical and political data that influence the treatment options. Because of the vast numbers of infected citizens relative to available treatment, not everyone can be cared for.

Implementation

You need to carefully analyze the outcomes of both theories for your decision making. There is no right or wrong answer. You just need to support your decision with an ethical theory.

Evaluation

Your evaluation needs to show logical sequencing of problem solving based on an ethical theory. There is no right or wrong response.

Chapter 4

I. Interpretation, Completion, and Comparison

MULTIPLE CHOICE

1. d
2. d
3. d
4. b
5. a
6. a
7. a
8. a
9. b
10. a
11. a

SHORT ANSWER

1. Significant factors are the availability of health care outside the conventional hospital setting, the employment of diverse health care providers to accomplish care management goals, and the increased use of alternative strategies.

2. People with chronic illness need as much health care information as possible to actively participate in and assume responsibility for the management of their own care. Health education can help the patient adapt to illness and cooperate with a treatment regimen. The goal of health education is to teach people to maximize their health potential.

3. Medication compliance, maintaining a healthy diet, daily exercise, self-monitoring for signs of illness, practicing good overall hygiene, health screenings and evaluations, and therapeutic, preventive measures.

4. Adherence implies that a patient makes one or more lifestyle changes to carry out specific activities to promote and maintain health.

5. Factors influencing adherence include demographic variables such as age, sex, and education; illness variables such as the severity of illness and the effects of therapy; psychosocial variables such as intelligence and attitudes toward illness; financial variables; and therapeutic regimen variables.

6. The variable of choice, establishment of agreed-upon goals, and the quality of the patient- provider relationship.

7. The teaching-learning process requires the active involvement of teacher and learner, in an effort to reach the desired outcome—a change in behavior. The teacher serves as a facilitator of learning.

8. The elderly have difficulty adhering to a therapeutic regimen because of increased sensitivity to medications, difficulty in adjusting to change and stress, financial constraints, forgetfulness, inadequate support systems, lifetime habits of self-medication, visual impairments, hearing deficits, and mobility limitations.

9. Increased age decreases the elderly's ability to draw inferences, apply information, and understand major teaching points.

10. The effects of a learning situation are influenced by a person's physical, emotional, and experiential readiness to learn. Physical readiness implies the physical ability of a person to attend to a learning situation. Basic physiologic needs are met so that higher-level needs can be addressed. Emotional readiness involves the patient's motivation to learn and can be encouraged by providing realistic goals that can be easily achieved so that self-esteem needs can be met. A person needs to be ready to accept the emotional changes (anxiety, stress) that accompany behavior modification

resulting from the learning process. Experiential readiness refers to a person's past experiences that influence his or her approach to the learning process. Previous positive feedback and improved self-image reinforce experiential readiness.

11. Lecture method, group teaching, demonstrations, teaching aids, reinforcement, and follow- up.

12. The two major goals from Healthy People 2010 are to increase the quality and years of healthy life for people and to eliminate health disparities among various segments of the population.

13. Self-responsibility, nutritional awareness, stress reduction and management, and physical fitness.

II. Critical Thinking Questions and Exercises

DISCUSSION AND ANALYSIS

1. Refer to Table 4-1.
2. Refer to chapter heading, "Health Promotion Exercises."

RECOGNIZING CONTRADICTIONS

1. Health education is an independent function of nursing practice that is a primary responsibility of the nursing profession.
2. Although diseases in children and those of an infectious nature are of utmost concern, the largest group of people today who need health education are those with chronic illness.
3. Patients are encouraged to adhere to their therapeutic regimen. Adherence connotes active, voluntary, collaborative patient efforts, whereas compliance is a more passive role.
4. Evaluation should be continuous throughout the teaching process so that the information gathered can be used to improve teaching activities.
5. The elderly usually experience significant gains from health promotion activities.
6. About 80% of those older than 65 years of age have one or more chronic illnesses.

EXAMINING ASSOCIATIONS

Refer to Table 4-1 in the text to complete the chart.

Chapter 5

I. Interpretation, Completion, and Comparison

MULTIPLE CHOICE

1. d	6. c
2. d	7. b
3. d	8. d (Chart 5-1)
4. b	9. b
5. b	10. a

11. d	14. a
12. a	15. a
13. a	

SHORT ANSWER

1. The responsibilities are obtaining a patient health history and performing a physical examination.
2. The nurse needs to establish rapport, put the patient at ease, encourage honest communication, make eye contact, and listen carefully.
3. When an atmosphere of mutual trust and confidence exists between an interviewer and a patient, the patient becomes more open and honest and is more likely to share personal concerns and problems.
4. The term chief complaint refers to that issue that brings the patient to seek help. When documenting a patient's chief complaint, exact words should be recorded in quotation marks.
5. Answer may include any of the following: cancer, hypertension, heart disease, diabetes, epilepsy, mental illness, tuberculosis, kidney disease, arthritis, allergies, asthma, alcoholism, and obesity.
6. Health-related behaviors include patterns of sleep, exercise, nutrition, recreation, and personal habits (e.g., smoking) and use of drugs, alcohol and caffeine.
7. The leading causes are heart disease, cancer, and stroke.
8. The values are 25 to 29 (overweight); 30 to 39 (obese); greater than 40 (extremely obese); below 24 (at risk for poor nutritional status). Refer to Figure 5-6.
9. Men, greater than 40 inches; women, greater than 35 inches.
10. Negative nitrogen balance occurs when nitrogen output (urine, feces, perspiration) exceeds nitrogen intake (food). When this happens, tissue is breaking down faster than it is being replaced.
11. The minerals often in deficit are iron, folate, and calcium.
12. Correlation

a. Inspection	e. Percussion
b. Inspection	f. Auscultation
c. Palpation	g. Auscultation
d. Palpation	h. Palpation

MATCHING

1. h	4. e
2. c	5. g
3. d	6. b

II. Critical Thinking Questions and Exercises

CLINICAL SITUATIONS

CASE STUDY: CALCULATE A HEALTHY DIET

Part I: Estimate Ideal Body Weight

1. b, medium frame (height-to-wrist circumference is 10.4)
2. IBW is 125 lb, needs to lose 50 lb (refer to Chart 5-6)
3. BMI is 29; overweight

Part II: Calculate a Balanced Diet Using the Food Guide Pyramid as a Reference (Fig. 5-7)

1. approximately 56 kilograms
2. 1418 cal
3. 1985 cal (1418–567)
4. 993 cal from carbohydrates, 595 cal from fat, 397 cal from protein (Fig. 5-6)
5. 248 g of carbohydrates, 66 g of fat, 99 g of protein

Part III

1. fruits; vegetables
2. whole grains
3. 2½ cups
4. meat; beans
5. low fat or fat-free
6. 2 cups

Chapter 6

I. Interpretation, Completion, and Comparison

MULTIPLE CHOICE

1. d	12. a	23. d
2. d	13. b	24. d
3. b	14. b	25. d
4. a	15. d	26. b
5. d	16. d	27. b
6. d	17. a	28. a
7. d	18. d	29. c
8. b	19. b	30. a
9. a	20. d	31. d
10. b	21. d	
11. c	22. c	

MATCHING

1. b	5. b
2. a	6. a
3. a	7. b
4. a	8. a

SHORT ANSWER

1. Four concepts are constancy, homeostasis, stress, and adaptation.
2. When the body suffers an injury, the response is mal-adaptive if the defense mechanisms have a negative effect on health.
3. Hyperpnea is the body's development of rapid breathing after intense exercise in response to an accumulation of lactic acid in muscle tissue and a deficit of oxygen.

4. Examples of acute, time-limited stressors include taking an examination, giving a speech, and driving in a snowstorm. Examples of chronic, enduring stressors include poverty, a handicap or disability, and living with an alcoholic.
5. Answer may include any of the following: traffic jam, sick child, missed appointment, car won't start, train is late (day-to-day stressors); earthquakes, wars, terrorism, events of history (major events that affect large groups of people); marriage, birth, death, retirement (infrequently occurring major stressors).
6. Adolph Meyer, in the 1930s, first showed a correlation between illness and critical life events. A Recent Life Changes Questionnaire (RLCQ) was developed by Holmes and Rahe which assigned numerical values to life events that require a change in an individual's life pattern. A correlation was seen between illness and the number of stressful events: the higher the numerical value, the greater the chance for becoming ill.
7. Cognitive appraisal refers to the evaluation of an event relative to what is at stake and what coping resources are available. External resources consist of money to purchase services and materials and social support systems that provide emotional and esteem support.
8. Hans Selye stated that "stress is essentially the rate of wear and tear on the body." He also defined stress as being a "nonspecific response" of the body regardless of the stimulus producing the response.
9. Bodily functions are blood pressure, acid-base balance, blood glucose levels, body temperature, and fluid and electrolyte balance.
10. The five signs are redness, heat, swelling, pain, and loss of function.
11. Answer can include anxiety, ineffective coping patterns, impaired thought processes, disrupted relationships, impaired adjustment, ineffective coping, social isolation, risk for spiritual distress, decisional conflict, and so on.

II. Critical Thinking Questions and Exercises

DISCUSSION AND ANALYSIS

1. Refer to chapter heading, "Stress and Function."
2. Refer to chapter heading, "Stress: Threats to the Steady State."
3. Refer to chapter heading, "Stress: Threats to the Steady State."
4. Refer to chapter heading, "Stress as a Stimulus for Disease."
5. Refer to chapter heading, " Psychological Responses to Stress."
6. Refer to chapter heading, "Selye's Theory of Adaptation."

CLINICAL SITUATIONS

FLOW CHART: THE SYMPATHETIC-ADRENAL MEDULLARY
RESPONSE TO STRESS

Refer to Table 6-1 for flow chart of physiologic reactions.

General body arousal		Rationale
↑ Norepinephrine =	↑ <u>blood coagulability</u>	↑ <u>cardiac output</u>
	↑ <u>heart rate</u>	↑ <u>myocardial contractility</u>
	↑ <u>blood pressure</u>	↑ <u>peripheral vasoconstriction</u>
	↑ <u>blood glucose levels</u>	↑ <u>glycogen breakdown</u>

Effects on:

Skeletal muscles	<u>increased tension</u>	↑ <u>increased excitation of muscles</u>
Pupils	<u>dilated</u>	<u>contraction of radial muscle of iris</u>
Ventilation	<u>rapid and shallow</u>	<u>stimulation of respiratory center in medulla</u>

CASE STUDY: HYPERTENSIVE HEART DISEASE

Refer to Figure 6-2 for nursing implications and
rationales.

Selected Compensatory Mechanisms	*Nursing Implications*	*Rationale*
Renal blood flow is decreased as a result of hypertensive heart disease	**Assessment**	
	A. Blood pressure	A. Changes in the cardiovascular system are reflected in the blood pressure
	B. Urinary output	
	1. Amount	1. Output decreased with decreased blood flow
	2. Characteristics	2. Color changes occur with increased blood flow
	3. Urine chemistry values	
	a. Osmolality	a. Osmolality increases with heart failure
	b. Electrolytes	b. Potassium increases with renal failure
	C. Ability to cope with stress	C. Stress results in increased resistance to cardiac output

Nursing Diagnoses/ Collaborative Problem

A. Fluid volume excess related to renin-angiotensin stimulation

A. Renin-angiotensin has a direct vasoconstriction effect on arterioles which leads to water retention

Planning

A. Plan time for assessment around patient's need for rest.
B. Plan an individual program of stress reduction

A. Rest lowers metabolic rate and facilitates the healing process

B. Compliance with a stress-management program will be higher if the program is individualized

Implementation

A. Teach various relaxation techniques

B. Develop specific ways to help the patient cope with and reduce stress
C. Modify diet to reduce sodium intake

A. Stress tends to increase epinephrine secretion, which causes vasoconstriction; this, in turn, increases the heart rate and resistance to cardiac output
B. Stress reduction tends to reduce epinephrine secretion

C. Lowered sodium levels tend to decrease fluid retention, which decreases the work load of the heart

Evaluation

A. Stress-reduction measures

B. Dietary compliance relative to lowered sodium intake

A. Blood pressure reduction may be indicative of successful stress-reduction measures
B. Weight estimates, serum sodium levels, and the presence of edema are indicators of fluid retention and possible excess intake of sodium.

IDENTIFYING PATTERNS

FLOW CHART: SYMPATHETIC-ADRENAL AND HYPOTHALAMIC-PITUITARY RESPONSE

Refer to Figure 6-3 and chapter heading, "Interpretation of Stressful Stimuli by the Brain."

Chapter 7

I. Interpretation, Completion, and Comparison

MULTIPLE CHOICE

1. d
2. d
3. d
4. b
5. c
6. b
7. d
8. b
9. a
10. b
11. c

SHORT ANSWER

1. 35% to 45%
2. The most common definition of a mental disorder is from the American Psychiatric Association: "a group of behavioral or psychological symptoms or a pattern which manifests itself in a significant distress, impaired functioning, or accentuated risk of enduring severe suffering or possible death."

3. Five significant family functions are (a) the use of power, decision making about resources, the establishment of rules, and provision of finances and future planning; (b) boundary setting; (c) communication; (d) education, family support, and appropriate modeling skills for living; and (e) socialization of acceptable behaviors for life.
4. Seven coping skills for families under stress are communication, spirituality, cognitive abilities, emotional strength, relationship capabilities, use of community resources, and personal talents and strengths.
5. Five common emotional responses to PTSD are anxiety, anger, aggression, depression, and fear of being threatened.
6. Physiologic responses that are increased are activity of the sympathetic nervous system, plasma catecholamine levels, and urinary epinephrine and norepinephrine levels.
7. Seven examples of life events that trigger PTSD are rape, family violence, torture, earthquake, terrorism, fire, and military combat.
8. Duration and severity are the two criteria.
9. Somatic complaints include headache, backache, abdominal pain, fatigue, malaise, anxiety, and sexual problems.

10. Intoxication and withdrawal are two common substance abuse problems.

MATCHING

1. e		6. a	
2. c		7. c	
3. a		8. a	
4. d		9. e	
5. b		10. c	

II. Critical Thinking Questions and Exercises

DISCUSSION AND ANALYSIS

1. Refer to Charts 7-3 and 7-4.

RECOGNIZING CONTRADICTIONS

1. Since the 1980s there has been an increase in the use of holistic health care.
2. The holistic approach to health care reconnects the mind and body traditionally separated by medicine.
3. Depression and its accompanying symptoms of sadness, anxiety, and fatigue is a common response to health problems and is not age specific. Clinical depression is distinguished from everyday feelings of sadness by duration and severity.
4. Almost 66% of people who were severely depressed and committed suicide had been seen by a health care practitioner within 4 weeks before death.
5. A diagnosis of clinical depression requires the presence of five out of nine diagnostic criteria.

CLINICAL SITUATIONS

CASE STUDY: HODGKIN'S DISEASE

1. a
2. b
3. d

CASE STUDY: RADICAL MASTECTOMY

1. a
2. b
3. b
4. d

Chapter 8

I. Interpretation, Completion, and Comparison

MULTIPLE CHOICE

1. d	3. d
2. d	4. d

5. a	10. a
6. d	11. c
7. b	12. c
8. a	13. b
9. a	

SHORT ANSWER

1. The founder is Madeleine Leininger.
2. The four basic characteristics of culture are the following: it is learned from birth through language and socialization; it is shared by all members of the same cultural group; it is influenced by specific environmental and technical factors; and it is dynamic and ever-changing.
3. Frequently differences in skin color, religion, and geographic area are the only elements used to identify diversity.
4. Four subcultures are African American, Hispanic/Latino, Asian/Pacific Islanders, and Native Americans.
5. Subcultures can also be grouped according to religion, occupation, age, sexual orientation, geographic location, and race.
6. Goals are to provide culture-specific care and culture-universal care.
7. Culturally competent or congruent nursing care refers to the delivery of interventions within the cultural context of the patient. It involves the integration of attitudes, knowledge, and skills to enable nurses to deliver care in a culturally sensitive manner.
8. Four strategies are changing the subject, nonquestioning, inappropriate laughter, and nonverbal cues.
9. Catholics, Mormons, Buddhists, Jews, and Muslims routinely abstain from eating as part of their religious practice.
10. The yin and yang theory of illness proposes that the seat of energy in the body is within the autonomic nervous system, where balance is maintained between the key opposing forces. Yin represents the female and negative forces, whereas yang represents the male and positive forces.

II. Critical Thinking Questions and Exercises

DISCUSSION AND ANALYSIS

1. The goal of Leininger's research-based theory is to provide culturally congruent nursing care to improve care to people of different or similar cultures. Her theory provides care through culture care accommodation and culture care restructuring.
2. Culture care accommodation refers to professional nursing actions and decisions to help patients of a designated culture achieve a beneficial outcome. Culture care restructuring refers to the professional actions that help patients reorder, change, or modify their lifestyles toward more beneficial health care.

3. Acculturation is the process by which members of a cultural group adapt to or learn how to take on the behaviors of another group. Cultural imposition is the tendency to impose one's cultural beliefs, values, and patterns of behavior on others from a different culture.
4. General polymorphism is the biologic variation in individuals' response to medications that is the result of differences in age, gender, size, and body composition.
5. Differences in the five categories of alternative medicine can be found under chapter heading, "Complementary and Alternative Therapies."

Chapter 9

I. Interpretation, Completion, and Comparison

MULTIPLE CHOICE

1. b	7. b
2. b	8. b
3. d	9. c
4. a	10. a
5. c	11. d
6. a	12. a

SHORT ANSWER

1. Genomic medicine encompasses the recognition that multiple genes work in concert with environmental influences, resulting in the appearance and expression of disease.
2. To integrate genetics into nursing practice, the nurse uses family history and the results of genetic tests, informs patients about genetic concepts, is aware of the personal and societal impact of genetic information, and values privacy and confidentiality.
3. genotype; phenotype
4. chromosomes; autosomes; sex chromosomes; X chromosomes; one X and one Y chromosome; one sex chromosome of each pair
5. Answer may include heart disease, high blood pressure, cancer, osteoarthritis, neural tube defects, spina bifida, and anencephaly.
6. Down syndrome
7. 1 in every 160; 50%
8. Pharmacogenetics involves the use of genetic testing to identify genetic variations that relate to the safety and efficacy of medications and gene-based treatments.
9. Hemochromatosis (iron overload)
10. The nursing activities are as follows: collect and help interpret relevant family and medical histories, identify patients and families who need genetic evaluation and counseling, offer genetics information and resources, collaborate with the genetic specialist, and participate in management of patient care.

MATCHING: GENETIC TERMS

1. e	5. g
2. h	6. d
3. f	7. b
4. a	8. c

MATCHING: ADULT-ONSET DISORDERS

1. b	5. a
2. c	6. a
3. e	7. d
4. d	8. f

II. Critical Thinking Questions and Exercises

DISCUSSION AND ANALYSIS

1. Refer to Chart 9-1.
2. Refer to chapter heading, "Inheritance Patterns"
3. Refer to chapter heading, "Specific Nursing Roles in Genetic Counseling"

Chapter 10

I. Interpretation, Completion, and Comparison

MULTIPLE CHOICE

1. b	8. a
2. c	9. b
3. b	10. b
4. d	11. b
5. b	12. a
6. a	13. b
7. b	

SHORT ANSWER

1. obesity, cardiac disease, and diabetes
2. Answer should include four of the following causes: decreased mortality from infectious disease; longer life spans due to advances in technology and pharmacology; improved screening, diagnosis, early detection, and treatment of diseases; prompt and aggressive management of acute conditions; increased longevity and lifestyle factors such as smoking, diet, and physical inactivity.
3. pain, fatigue, and some degree of disability
4. Inability to shower or bathe because of a fear of falling and inability to get to the bathroom are the two most frequent interferences with daily activities that occur in chronic illnesses.

5. Answers may include preventing the occurrence of other chronic conditions; alleviating and managing symptoms; preventing, adapting to, and managing disabilities; preventing and managing crises and complications; adapting to repeated threats and progressive functional loss; and living with isolation and loneliness.

6. The Trajectory Model refers to the path or course of action taken by the ill person, his family, health professionals, and others to manage the course of the illness.

II. Critical Thinking Questions and Exercises

DISCUSSION AND ANALYSIS

1. A disability is a physical or mental impairment that substantially limits one or more major life events. A handicap is a disadvantage experienced because of society-imposed barriers.
2. Refer to chapter heading, "Overview of Chronicity."
3. Refer to chapter heading, "Implications of Managing Chronic Conditions."
4. Refer to chapter heading, "Federal Legislation."

EXAMINING ASSOCIATIONS

1. Explain that medical conditions are associated with psychological and social problems which can affect body image and alter lifestyles. Give examples.
2. Explain that chronic conditions have acute, stable, and unstable periods, flare-ups, and remissions. Each phase requires different types of management. Give examples.
3. Explain that complying with a therapeutic treatment plan requires time, knowledge, and a long-term commitment to prevent the incidence of complications.
4. Explain that the whole family experiences stress and caretaker fatigue. Social changes that can occur include loss of income, role reversals, and altered socialization activities.

CLINICAL SITUATIONS

CASE STUDY: APPLYING THE NURSING PROCESS TO THE TRAJECTORY MODEL OF CHRONIC ILLNESS.

1. Step 1. The nurse uses assessment to determine specific problems and the Trajectory phase of the chronic illness. For example, the nurse determines whether any musculoskeletal deficiencies are evident, whether fatigue is interfering with activities of daily living, and whether the patient is emotionally capable of coping with the diagnosis.
2. Step 2. The nurse interacts with the family and the medical team to establish and prioritize specific collaborative goals of management and support. For

example, the nurse, working with the physician and physical therapist, designs an exercise program that will maximize current musculoskeletal strength while preventing excessive stress on major joints.

3. Step 3. The nurse can help the patient and family define a plan of action (e.g., draft a list of activities, exercises periods, and rest periods that can support established goals). The nurse can also identify specific criteria to be used to measure progress toward goal attainment. For example, the patient can keep a daily record of pain and joint stiffness, participation in work activities, and time allocated for recreation. The nurse can review the plan periodically with the patient.
4. Step 4. The nurse plans specific interventions to provide care. The nurse can help with direct care (e.g., range of motion exercises, applications of warm compresses, adjustments to the environment). The nurse can recommend referrals to counseling or agencies that can help provide services. The nurse can help the family work together to determine a lifelong approach to treatment and support.
5. Step 5. The nurse follows up to determine how the problem, along with treatment and management interventions, is being resolved and whether there is adherence to the plan. The nurse identifies environmental, social, and psychological factors that may facilitate or hinder goal achievement. For example, the nurse could explore the time commitment and types of activities required for child care and how they affect the patient. Does the patient have support from extended family members? Can the patient adjust his or her work schedule if necessary? Are there any associated systemic conditions that may compromise a plan of care, such as renal problems or swollen joints?

Chapter 11

I. Interpretation, Completion, and Comparison

MULTIPLE CHOICE

1. d	8. c	15. d
2. b	9. d	16. d
3. b	10. d	17. a
4. b	11. c	18. d
5. a	12. a	19. d
6. a	13. a	20. d
7. b	14. b	

SHORT ANSWER

1. The goal of rehabilitation is to restore the patient's ability to function independently or at a preillness or preinjury level and to maximize independence and prevent secondary disability.
2. Refer to chapter heading, "Nursing Process: The Patient with Self-Care Deficits in Activities of Daily Living."

3. Answer should include four of the following eight diagnoses: impaired physical mobility, activity intolerance, risk for injury, risk for disuse syndrome, impaired walking, impaired wheelchair mobility, and impaired bed mobility. Answer should also include four of the following five goals: absence of contracture and deformity, maintenance of muscle strength and joint mobility, independent mobility, increased activity tolerance and prevention of further disability.
4. "reasonable accommodations" and "without undue hardship"
5. A contracture is a shortening of the muscle and tendon that leads to deformity. Contractures limit joint mobility.
6. Weakened muscles, joint contractures, and deformity are common complications associated with prolonged immobility.
7. external rotation of the hip and plantar flexion of the foot (footdrop)
8. prolonged bed rest, lack of exercise, incorrect positioning in bed, and the weight of the bedding
9. three
10. right; right
11. braces, splints, collars, corsets, supports, and calipers
12. Refer to Figure 11-3.
13. sepsis, osteomyelitis, pyarthrosis, and septic shock
14. does not permit free drainage of the tissue

MATCHING

1. e
2. a
3. b
4. d
5. f
6. c

II. Critical Thinking Questions and Exercises

DISCUSSION AND ANALYSIS

1. Refer to Chart 11-2.
2. Refer to chapter heading, "Assessment of Functional Ability."
3. Refer to chapter heading, "Nursing Process: The Patient with Self-Care Deficits in Activities of Daily Living."
4. Pressure ulcers occur when pressure on the skin is greater than normal capillary closure pressure (32 mm Hg). The initial sign of pressure is erythema caused by reactive hyperemia which, if unrelieved after 1 hour, results in tissue ischemia or anoxia.
5. Refer to chapter heading, "Promoting Pressure Ulcer Healing"
6. For example, define the goal of the activity. The goal would be to demonstrate independent self-care in bathing/hygiene with assistance. The nurse would assess the home environment and family support and then design a realistic plan of care for 1 to 2 weeks.
7. Answer may include impaired physical mobility, activity intolerance, risk for injury, risk for disuse syndrome, impaired walking, and impaired mobility.

CLINICAL SITUATIONS

1. Pressure ulcers are localized areas of infarcted soft tissue that occur when pressure applied to the skin over time is greater than normal capillary closure pressure, approximately 32 mm Hg.
2. erythema; reactive hyperemia
3. sacrum and heels
4. c
5. b
6. Pascal's law; As the body sinks into the fluid, more surface area becomes available for weight bearing, thus decreasing body weight per unit area.
7. Increased elevation increases the downward-pulling force of body weight, which increases pressure on the skin, which results in localized blood flow reduction.

CASE STUDY: TRAUMATIC AMPUTATION—PSYCHOSOCIAL PERSPECTIVE

1. c
2. c
3. b
4. d

CASE STUDY: BUCK'S EXTENSION TRACTION

1. b
2. a
3. a

CASE STUDY: ASSISTED AMBULATION: CRUTCHES

1. b
2. b
3. c
4. b

Chapter 12

I. Interpretation, Completion, and Comparison

MULTIPLE CHOICE

1. b
2. b
3. d
4. b
5. b
6. d
7. a
8. a
9. b
10. a
11. c
12. c
13. a
14. b
15. d
16. c
17. c
18. d
19. b
20. a
21. a

SHORT ANSWER

1. 28 years; 22%; 21%
2. 87 years
3. chronic disease
4. heart disease; cancer; and stroke
5. The six tasks are maintenance of self-worth, conflict resolution, adjustment to loss of dominant roles, adjustment to deaths of significant others, environmental adaptation, and maintenance of optimal levels of wellness.
6. macular degeneration
7. 70 years

8. memory, abstract reasoning, judgment, and language
9. multi-infarct dementia
10. pneumonia, urinary tract infections, tuberculosis, gastrointestinal infections, and skin infections

II. Critical Thinking Questions and Exercises

INTERPRETING DATA

1. 4.7%
2. 13.8%; two
3. greater rate; 16.2%
4. 9%; 1960–1980; 1980–2000
5. 70 million

RECOGNIZING CONTRADICTIONS

1. The muscles, composed of postmitotic cells, diminish in size and lose strength, flexibility, and endurance with decreased activity and advanced age.
2. Osteoporosis can be arrested or prevented, but not reversed.
3. If the symptoms of delirium go untreated and the underlying cause is not treated, permanent, irreversible brain damage or death can occur.
4. It is a myth that older people should avoid vigorous activity. Activity is a desired state in older adults.
5. In the older person, the baseline body temperature is usually 1°F lower than in a younger person. Therefore, a temperature elevation should be considered serious.

DISCUSSION AND ANALYSIS

1. The activity theory proposes that life satisfaction in normal aging requires maintaining the active lifestyle of middle age. The continuity theory proposes that successful adjustment to old age requires continuing life patterns across a lifetime.
2. Refer to chapter heading, "Health Care Costs of Aging."
3. Refer to chapter heading, "Ethical and Legal Issues Affecting the Older Adult."
4. Refer to chapter heading, "Ethical and Legal Issues Affecting the Older Adult."

CLINICAL SITUATIONS

CASE STUDY: LONELINESS

1. d	4. d
2. d	5. d
3. a	

CASE STUDY: ALZHEIMER'S DISEASE

1. a
2. acetylcholine; cerebral cortex; brain size
3. c
4. d

5. d
6. pneumonia, malnutrition, and dehydration

CASE STUDY: DEHYDRATION

1. d	3. d
2. c	4. d

Chapter 13

I. Interpretation, Completion, and Comparison

MULTIPLE CHOICE

1. d	8. a	15. c
2. b	9. a	16. b
3. d	10. a	17. d
4. b	11. d	18. d
5. c	12. d	19. c
6. c	13. d	20. d
7. b	14. c	

SHORT ANSWER

1. "whatever the person says it is, existing whenever the experiencing person says it does"
2. duration, location, and etiology
3. the suppression of immune function that promotes tumor growth
4. histamine, bradykinin, acetylcholine, serotonin, and substance P
5. past experience, anxiety, depression, culture, gender, and genetics
6. A placebo effect occurs when a person responds to a medication or treatment because of an expectation that the treatment will work rather the treatment's actually effectiveness.
7. Factors include intensity, timing, location, quality personal meaning of pain, aggravating and alleviating factors, and pain behaviors.
8. Physiologic responses are tachycardia, hypertension, tachypnea, pallor, diaphoresis, mydriasis, hyper vigilance, and increased muscle tone.
9. Balanced analgesia refers to the use of more than one form of analgesia concurrently to obtain more pain relief with fewer side effects.
10. opioids, NSAIDs, and local anesthetics
11. transcutaneous electrical nerve stimulation (TENS) and dorsal spinal cord stimulation.

CROSSWORD PUZZLE

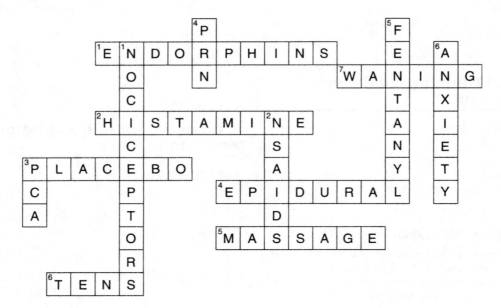

II. Critical Thinking Questions and Exercises

DISCUSSION AND ANALYSIS

1. Refer to Chart 13-1.
2. Acute pain, which lasts from seconds to 3 to 6 weeks (e.g., appendectomy, ankle sprain). Chronic, persistent, nonmalignant pain lasts 6 months or longer (e.g., rheumatoid arthritis, fibromyalgia). Cancer-related pain can be directly associated with the cancer and/or the result of cancer treatment (e.g., ovarian and lung cancer).
3. Refer to Figure 13-3.
4. The classic Gate Control Theory proposes that stimulation of the skin evokes nervous impulses which are then transmitted by three systems located in the spinal cord. The noxious impulses are influenced by a "gating mechanism." The concept proposed is that stimulation of the large-diameter fibers inhibits the transmission of pain, thus "closing the gate." Conversely, when smaller fibers are stimulated, the gate is opened. This mechanism is influenced by nerve impulses that descend from the brain. This theory also proposes a specialized system of large-diameter fibers that activate selective cognitive processes via the modulating properties of the spinal gate. (Refer to Fig. 13-4.)
5. Refer to Table 13-3.
6. COX-1 and COX-2 inhibitors (e.g., Advil, Motrin, Celebrex, Vioxx) inhibit the enzyme (cyclo-oxygenase) that is involved in the production of prostaglandin in response to traumatized or inflamed tissues.
7. Distraction, which involves focusing the patient's attention on something other than the pain, reduces the perception of pain by stimulating the descending control system. This results in transmission of fewer painful stimuli to the brain.

CLINICAL SITUATIONS

CASE STUDY: PAIN EXPERIENCE

1. a	3. d
2. c	4. d

Chapter 14

I. Interpretation, Completion, and Comparison

MULTIPLE CHOICE

1. c	13. b	25. b
2. b	14. a	26. d
3. b	15. c	27. b
4. c	16. a	28. c
5. d	17. b	29. d
6. a	18. c	30. d
7. b	19. c	31. c
8. a	20. a	32. a
9. d	21. b	33. c
10. b	22. d	34. b
11. c	23. d	35. a
12. b	24. c	36. d

SHORT ANSWER

1. 66%; potassium; compartments are intravascular, interstitial and transcellular; sodium; 50%; 6 liters; plasma

2. Colloidal osmotic pressure refers to the pressure exerted by plasma proteins to hold fluid within vessels. The osmotic pressure is a pulling force.
3. Urine specific gravity measures the kidney's ability to excrete or conserve water. BUN, made up of urea, is an end product of protein (muscle and dietary) metabolism. Creatinine, as the end product of muscle metabolism, is a better indicator of renal function.
4. Baroreceptors, which are responsible for monitoring the circulating volume, are small nerve receptors that detect changes in pressure within blood vessels. Osmoreceptors sense changes in sodium concentration.
5. bones; soft tissue
6. the combined actions of parathyroid hormone and vitamin D
7. metastatic calcification of soft tissue, joints, and arteries
8. 7.35 to 7.45
9. upper, 7.8; lower, 6.8
10. a. Low   g. High
    b. Low   h. Low
    c. High   i. Low
    d. High   j. High
    e. High   k. High
    f. Low   l. Low
11. a. Low   g. Low
    b. High   h. Low
    c. Low   i. Low
    d. Low   j. High
    e. High   k. Low
    f. Low   l. High
12. a. High   e. Low
    b. Low   f. High
    c. High   g. High
    d. High   h. Low
13. a. Low   d. Low
    b. High   e. Low
    c. Low
14. a. Low   d. Low
    b. High   e. High
    c. Low
15. a. R-ACID   f. R-ACID
    b. M-ACID   g. M-ACID
    c. M-ACID   h. M-ALKA
    d. R-ACID   i. M-ALKA
    e. R-ALKA   j. R-ALKA
16. Intense supervision is required because only small volumes are needed to elevate the serum sodium from dangerously low levels.
17. dyspnea, cyanosis, a weak pulse, hypotension, and unresponsiveness
18. infection and septicemia

II. Critical Thinking Questions and Exercises

DISCUSSION AND ANALYSIS

1. An early indicator of a third space fluid shift is a decrease in urinary output despite adequate fluid intake. This occurs because fluid shifts out of the intravascular space. The kidneys, receiving less blood, attempt to compensate by decreasing urine output.
2. Hydrostatic pressure (pressure exerted by fluid on the walls of the blood vessels) affects the movement of fluids through the capillary walls of the blood vessels. Osmotic pressure is pressure exerted by proteins in the plasma. Both pressures help maintain a high extracellular concentration of sodium and a high intracellular concentration of potassium.
3. The usual daily urine output is 1.0 L per kilogram of body weight per hour. The outputs per hour would be 50 mL (110 lb), 60 mL (132 lb), and 80 mL (176 lb).
4. Osmolality refers to the concentration of fluid that affects the movement of water between the fluid compartments by osmosis. It measures the solute concentration per kilogram in the blood and urine. Osmolarity describes the concentration of solutions and is measured in milliosmoles per liter (mOsm/L).
5. Refer to chapter heading, "Fluid Volume Disturbances," and Tables 14-3 and 14-4.
6. Refer to chapter heading, "Types of Intravenous Solutions."
7. Refer to chapter heading, "Nursing Management of the Patient Receiving Intravenous Therapy."
8. Refer to chapter heading, "Managing Local Complications."

APPLYING CONCEPTS: OSMOSIS

1. Osmosis is the movement of fluid, through a semipermeable membrane, from an area of low solute concentration to an area of high solute concentration until the solutions are of equal concentration. Diffusion is the movement of a substance from an area of higher concentration to one of lower concentration. The concentration of dissolved substances (fluid concentration gradient) draws fluid in that direction.
2. The number of dissolved particles within a unit of fluid determines the osmolality of a solution. It is the osmolality that influences the movement of fluid between compartments.
3. Tonicity is the osmotic driving force of all the solutes. Tonicity determines cellular size and hydration.
4. Osmotic pressure, determined by the concentration of solutes, is the amount of hydrostatic pressure needed to stop the flow of water by osmosis. Oncotic pressure is the osmotic pressure exerted by proteins. Osmotic diuresis is urine output caused by the excretion of substances such as glucose and mannitol.
5. Diffusion is the movement of a substance from an area of higher concentration to one of lower concentration. Filtration is the movement of water and solutes from an area of high hydrostatic pressure to an area of low hydrostatic pressure.
6. Osmosis: the oncotic pressure of plasma proteins (albumin)
Filtration: the filtration of water and electrolytes by the kidneys

Diffusion: the exchange of oxygen and carbon dioxide between the pulmonary capillaries and the alveoli

EXAMINING ASSOCIATIONS

1. Refer to chapter heading, "Sodium-Potassium Pump."
2. Refer to Figure 14-2 for an illustration of the fluid regulation cycle.
3. Three-Column Matching: Body Fluid Compartments

   1. d   a. V
   2. e   b. IV
   3. f   c. III
   4. a   d. II
   5. b   e. VI
   6. c   f. I

EXTRACTING INFERENCES

1. osmolality; affects the movement of water between fluid compartments
2. thirst, antidiuretic hormone (ADH), and the renin-angiotensin aldosterone system
3. muscle contraction and the transmission of nerve impulses
4. a
5. c
6. b
7. b
8. c

CLINICAL SITUATIONS

CASE STUDY: EXTRACELLULAR FLUID VOLUME DEFICIT

1. b   3. a
2. b   4. b

CASE STUDY: CONGESTIVE HEART FAILURE

1. b   3. d
2. d   4. b

CASE STUDY: DIABETES MELLITUS

1. a   3. a
2. a   4. c

Chapter 15

I. Interpretation, Completion, and Comparison

MULTIPLE CHOICE

1. d	10. a	19. d
2. c	11. d	20. d
3. d	12. d	21. a
4. b	13. b	22. d
5. a	14. c	23. d
6. a	15. a	24. a
7. d	16. b	25. a
8. d	17. c	26. a
9. b	18. c	27. d

FILL-IN

1. inadequate tissue perfusion; poor oxygen and nutrient delivery, cellular starvation, cell death, organ dysfunction leading to organ failure, and eventual death
2. distributive and vasoactive
3. glucose; adenosine triphosphate (ATP)
4. Mean arterial pressure is the average pressure at which blood flows through the vasculature. MAP must exceed 65 mmHg.
5. carotid sinus and aortic arch; aortic arch and carotid arteries
6. Stage 1 is compensatory, stage 2 is progressive, and stage 3 is irreversible.
7. B-type natriuretic peptide (BNP)
8. lactated Ringer's solution and 0.9% sodium chloride solution
9. loss of sympathetic tone and release of biochemical mediators from cells
10. spinal cord injury, spinal anesthesia, or nervous system damage

SCRAMBLEGRAM

1. shock
2. ATP
3. renin
4. ADH
5. hypoxemia
6. preload
7. oliguria
8. albumin
9. dopamine
10. septic
11. CVP
12. pulmonary edema
13. colloids
14. lungs
15. Tridil

D	A	O	L	E	R	P	B	D	F	H	R
B	L	C	F	I	L	U	M	P	R	E	E
C	B	A	J	A	R	L	D	G	N	H	G
Y	U	D	K	S	E	M	J	I	L	F	K
L	M	G	W	F	B	O	N	E	D	N	O
M	I	S	P	T	G	N	S	G	N	U	L
A	N	D	T	C	R	A	R	M	T	H	I
I	V	I	A	D	H	R	I	R	R	D	G
M	L	O	R	O	C	Y	P	J	I	K	U
E	A	L	T	P	X	E	L	S	D	O	R
X	C	L	B	A	I	D	M	N	I	M	I
O	S	O	K	M	W	E	S	O	L	P	A
P	V	C	O	I	L	M	A	H	K	I	F
Y	R	A	Q	N	F	A	N	T	O	C	P
H	T	R	C	E	S	E	P	T	I	C	J
C	K	G	P	N	W	T	U	C	M	B	K
F	H	J	M	E	S	B	M	E	D	I	A
H	A	D	G	K	O	R	H	L	O	B	F

MATCHING

1. c	6. d
2. a	7. c
3. a	8. b
4. e	9. b
5. f	10. e

II. Critical Thinking Questions and Exercises

IDENTIFYING PATTERNS

FLOW CHART: BLOOD PRESSURE REGULATION: SHOCK

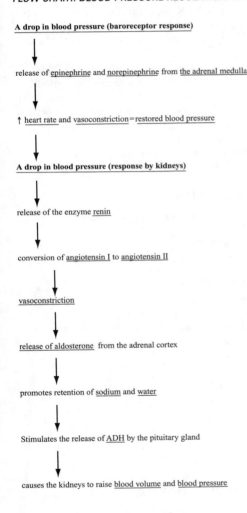

A drop in blood pressure (baroreceptor response)

↓

release of epinephrine and norepinephrine from the adrenal medulla

↓

↑ heart rate and vasoconstriction = restored blood pressure

↓

A drop in blood pressure (response by kidneys)

↓

release of the enzyme renin

↓

conversion of angiotensin I to angiotensin II

↓

vasoconstriction

↓

release of aldosterone from the adrenal cortex

↓

promotes retention of sodium and water

↓

Stimulates the release of ADH by the pituitary gland

↓

causes the kidneys to raise blood volume and blood pressure

FLOW CHART: HYPOVOLEMIC SHOCK

↓ intravascular volume from hemorrhage or severe dehydration

results in

↓ venous blood return and ↓ ventricular filling

which causes

↓ stroke volume and ↓ cardiac output

which leads to

↓ blood pressure and inadequate tissue perfusion

CLINICAL SITUATIONS

CASE STUDY: HYPOVOLEMIC SHOCK

1. d
2. 20 mm Hg
3. rise; decline
4. 90
5. 30
6. a. colloids
   b. Ringer's lactate
   c. normal saline

CASE STUDY: SEPTIC SHOCK

1. *Escherichia coli*
2. between 40% and 90%
3. urine, blood, sputum, and wound drainage
4. aggressive fluid replacement, antibiotic pharmacotherapy, crystalloids, and colloids
5. cardiovascular overload and pulmonary edema
6. 4 to 12 cm H_2O

Chapter 16

I. Interpretation, Completion, and Comparison

MULTIPLE CHOICE

1. b	9. c	17. a
2. a	10. b	18. d
3. d	11. c	19. d
4. d	12. b	20. a
5. d	13. a	21. a
6. c	14. d	22. d
7. a	15. b	23. d
8. d	16. a	

DEFINE

1. Anaplasia: cells that lack normal cellular characteristics and differ from other cells in shape and organization. Anaplastic cells are usually malignant
2. Alopecia: hair loss
3. Carcinogenesis: the process of transforming normal cells into malignant cells
4. Cytokines: substances produced by immune system cells to enhance the immune system
5. Metastasis: the spread of cancer cells from the primary tumor to distant sites
6. Nadir: the lowest point of white blood cell depression
7. Vesicant: a substance that can cause tissue necrosis
8. Xerostomia: a dry oral cavity caused by dysfunction of the salivary glands

SHORT ANSWER

1. Men: lung, prostate, colorectal; women: lung, breast, colorectal

2. Cancer begins when an abnormal cell, after being transformed by the genetic mutation of DNA, forms a clone and begins to proliferate abnormally.

3. carcinoembryonic antigen (CEA) and prostate-specific antigen (PSA)

4. 75%

5. tobacco smoke (accounts for at least 30% of cancer deaths)

6. Answer should include any of the following: nephroblastomas, retinoblastomas, pheochromocytomas, malignant neurofibromatosis and cancer of the breast, ovaries, stomach, colon, prostate, and lung.

7. Cruciferous vegetables include cabbage, broccoli, cauliflower, Brussels sprouts, and kohlrabi; fats, alcohol, salt-cured and smoked meats (ham), and nitrite/nitrate-containing foods (bacon) tend to increase the risk of cancer.

8. Five substances are antibodies produced by B lymphocytes, lymphokines, macrophages, natural killer (NK) cells, and T lymphocytes.

9. Answer may include the following:
   a. Skin: alopecia, erythema, desquamation
   b. Oral mucosal membrane: xerostomia, stomatitis, decreased salivation, loss of taste
   c. Stomach or colon: anorexia, nausea, vomiting, diarrhea
   d. Bone marrow-producing sites: anemia, leukopenia, thrombocytopenia

10. An extravasation of an infusion of a cancer chemotherapeutic agent is believed to have occurred if there is redness, pain, swelling, a mottled appearance, phlebitis, loss of blood return, resistance to flow, tissue necrosis, or damage to underlying tendons, nerves, and blood vessels.

11. nausea and vomiting.

MATCHING

1. b
2. a
3. a
4. b
5. b

MATCHING

1. e; bone marrow suppression
2. c; nausea, vomiting, and diarrhea
3. a; stomatitis and alopecia
4. f; masculinization and feminization
5. a ; bone marrow suppression
6. b; delayed and cumulative myelosuppression
7. d; bone marrow suppression
8. a; nausea, vomiting, and cystitis
9. c; proctitis, stomatitis, and renal toxicity
10. g; hepatotoxicity

II. Critical Thinking Questions and Exercises

DISCUSSION AND ANALYSIS

1. Invasion is the growth of the primary tumor into surrounding host tissues in a variety of ways. Metastasis is the direct spread of tumor cells to body cavities or through lymphatic and blood circulation.

2. Primary prevention is concerned with reducing the risk or preventing the development of cancer in healthy people. An example is teaching people the importance of stopping smoking to decrease the incidence of lung cancer. Secondary prevention involves detection and screening efforts to achieve early diagnosis and prompt intervention to halt the cancerous process. An example is teaching principles of breast self-examination to facilitate the early detection of breast cancer

3. Refer to Table 16-4.

4. Cell cycle–specific agents destroy cells in specific phases of the cell cycle by interfering with DNA and RNA synthesis or by halting mitosis. Cell cycle–nonspecific agents exert prolonged effects on cells, independent of cell cycle phases, which lead to cell damage or death.

5. Interferons are biologic response modifiers (BRMs) with antiviral and antitumor properties that stimulate an immune response. It is believed that the stimulated immune system will eradicate the malignant growth.

6. Refer to chapter heading, "Administration of Chemotherapeutic Agents."

7. Refer to chapter heading, "Nursing Process: The Patient with Cancer."

EXAMINING ASSOCIATIONS

1. detection and screening for an early diagnosis and treatment
2. tumor cell classification
3. incisional
4. palliative
5. an identical twin donor
6. interleukins
7. the thinning or complete loss of hair
8. appetite failure resulting in a wasting syndrome
9. *Pseudomonas aeruginosa*
10. acute leukemia

CLINICAL SITUATIONS

CASE STUDY: CANCER OF THE BREAST

1. b
2. d
3. a
4. d
5. d
6. c
7. a
8. d
9. b

CASE STUDY: CANCER OF THE LUNG

1. d
2. disease progression, immune competence, increased incidence of infection, delayed tissue repair, and diminished functional ability

3. fear, apprehension, fatigue, anger, and social isolation
4. c
5. answer questions and concerns; identify resources and support persons; communicate and share concerns; help frame questions for the physician
6. infection
7. *Pseudomonas aeruginosa* and *Escherichia coli*
8. b

Chapter 17

I. Interpretation, Completion, and Comparison

MULTIPLE CHOICE

1. b
2. c
3. c
4. b
5. b
6. d
7. d
8. d
9. d

SHORT ANSWER

1. Kubler-Ross; *On Death and Dying*
2. Assisted suicide refers to providing another person the means to end his or her own life. Physician-assisted suicide involves a prescription by a physician of a lethal dose of medication to end life.
3. Palliative care and hospice care involve coordinated programs of interdisciplinary services provided by professional caregivers and trained volunteers to patients with serious, progressive illnesses that are not responsive to curative treatments. However, palliative care does not focus primarily on preparation for death, as hospice care does.
4. England; Dr. Cicely Saunders; St. Christopher's Hospital
5. Connecticut; 1974
6. 2004
7. bronchodilators and corticosteroids
8. Decadron (dexamethasone), Periactin (cyprohepta-dine), Megace (megestrol), and Marinol (dronabinol).

II. Critical Thinking Questions and Exercises

DISCUSSION AND ANALYSIS

1. Refer to chapter heading, "Technology and End-Of-Life Care."
2. Refer to chapter heading, "Clinicians' Attitudes Toward Death."
3. Refer to chapter heading, "Assisted Suicide," and the ANA's Position Statement (ANA, 1994).
4. Refer to Chart 17-5.
5. Refer to Chart 17-6 as an outline for discussion and analysis.
6. Refer to chapter heading, "Goal Setting in Palliative Care at the End of Life."
7. Refer to Table 17-4 as a resource to personalize your responses.

Chapter 18

I. Interpretation, Completion, and Comparison

MULTIPLE CHOICE

1. a
2. d
3. a
4. d
5. c
6. a
7. a
8. a
9. c
10. a
11. d
12. b
13. a
14. d
15. d
16. d
17. c
18. a
19. a
20. a
21. d
22. d
23. a
24. c
25. c

SHORT ANSWER

1. when the decision to do surgery is made; is transferred onto the operating room table
2. is transferred to the operating room table; the patient is admitted to the PACU
3. it is invasive, it requires anesthesia, it involves radiation, and/or it carries more than a slight risk of potential harm
4. hypoglycemia, hyperglycemia, acidosis, and glucosuria
5. 7 to 10 days; inhibiting platelet aggregation
6. dehydration, hypovolemia, and electrolyte imbalances
7. improve circulation, prevent venous stasis, and promote optimal respiratory function
8. Refer to Chart 18-5.

MATCHING

1. d
2. a
3. e
4. c
5. b

II. Critical Thinking Questions and Exercises

EXAMINING ASSOCIATIONS

1. Medication Administration: Refer to Table 18-3.
2. Preoperative Nursing: Refer to chapter heading, "Preparation for Surgery."

CLINICAL APPLICATIONS

1. Splinting When Coughing: Refer to Chart 18-4.
2. Leg Exercises: Refer to Chart 18-4.

Chapter 19

I. Interpretation, Completion, and Comparison

MULTIPLE CHOICE

1. b	6. b	11. d
2. d	7. c	12. b
3. a	8. c	13. c
4. d	9. a	14. d
5. c	10. d	15. b

SHORT ANSWER

1. Anesthesia is reduced with age because the percentage of fatty tissue increases. Fatty tissue has an affinity for anesthetic agents.
2. Answer should include handling tissue, providing exposure at the operative field, suturing, and maintaining hemostasis.
3. Health hazards include exposure to blood and body fluids, hazards associated with laser beams, exposure to latex and adhesive substances, exposure to radiation, and exposure to toxic agents.
4. moderate sedation; Versed and Valium
5. thiopental sodium (Pentothal); respiratory depression
6. the subarachnoid space at the lumbar level (usually at L2)
7. epidural
8. Complete return of sensation in the patient's toes, in response to a pinprick, indicates recovery.
9. nausea and vomiting, anaphylaxis, hypoxia, hypothermia, malignant hypothermia, and disseminated intravascular coagulation (DIC)
10. 104°F

MATCHING: INHALATION ANESTHETIC AGENTS

1. d	4. c
2. b	5. e
3. a	

MATCHING: COMMON INTRAVENOUS MEDICATIONS

1. d	4. c
2. b	5. e
3. a	

II. Critical Analysis Questions

DISCUSSION AND ANALYSIS

1. Refer to Chart 19-1
2. The elderly have a variety of age-related cardiovascular and pulmonary changes as well as changes in the liver and kidneys. Refer to chapter heading, "The Surgical Team: Gerontological Considerations."
3. Refer to chapter heading, "Basic Guidelines for Maintaining Surgical Asepsis."

4. Anesthesia awareness is a condition whereby patients are partially awake while under general anesthesia. Cardiac, obstetric, and major trauma patients are most at risk.
5. Refer to chapter heading, "Nursing Process: The Patient During Surgery."

RECOGNIZING CONTRADICTIONS

1. Older patients require less anesthesia and take longer to eliminate anesthetic drugs.
2. The circulating nurse controls the environment, coordinates the activities of other personnel, and monitors aseptic techniques.
3. Whenever sterility is in question, an item is considered unsterile.
4. Only the top of a table that is draped is considered sterile. Drapes hanging over the edge are clean but not sterile.
5. The unsterile arm of the circulating nurse should never extend over a sterile area.

CLINICAL SITUATIONS

CASE STUDY: GENERAL ANESTHESIA

1. b
2. b
3. c

CASE STUDY: INTRAVENOUS ANESTHESIA

1. d
2. a
3. b

Chapter 20

I. Interpretation, Completion, and Comparison

MULTIPLE CHOICE

1. c	9. a	17. d
2. d	10. c	18. c
3. d	11. b	19. d
4. a	12. c	20. a
5. d	13. c	21. d
6. c	14. d	22. d
7. a	15. d	23. c
8. d	16. a	

SHORT ANSWER

1. The answer may include any of the following: medical diagnosis; type of surgery performed; patient's general condition (age, airway patency, vital signs); anesthetic and other medications used; any intraoperative problems that might influence postoperative care (shock, hemorrhage, cardiac arrest); any pathology

encountered; fluid administered, blood loss, and replacement; tubing, drains, catheters, or other supportive aids; and specific information about which surgeon or anesthesiologist wishes to be notified.

2. respiratory function and patency of the airway.

3. Primary hemorrhage occurs at the time of the operation. Intermediary hemorrhage occurs within the first few hours after an operation and is caused by the return of blood pressure to its normal level. Secondary hemorrhage occurs some time after the operation as a result of the slipping of a ligature, which may happen because of infection, insecure tying, or erosion of a vessel by a drainage tube.

4. respiratory

5. Answer should include five of the following: atelectasis, pneumonia, deep vein thrombosis, pulmonary embolism, bleeding, constipation, paralytic ileus, and wound infections.

6. self-perception, personality, learning, ethnic and cultural factors, and environment

7. Patient-controlled analgesia refers to self-administration of pain medication by way of intravenous or epidural routes within prescribed time/dosage limits.

8. Atelectasis and hypostatic pneumonia are reduced with early ambulation because ventilation is increased and the stasis of bronchial secretions in the lungs is reduced.

9. absence of nausea, absence of vomiting, and presence of bowel sounds

10. bowel sounds and passage of flatus

11. Wound dehiscence refers to the disruption of the wound or surgical incision. Wound evisceration refers to the protrusion of wound contents.

II. Critical Thinking Questions and Exercises

DISCUSSION AND ANALYSIS

1. Refer to Figure 20-3 and chapter heading, "Determining Readiness for Discharge from the PACU."

2. Refer to Table 20-3.

3. Refer to chapter heading, "Nursing Process: The Hospitalized Patient Recovering from Surgery."

4. The respiratory depressive effects of opioids, decreased lung expansion secondary to pain, and decreased mobility are three conditions that put patients at risk for atelectasis, pneumonia, and hypoxemia.

5. The nurse should tilt the postoperative patient's head back and push forward on the angle of the lower jaw. This maneuver pulls the tongue forward and closes the air passages.

IDENTIFYING PATTERNS

CASE STUDY: POSTOPERATIVE PAIN

Pain stimulates <u>the stress response</u> ⟶ which increases <u>muscle tension</u>
and
<u>local vasoconstriction</u>

Noxious impulses stimulate <u>sympathetic activity</u> ⟶ which increases <u>myocardial demand</u>
and
<u>oxygen consumption</u>
<u>blood viscosity</u>
and
<u>platelet aggregation</u>

Hypothalmic stress responses increase ⟶
Which can lead to <u>phlebothrombosis</u>
and
<u>pulmonary embolism</u>

CLINICAL SITUATIONS

CASE STUDY: HYPOVOLEMIC SHOCK

1. b   4. a
2. b   5. b
3. a

CASE STUDY: HYPOPHARYNGEAL OBSTRUCTION

1. d   3. d
2. b   4. c

CASE STUDY: WOUND HEALING

1. b   3. d
2. a   4. b

Chapter 21

I. Interpretation, Completion and Comparison

MULTIPLE CHOICE

1. d	12. a	23. a
2. b	13. a	24. d
3. c	14. a	25. a
4. a	15. b	26. a
5. c	16. d	27. c
6. a	17. c	28. b
7. b	18. a	29. b
8. b	19. d	30. b
9. b	20. c	31. c
10. d	21. d	32. d
11. b	22. d	33. d

SHORT ANSWER

1. Ventilation refers to the movement of air in and out of the airways, whereas respiration refers to gas exchange between atmospheric air and blood and between the blood and the cells of the body.
2. The epiglottis is a flap of cartilage that covers the opening of the larynx during swallowing.
3. Compliance refers to the ability of the lungs and thorax to stretch and distend with ventilation. Low or decreased compliance exists with certain pathology, such as atelectasis, pneumothorax, hemothorax, and pulmonary fibrosis.
4. Partial pressure is the pressure exerted by each type of gas (e.g., oxygen, carbon dioxide) in a mixture of gases.
5. the apneustic center in the lower pons and the pneumotaxic center in the upper pons
6. age 50 years
7. Answer can include dyspnea, cough, sputum production, chest pain, wheezing, clubbing of the fingers, hemoptysis, and cyanosis.
8. Cheyne-Stokes respirations are characterized by alternating episodes of apnea (cessation of breathing) and periods of deep breathing. It is usually associated with heart failure and damage to the respiratory center.

II. Critical Thinking Questions and Exercises

DISCUSSION AND ANALYSIS

1. Refer to Chart 21-1.
2. Diffusion is the exchange of oxygen and carbon dioxide at the air–blood interface. Pulmonary perfusion is the actual flow of blood through the pulmonary circulation.
3. Oxygen is carried in the blood dissolved in plasma or combined with hemoglobin. The higher the PaO_2, the greater the amount of dissolved oxygen.

CLINICAL SITUATIONS

CASE STUDY: BRONCHOSCOPY

1. c	4. d
2. d	5. a
3. b	

CASE STUDY: THORACENTESIS

1. d	4. d
2. b	5. c
3. b	

INTERPRETING DATA

For an explanation of the oxyhemoglobin dissociation curve, see Chart 21-4 in the text.

Chapter 22

I. Interpretation, Completion, and Comparison

MULTIPLE CHOICE

1. a	9. d	16. d
2. d	10. d	17. b
3. c	11. a	18. b
4. a	12. c	19. b
5. a	13. d	20. a
6. d	14. a	21. d
7. b	15. a	22. d
8. a		

SHORT ANSWER

1. Rhinitis causes the nasal passages to become inflamed, congested, and edematous. The swollen conchae block the sinus openings and cause sinusitis.
2. *Streptococcus pneumoniae, Haemophilus influenzae,* and *Moraxella catarrhalis*
3. meningitis, brain abscess, ischemic infarction, and osteomyelitis
4. hemorrhage
5. viral; hoarseness, aphonia, and severe cough
6. Refer to chapter heading, "Nursing Process: The Patient with an Upper Airway Infection."
7. Complications may include sepsis, a peritonsillar abscess, otitis media, sinusitis, and meningitis.
8. Obstructive sleep apnea is defined as frequent loud snoring and breathing cessation for 10 seconds or longer with five or more episodes per hour. This is followed by awakening abruptly with a loud snort when the blood oxygen level drops.
9. esophageal speech, an artificial larynx, and tracheoesophageal puncture

II. Critical Thinking Questions and Exercises

CLINICAL SITUATIONS

CASE STUDY: TONSILLECTOMY AND ADENOIDECTOMY

1. d
2. c
3. a
4. c

CASE STUDY: EPISTAXIS

1. Gilberta should sit upright with her head tilted forward to prevent swallowing and aspiration of blood. She should also pinch the soft outer portion of the nose against the midline spectrum for 5 to 10 continuous minutes.
2. d
3. b
4. d

CASE STUDY: CANCER OF THE LARYNX

1. Refer to Chart 22-7.
2. squamous cell carcinoma
3. b
4. 50%; 75% to 95%
5. radiation therapy or surgery
6. 2 to 3 years

CASE STUDY: LARYNGECTOMY

1. b
2. d
3. d
4. respiratory distress, hypoxia, hemorrhage, infection, wound breakdown, and aspiration
5. d
6. Answer should include at least four of the following: increase in temperature, tachycardia, purulent drainage, odor, redness or tenderness at the surgical site, and increased WBCs.
7. d
8. carotid artery rupture

APPLYING CONCEPTS: PERFORMING AN ABDOMINAL THRUST MANEUVER

Refer to Chart 22-6 in the text.

Chapter 23

I. Interpretation, Completion, and Comparison

MULTIPLE CHOICE

1. d
2. a
3. c
4. d
5. d
6. c
7. a
8. a
9. c
10. d
11. d
12. d
13. a
14. a
15. d
16. c
17. a
18. d
19. b
20. b
21. d
22. b
23. c
24. a
25. a
26. a
27. a
28. b
29. a
30. b
31. c

SHORT ANSWER

1. Refer to Figure 23-1 and chapter heading, "Atelectasis."
2. cough, sputum production, low-grade fever, dyspnea, tachycardia, tachypnea, pleural pain, and central cyanosis
3. frequent turning, early mobilization, deep breathing maneuvers, assistance with the use of spirometry, suctioning, postural drainage, aerosol nebulizer treatments, and chest percussion
4. impaired host defenses, an inoculum of organisms that reach the lower respiratory tract, and the presence of a highly virulent organism
5. *Streptococcus pneumoniae, Haemophilus influenzae,* and *Staphylococcus aureus*
6. alcoholism, COPD, AIDS, diabetes, and heart failure
7. hypotension, shock, and respiratory failure
8. Superinfection is suspected when a subsequent infection occurs with another bacteria during antibiotic therapy.
9. *Mycobacterium tuberculosis*
10. alveolar hypoventilation, diffusion abnormalities, ventilation–perfusion mismatching, and shunting
11. 60%; multiple-system organ failure
12. hypoxemia that does not respond to supplemental oxygen
13. enlargement of the right ventricle of the heart because of diseases affecting the structure or functions of the lung

II. Critical Thinking Questions and Exercises

DISCUSSION AND ANALYSIS

1. Refer to chapter heading, "Atelectasis."
2. Refer to Table 23-2.
3. Inadequate left ventricular function leads to a backup of blood into the pulmonary vasculature, which causes increased microvascular pressure. Fluid leaks into the interstitial space and alveoli.
4. Refer to Chart 23-5.
5. Refer to Chart 23-7.
6. Refer to chapter headings, "Sarcoidosis" and "Pneumoconioses."

INTERPRETING PATTERNS

FLOW CHART: THE PATHOPHYSIOLOGY OF PNEUMONIA

Inflammation in alveoli ——————————→ Neutrophils fill alveoli

↓   ↓

Exudate formation ——————————→ ⎰ Partial occlusion of alveoli and bronchi ↓

↓   ↓ alveolar oxygen tension

                                                                              ↓

Interference with diffusion of ——————→ ⎰ Bronchospasm and hypoventilation ↓
oxygen and carbon dioxide   ventilation-perfusion mismatch ↓
                                                                arterial hypoxemia

FLOW CHART: THE PATHOPHYSIOLOGY OF ACUTE RESPIRATORY DISTRESS SYNDROME (ARDS)

Inflammatory event

↓   → Alveolar collapse

Release of cellular and chemical mediators   ↓

↓   Airways narrow with bronchial obstruction

Injury to alveolar capillary membrane   ↓

↓   Decreased functional residual
                                                capacity; stiff lungs and severe hypoxemia
Leaks fluid into alveolar interstitial spaces

CLINICAL SITUATIONS

CASE STUDY: COMMUNITY-ACQUIRED PNEUMONIA

1. d   4. d
2. b   5. b
3. d   6. d

CASE STUDY: TUBERCULOSIS

1. b   4. b
2. b   5. c
3. d

CASE STUDY: ADULT RESPIRATORY DISTRESS SYNDROME (ARDS)

1. d   4. d
2. d   5. d
3. c

CASE STUDY: PULMONARY EMBOLISM

1. c   5. b
2. a   6. c
3. b   7. d
4. a

APPLYING CONCEPTS: PNEUMONIA

1. Refer to Figure 23-2 in the text.
2. Refer to Figure 23-2 in the text.

Chapter 24

I. Interpretation, Completion, and Comparison

MULTIPLE CHOICE

1. c   8. d   15. a
2. d   9. b   16. c
3. d   10. d   17. c
4. d   11. b   18. c
5. b   12. d   19. d
6. b   13. c   20. d
7. d   14. b

SHORT ANSWER

1. narrowing of the small peripheral airways
2. Emphysema is an abnormal distention of the air spaces, beyond the terminal bronchioles, that results in destruction of the walls of the alveoli.
3. cigarette smoking
4. a deficiency in alpha-antitrypsin, an enzyme inhibitor that protects the lungs
5. chronic cough, sputum production, and dyspnea on exertion
6. Answer should include five of the following: history of cigarette smoking, passive smoking exposure, age, rate of decline of FEV_1, hypoxemia, weight loss, and reversibility of airflow obstruction
7. cessation of smoking
8. tracheobronchial infection and air pollution
9. Refer to chapter heading, "Nursing Process: The Patient with COPD."
10. allergy; cough, wheezing, and dyspnea
11. status asthmaticus, respiratory failure, pneumonia, and atelectasis

II. Critical Thinking Questions and Exercises

DISCUSSION AND ANALYSIS

1. Refer to Charts 24-1 and 24-2 and chapter heading, "Risk Factors: COPD."
2. Refer to chapter heading, "Oxygen Therapy."
3. Refer to chapter heading, "Asthma."

IDENTIFYING PATTERNS

The Pathophysiology of Chronic Bronchitis

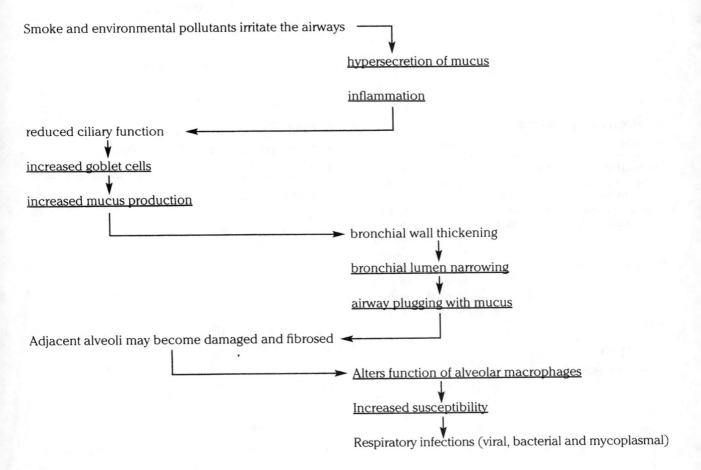

Smoke and environmental pollutants irritate the airways

hypersecretion of mucus

inflammation

reduced ciliary function

increased goblet cells

increased mucus production

bronchial wall thickening

bronchial lumen narrowing

airway plugging with mucus

Adjacent alveoli may become damaged and fibrosed

Alters function of alveolar macrophages

Increased susceptibility

Respiratory infections (viral, bacterial and mycoplasmal)

The Pathophysiology of Emphysema

Alveolar walls are destroyed causing an increase in dead space ⟶ { <u>Impaired oxygen diffusion</u>

<u>Hypoxemia</u>

In later stage emphysema, carbon dioxide elimination is impaired ⟶ { <u>Hypercapnia</u>

<u>Respiratory acidosis</u>

As the alveolar walls breakdown, the pulmonary capillary bed is reduced, causing increased pulmonary blood flow

↓

<u>Right-sided heart failure</u> ⟶ { <u>Congestion</u>

<u>Dependent edema</u>

↓

Cardiac failure

EXAMINING ASSOCIATIONS

Panlobular	*Centrilobular*
Destruction of respiratory bronchioles, alveolar ducts, and alveoli	Altered ventilation-perfusion ratios
Minimal inflammatory disease	Chronic hypoxemia
Hyperinflated chest (barrel chest)	Hypercapnia, polycythemia, and right-sided heart failure
Dyspnea on exertion	Central cyanosis, peripheral edema, and respiratory failure
Weight loss	

CLINICAL SITUATIONS

CASE STUDY: EMPHYSEMA

1. c		4. d
2. b		5. b
3. a		6. d

Chapter 25

I. Interpretation, Completion, and Comparison

MULTIPLE CHOICE

1. a	11. c	21. c
2. b	12. d	22. a
3. a	13. d	23. c
4. b	14. d	24. d
5. d	15. a	25. c
6. d	16. c	26. c
7. b	17. a	27. b
8. c	18. d	28. d
9. d	19. a	29. d
10. a	20. d	

SHORT ANSWER

1. cardiac output, arterial oxygen content, hemoglobin concentration, and metabolic requirements
2. more than 50%; 48 hours
3. Answer may include substernal discomfort, paresthesias, dyspnea, restlessness, fatigue, malaise, progressive respiratory difficulty, refractory hypoxemia, alveolar atelectasis, and alveolar infiltrates on x-ray.

4. decreased blood oxygen rather than elevated carbon dioxide levels
5. nasal cannula, simple mask, partial-rebreather mask, and non-rebreather mask
6. 6 to 8 L/min
7. Goals of CPT are to remove bronchial secretions, to improve ventilation, and to increase the efficiency of the respiratory muscles.
8. 15 and 20 mm Hg
9. iron lung, body wrap, and chest cuirass
10. inflating the lungs by exerting pressure on the airway, forcing the alveoli to expand during inspiration

11. A patient "bucks the ventilator" when his or her breathing is out of phase with the machine. This occurs when the patient attempts to breathe out during the ventilator's mechanical inspiratory phase or when there is jerky and increased abdominal muscle effort.
12. 10 to 15 mL/kg; 6 L/min; 3.5 mL/kg
13. respiratory failure, dysrhythmias, bronchopleural fistula, hemorrhage, shock, atelectasis, and pulmonary infection

COMPLETE THE CHART

II. Critical Thinking Questions and Exercises

EXAMINING ASSOCIATIONS

1. decreased arterial oxygen tension in the blood
2. 80% to 98%
3. 12 L/min; 80% to 100%
4. inadequate capillary circulation
5. 12 to 16 breaths/min

DISCUSSION AND ANALYSIS

1. Refer to chapter heading, "Oxygen Therapy."
2. Refer to chapter heading, "Suppression of Ventilation."
3. Refer to Figure 25-4 and chapter heading, "Chest Percussion and Vibration."

4. Refer to Charts 25-4 and 25-5.
5. Refer to Chart 25-6.
6. Refer to Chart 25-10.
7. Refer to Chart 25-15.
8. Refer to Chart 25-18.

APPLYING CONCEPTS: CARE OF A PATIENT WITH AN ENDOTRACHEAL TUBE

Refer to Charts 25-7, 25-8, 25-9 and 25-10.

CLINICAL SITUATIONS

CASE STUDY: PNEUMONECTOMY: PREOPERATIVE CONCERNS

1. d   3. d
2. a   4. a

CASE STUDY: PNEUMONECTOMY: POSTOPERATIVE CONCERNS

1. a	3. d
2. b	4. a

CASE STUDY: VENTILATOR PATIENT

1. d	3. d
2. a	4. d

CASE STUDY: WEANING FROM VENTILATOR

1. d	3. d
2. d	

Chapter 26

I. Interpretation, Completion, and Comparison

MULTIPLE CHOICE

1. a	7. d	12. c
2. a	8. d	13. a
3. d	9. c	14. b
4. d	10. c	15. d
5. c	11. a	16. d
6. c		

SHORT ANSWER

1. hypertension, coronary artery disease, heart failure, stroke, and congenital cardiovascular defects
2. The atrioventricular (AV) valves separate the atria from the ventricles. The tricuspid separates the right atrium and ventricle; the bicuspid separates the left atrium and ventricle. The AV valves permit blood to flow from the atria into the ventricles. The semilunar valves are situated between each ventricle and its corresponding artery. The pulmonic valve is between the right ventricle and the pulmonary artery; the aortic valve is between the left ventricle and the aorta. These valves permit blood to flow from the ventricles into the arteries.
3. Depolarization is said to have occurred when the electrical difference between the inside and the outside of the cell is reduced. The inside of the cell becomes less negative, membrane permeability to calcium is increased, and muscle contraction occurs.
4. Cardiac output would equal 5320 mL.
5. Starling's law of the heart refers to the relationship between increased stroke volume and increased ventricular end-diastolic volume for a given intrinsic contractility.
6. Physiologic effects of the aging process may include reduction in the size of the left ventricle, decreased elasticity and widening of the aorta, thickening and rigidity of cardiac valves, and increased connective tissue in the sinoatrial and atrioventricular nodes and bundle branches.
7. hyperlipidemia, hypertension, and diabetes mellitus
8. LDL, less than 70 mg/dL; BP, less than 140/90 mm Hg; serum glucose, less than 110 mg/dL; BMI, 18.5 to 24.9 Kg/m^2
9. below the fifth intercostal space and lateral to the midclavicular line
10. creatine kinase (CK) and isoenzyme CK-MB; troponin T and troponin I
11. Cardiac catheterization is used most frequently to assess the patency of the patient's coronary arteries and to determine readiness for coronary bypass surgery. It is also used to measure pressures in the various heart chambers and to determine oxygen saturation of the blood by sampling specimens.
12. Selective angiography refers to the technique of injecting a contrast medium into the vascular system to outline a particular heart chamber or blood vessel.
13. A lowered central venous pressure reading indicates that the patient is hypovolemic. Serial measurements are more reflective of a patient's condition and should be correlated with the patient's clinical status.
14. Complications of pulmonary artery monitoring include infection, pulmonary artery rupture, pulmonary thromboembolism, pulmonary infarction, catheter kinking, dysrhythmias, and air embolism.

MATCHING

1. c		4. d
2. e		5. b
3. a		6. f

CROSSWORD PUZZLE: TERMS ASSOCIATED WITH CORONARY ATHEROSCLEROSIS

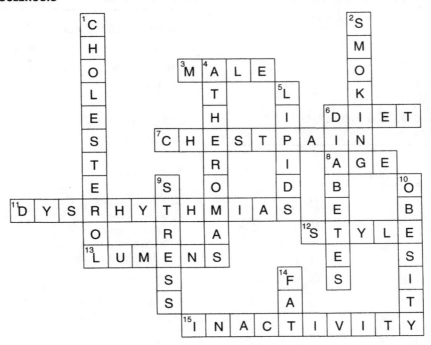

II. Critical Thinking Questions and Exercises

DISCUSSION AND ANALYSIS

1. Refer to chapter heading, "Coronary Artery Disease."
2. Refer to Table 26-2.
3. Refer to Chart 26-1.
4. Type A personalities are competitive, hard-driving, and exhibit a sense of time urgency. This type personality tends to react to frustrating events with increased blood pressure, heart rate, and neuroendocrine responses. This physiologic activation, which is believed to cause cardiovascular events, is known as " cardiac reactivity."
5. Refer to chapter heading, "Gallop Sounds."

EXAMINING ASSOCIATIONS

Refer to Table 26-2 in the text.

INTERPRETING DATA

1. Assessment

Myocardial Infarction:
Substernal pain or pain over precordium. May spread widely throughout chest. Painful disability of shoulders and hands may be present. Pain lasting longer than 15 minutes.

Angina Pectoris:
Substernal or retrosternal pain spreading across chest. May radiate to inside of arm, neck, or jaws.
Pain lasting 5 to 10 minutes.

2. Precipitating Events

Myocardial Infarction:
Occurs spontaneously but may be sequela of unstable angina

Angina Pectoris:
Usually related to exertion, emotion, eating or cold.

3. Nursing Intervention

Myocardial Infarction:
Morphine sulfate, successful reperfusion of blocked coronary artery

Angina Pectoris:
Rest, nitroglycerin, oxygen

CLINICAL APPLICATIONS

CASE STUDY: CARDIAC ASSESSMENT FOR CHEST PAIN

1. c
2. d
3. c
4. d
5. b

Chapter 27

I. Interpretation, Completion, and Comparison

MULTIPLE CHOICE

1. d	8. d	14. d
2. b	9. c	15. d
3. c	10. b	16. c
4. b	11. a	17. a
5. d	12. d	18. d
6. a	13. c	19. d
7. b		

SHORT ANSWER

1. atria, atrioventricular node or junction, sinus node, and ventricles
2. Electrical conduction through the heart begins in the sinoatrial node (SA), travels across the atria to the atrioventricular node (AV), and then travels down the right and left bundle branches and Purkinje fibers to the ventricular muscle.
3. Answer may include any of the following: fever, hypovolemia, anemia, exercise, pain, congestive heart failure, anxiety, and sympathomimetic or parasympatholytic drugs.
4. 100 bpm
5. Ventricular tachycardia occurs when there are more than three PVCs in a row and the rate exceeds 100 bpm
6. a thromboembolic event, heart failure, and cardiac arrest
7. The difference is in the timing of the electrical current. With cardioversion, the current is synchronized with the patient's electrical events; with defibrillation, the current is unsynchronized and immediate.
8. The standard procedure is to place one paddle to the right of the upper sternum below the right clavicle and the other paddle just to the left of the cardiac apex.
9. A demand pacemaker is set for a specific rate and stimulates the heart when normal ventricular depolarization does not occur; the fixed rate pacemaker stimulates the ventricle at a preset constant rate, independently of the patient's rhythm.

SCRAMBLEGRAM

1. dysrhythmic
2. automaticity
3. conductivity
4. depolarization
5. diastole
6. ablation

II. Critical Thinking Questions and Exercises

EXAMINING ASSOCIATIONS

1. ventricular muscle
2. repolarization
3. t-wave
4. sinus bradycardia
5. Norpace
6. 3:2 or 4:3

CLINICAL SITUATIONS

GRAPH ANALYSIS

1. a. T wave
   b. P-R interval
   c. P wave
   d. QRS complex
   e. ST segment
2. a. Q wave is larger.
   b. ST segment is elevated.
   c. T wave is inverted.

GRAPHIC RECORDINGS

1. *Premature atrial complexes (PACs):* P waves come early in cycle and close to T wave of previous heartbeat.
2. *Premature ventricular complexes (PVCs):* QRS complex is bizarre; P waves are hidden in QRS complexes.
3. *Ventricular tachycardia:* There are three or more PVCs in a row, occurring at a rate greater than 100 bpm.

CASE STUDY: PERMANENT PACEMAKER

1. Yes. Heart rate can vary as much as 5 bpm faster or slower than the preset rate.
2. bleeding, hematoma formation, and infection
3. hemothorax; ventricular ectopy and tachycardia; dislocation of the lead; and phrenic nerve, diaphragmatic, or skeletal muscle stimulation
4. dislodgment of the pacing electrode
5. a. pacemaker model
   b. date and time of insertion
   c. stimulation threshold
   d. pacer rate
   e. incision appearance
   f. patient tolerance
6.

Goals	Nursing Activities	Expected Outcomes
a. absence of infection	a. sterile wound care	a. free from infection
b. adherence to a self-care program	b. patient teaching	b. adheres to a self-care program
c. maintenance of pacemaker function	c. patient teaching	c. maintains pacemaker function

7. a. has a normal temperature, white blood cells within normal range, and no evidence of redness or swelling at insertion site
   b. understands signs and symptoms of infection and knows when to seek medical attention
   c. assesses pulse rate at regular intervals and experiences no abrupt changes in pulse rate or rhythm

Chapter 28

I. Interpretation, Completion, and Comparison

MULTIPLE CHOICE

1. b	12. b	23. c
2. d	13. a	24. d
3. a	14. b	25. b
4. c	15. a	26. d
5. d	16. b	27. a
6. c	17. a	28. d
7. a	18. b	29. b
8. d	19. c	30. b
9. a	20. d	31. c
10. c	21. c	32. a
11. a	22. d	33. d

SHORT ANSWER

1. cardiovascular disease
2. atherosclerosis
3. chest pain, referred to as angina pectoris
4. age (more than 50% are older than 65 years of age)
5. Answer can include hyperlipidemia, cigarette smoking, obesity, hypertension, diabetes mellitus, and physical activity.
6. less than 200 mg/dL; 3.5:1.0; less than 160 mg/dL; greater than 35mg/dL
7. 30%
8. severe and incapacitating
9. Answer should include five of the following: fever, pericardial pain, pleural pain, dyspnea, pericardial effusion, pericardial friction rub, and arthralgia.

II. Critical Thinking Questions and Exercises

DISCUSSION AND ANALYSIS

1. Atherosclerosis, the abnormal accumulation of lipid substances, causes a repetitive inflammatory response that alters the artery walls.
2. Cigarette smoking contributes to coronary heart disease in three ways. Smoke inhalation increases the level of blood carbon monoxide by causing hemoglobin to combine more readily with carbon monoxide

than with oxygen. Nicotine triggers the release of catecholamines, which raise heart rate and blood pressure and cause the coronary arteries to constrict. Smoking causes a detrimental vascular response and increases platelet adhesion, increasing the probability of thrombus formation.

EXAMINING ASSOCIATIONS

1. the profile of those at highest risk for a cardiac event in 10 years
2. metabolic syndrome, a significant risk factor for coronary artery disease
3. factors, weighted by points, that indicate increased risk of having a cardiac event
4. modifiable risk factors for coronary artery disease
5. four primary factors of fat metabolism that affect the development of heart disease

IDENTIFYING PATTERNS

1. Arterial lumen narrowing begins with the deposit of fatty streaks (lipids) on the intima (inner vessel wall). Some develop into advanced lesions as atherosclerosis advances. An inflammatory response occurs, and T lymphocytes and monocytes infiltrate the area, ingest lipids, and die. Smooth muscle cells then proliferate and form a fibrous cap around a dead fatty core. These deposits narrow and obstruct blood flow.
2. An atheroma is a fatty thickening or degeneration of the walls of the arteries that results from an atherosclerotic response to lipid deposits.
3. formation of a thrombus
4. A thrombus can obstruct blood flow, cause an acute myocardial infarction, or result in sudden death.

SUPPORTING ARGUMENTS

1. a. *Increased CO levels:* Hemoglobin combines more readily with CO than with O_2, thereby limiting the oxygen being supplied to the heart.
   b. *Increased catecholamines:* Nicotine triggers the release of catecholamines, which cause arterial constriction and decreased oxygenation.
   c. *Increased platelet adhesion:* Smoking increases platelet adhesion, which increases thrombus formation.
2. Calcium channel blockers increase myocardial oxygen supply by dilating the smooth muscle wall of the coronary arterioles, by decreasing myocardial oxygen demands, and by decreasing systemic arterial pressure.

CLINICAL SITUATIONS

CASE STUDY: ANGINA PECTORIS

1. b	3. b
2. c	4. c

CASE STUDY: DECREASED MYOCARDIAL TISSUE PERFUSION

1. c	3. a	5. a
2. a	4. b	6. d

Chapter 29

I. Interpretation, Completion, and Comparison

MULTIPLE CHOICE

1. d	8. c	14. a
2. b	9. c	15. d
3. c	10. a	16. b
4. b	11. c	17. a
5. a	12. b	18. b
6. a	13. a	19. a
7. d		

SHORT ANSWER

1. Mitral valve prolapse syndrome is a dysfunction of the mitral valve leaflets that results in valve incompetency and regurgitation. Valve dysfunction progresses, and symptoms of heart failure ensue.
2. caffeine, alcohol, and smoking
3. at the third and fourth intercostal spaces at the left sternal border; a blowing diastolic murmur
4. prophylactic antibiotics
5. Answer should include four of the following: congestive heart failure, ventricular dysrhythmias, atrial dysrhythmias, cardiac conduction defects, pulmonary or cerebral embolism, and valvular dysfunction.
6. cardiomyopathy, ischemic heart disease, valvular disease, rejection of previously transplanted hearts, and congenital heart disease
7. penicillin therapy; rheumatic fever
8. An inflamed endothelium causes a fibrin clot to form (vegetation), which converts to scar tissue that thickens, contracts, and causes deformities. The result is leakage or valvular regurgitation and stenosis.
9. streptococci, enterococci, pneumococci, and staphylococci
10. Myocarditis is an inflammatory process that usually results from an infection. The infectious process can cause heart dilation, thrombi formation, infiltration of blood cells around the coronary vessels and between the muscle fibers, and eventual degeneration of the muscle fibers themselves.

11. Listen at the left sternal edge of the thorax in the fourth intercostal space, where the pericardium comes in contact with the left chest wall.

MATCHING

1. a	4. b
2. e	5. c
3. d	

II. Critical Thinking Questions and Exercises

DISCUSSION AND ANALYSIS

1. On auscultation, an extra heart sound will be heard. This mitral click is an early sign that the valve leaflet is ballooning into the left atrium. Sometimes a murmur can be heard if the valve leaflet has stretched and regurgitation has occurred.
2. Left ventricular hypertrophy develops with mitral valve insufficiency because incomplete valve closure allows a regurgitation of blood from the left ventricle to the atrium during ventricular systole. This regurgitated blood is returned to the left ventricle, increasing the volume of blood that the left ventricle must handle. Hypertrophy of the left atrium and the left ventricle develops.
3. In aortic regurgitation, blood from the aorta returns to the left ventricle during diastole. Left ventricular dilation occurs. Left ventricular hypertrophy occurs, raising systolic blood pressure. Reflex vasodilation results as a compensatory measure. Peripheral arterioles relax, reducing peripheral resistance and diastolic blood pressure.
4. The characteristic sound is a systolic crescendo–decrescendo murmur which is low-pitched, rough, rasping, and vibrating.
5. Refer to Figure 29-3 and chapter heading, "Balloon Valvuloplasty."
6. Refer to Figure 29-6 and chapter heading, "Valve Replacement."
7. Refer to chapter heading, "Nursing Management: Valvuloplasty and Replacement."
8. All cardiomyopathies result in impaired cardiac output. The decrease in stroke volume stimulates the sympathetic nervous system and the renin–angiotensin–aldosterone response, resulting in increased systemic vascular resistance and increased sodium and fluid retention.
9. Refer to chapter heading, "The Patient with Cardiomyopathy."
10. Refer to Chart 29-3 and chapter heading, "Pericarditis."

Mitral valve stenosis

↓

resistance to aortic blood flow through narrowed orifice

↓

dilation and hypertrophy of the left atrium

↓

congested pulmonary circulation

↓

excessive strain on the right ventricle

↘ right ventricular failure

IDENTIFYING PATTERNS
FLOW CHART: MITRAL VALVE STENOSIS

CLINICAL SITUATIONS
CASE STUDY: INFECTIVE ENDOCARDITIS

1. toxicity of the infection, heart valve destruction, or embolization of fragments of vegetative growth on the heart
2. a
3. headache, transient cerebral ischemia, focal neurologic lesions, and strokes
4. total eradication of the invading organism
5. c
6. congestive heart failure, strokes, valvular stenosis, and myocardial erosion
7. d

CASE STUDY: ACUTE PERICARDITIS

1. a
2. pain related to inflammation of the pericardium
3. d
4. analgesics, antibiotics, and corticosteroids
5. left sternal edge in the fourth intercostal space
6. freedom from pain and absence of complications

Chapter 30

I. Interpretation, Completion, and Comparison

MULTIPLE CHOICE

1. a	9. b	17. d
2. a	10. c	18. d
3. d	11. d	19. b
4. b	12. a	20. b
5. b	13. b	21. d
6. c	14. a	22. d
7. b	15. d	23. b
8. d	16. a	24. a

25. d	27. a	29. c
26. c	28. b	

MATCHING

1. a	6. a
2. b	7. a
3. a	8. b
4. b	9. a
5. b	10. b

SHORT ANSWER

1. Cardiac output equals the heart rate times the stroke volume (the amount of blood pumped out with each contraction).
2. Preload is the amount of myocardial stretch created by the volume of blood within the ventricle before systole. Afterload refers to the amount of resistance to the ejection of the blood from the ventricle.
3. Venous return and ventricular compliance determine preload and the diameter/distensibility of the great vessels. The opening/competence of the semilunar valves determine afterload.
4. jugular venous distention; mean arterial blood pressure; a positive hepatojugular test
5. coronary artery disease, cardiomyopathy, hypertension, and valvular disorders
6. hypoxia and acidosis result from the accumulation of lactic acid
7. dilated, hypertrophic, and restrictive; dilated
8. dyspnea, cough, pulmonary crackles, low oxygen saturation, and a probable extra heart sound (ventricular gallop)
9. dependent edema, hepatomegaly, ascites, anorexia, nausea, weakness, and weight gain (fluid retention)
10. ACE inhibitors, beta-blockers, diuretics, and digitalis
11. symptomatic hypotension, hyperuricemia, ototoxicity, and electrolyte imbalances
12. weak pulse, faint heart sounds, hypotension, muscle flabbiness, diminished deep tendon reflexes, and generalized weakness
13. pulmonary embolism

II. Critical Thinking Questions and Exercises

DISCUSSION AND ANALYSIS

1. The ejection factor (EF), an indication of the volume of blood ejected with each contraction, is calculated by subtracting the amount of blood at the end of systole from the amount of blood at the end of diastole and calculating the percentage of blood that is ejected. A normal EF is 55% to 65% of ventricular volume.
2. Refer to Figure 30-2 and chapter heading, "Pathophysiology: Heart Failure."
3. Refer to Figure 30-3 and chapter headings, "Left-Sided Heart Failure" and "Right-Sided Heart Failure."
4. Refer to chapter heading, "Other Interventions: Cardiac Resynchronization Therapy."
5. Refer to Figure 30-4 and chapter heading, "Cardiogenic Shock."
6. Refer to Figures 30-7 and 30-8 and chapter heading, "Emergency Management: 7. Cardiopulmonary Resuscitation."

IDENTIFYING PATTERNS

FLOW CHART: THE PATHOPHYSIOLOGY OF PULMONARY EDEMA

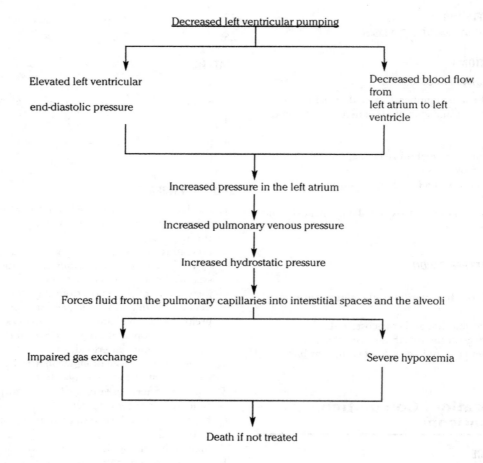

CLINICAL SITUATIONS

CASE STUDY: PULMONARY EDEMA

1. cardiac disease   4. b
2. a   5. d
3. d   6. d

Chapter 31

I. Comprehension and Interpretation

MULTIPLE CHOICE

1. d   3. b   5. a
2. b   4. a   6. b

7. b	13. b	19. c
8. c	14. d	20. d
9. b	15. d	21. d
10. d	16. a	22. b
11. d	17. d	23. a
12. b	18. d	

MATCHING

1. a   5. b
2. b   6. b
3. a   7. a
4. a   8. b

II. Critical Thinking Questions and Exercises

DISCUSSION AND ANALYSIS

1. The rate of blood flow through a vessel is determined by dividing the pressure difference (ΔP) (arterial minus venous) by the resistance to flow (R).
2. The pain in intermittent claudication is caused by the inability of the arterial system to provide adequate blood flow to the tissues in the face of increased demands for oxygen and nutrients during exercise.
3. Refer to Chart 31-1.
4. Refer to the Plan of Nursing Care in Chart 31-3.
5. Refer to chapter headings, "Thoracic Aortic Aneurysm" and "Abdominal Aortic Aneurysm."
6. Refer to Chart 31-7.
7. Refer to chapter heading, "Leg Ulcers."
8. Refer to chapter heading, "Varicose Veins."

EXAMINING ASSOCIATIONS

1. atherosclerosis
2. intermittent claudication
3. ratio of ankle to arm systolic pressure

4. the adventitia
5. lymphatic delivery to the remainder of the body
6. approximately 4 mm Hg
7. force generated by plasma proteins
8. inflammatory arterial aneurysm
9. lymphangitis

CLINICAL SITUATIONS

CASE STUDY: PERIPHERAL ARTERIAL OCCLUSIVE DISEASE

1. a
2. a
3. d
4. one joint level below the stenosis or occlusion
5. muscle metabolites and lactic acid
6. d
7. b
8. b
9. d

APPLYING CONCEPTS

Refer to Figure 31-1 and chapter heading, "Anatomic and Physiologic Overview."

Chapter 32

I. Interpretation, Completion, and Comparison

MULTIPLE CHOICE

1. d	7. d
2. d	8. b
3. c	9. c
4. b	10. c
5. b	11. b
6. c	

SHORT ANSWER

1. cardiac output; peripheral resistance
2. heart rate; stroke volume
3. 90% to 95% of the 30% who have hypertension
4. heart, kidneys, brain, and eyes
5. myocardial infarction, heart failure, renal failure, stroke, impaired vision, and left ventricular hypertrophy
6. accumulation of atherosclerotic plaques, fragmentation of arterial elastins, increased collagen deposits, and impaired vasodilation

7. acute myocardial infarction, a dissecting aortic aneurysm, an intracranial hemorrhage, and hypertension associated with pregnancy

MATCHING

1. d	4. a
2. b	5. c
3. f	6. e

II. Critical Thinking Questions and Exercises

DISCUSSION AND ANALYSIS

1. Refer to chapter heading, "Hypertension: Pathophysiology."
2. The control of hypertension is multifaceted. Discuss the roles of diet, exercise, smoking cessation, medication regimen compliance, and stress reduction in this process.
3. Refer to Chart 32-1.
4. Refer to Tables 32-2 and 32-3.

IDENTIFYING PATTERNS

FLOW CHART: THE PATHOPHYSIOLOGY OF PRIMARY ESSENTIAL HYPERTENSION

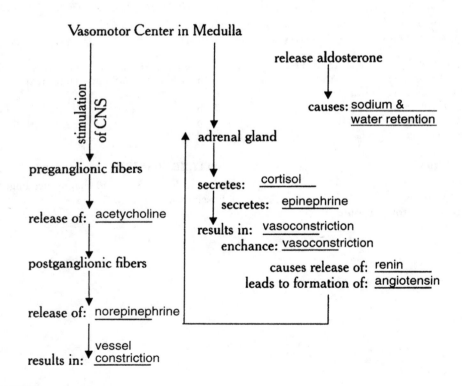

CLINICAL APPLICATIONS

CASE STUDY: SECONDARY HYPERTENSION

1. b	3. c
2. d	4. d

Chapter 33

I. Interpretation, Completion, and Comparison

MULTIPLE CHOICE

1. d	13. b	24. d
2. c	14. b	25. d
3. d	15. a	26. b
4. b	16. d	27. b
5. a	17. a	28. a
6. d	18. d	29. c
7. c	19. d	30. c
8. c	20. d	31. d
9. a	21. d	32. d
10. c	22. b	33. d
11. d	23. b	34. c
12. d		

SHORT ANSWER

1. 5 to 6
2. bone marrow
3. ribs, vertebrae, pelvis, and sternum
4. hemoglobin; transport oxygen between the lungs and the tissues
5. 15
6. 2 mg
7. Vitamin C
8. protect the body from invasion by bacteria and other foreign entities (phagocytosis)
9. albumin and globulins
10. the sternum and the iliac crest
11. Primary polycythemia, or polycythemia vera, is a proliferative disorder in which all cells are nonresponsive to normal control mechanisms; secondary polycythemia is caused by excessive production of erythropoietin.
12. hypochromia, microcytosis, hemolysis, and anemia
13. erythropoietin; reduced oxygen

SCRAMBLEGRAM: HEMATOLOGIC TERMS

```
F I B R I N O G E N A N O E L
B D H E M O S T A S I S P R M
F R S S C M P R H S G T H Y I
I E W C V R T C E L L S A T P
B E A B B T L D E F I J G H R
R S W A O H O A S V T S O R K
I F T P N R K L B J N M C O L
N E U T R O P H I L S K Y C B
F W O D C M F N K G H A T Y O
A H B E R B S J C T C B O T N
H E M A T O P O I E S I S E E
E M N E E C F M F G P S I S M
M O N O C Y T E S P L A S M A
O S C G D T K L A I E L K A R
G T O A H E E I J B E B A J R
L A G P E S F R M C N U L B O
O S G T I J D S A N M M S L W
B I H E O A G H H D O I I T L
I S D A U O U L M E S N P U M
N A S E L Y M P H O C Y T E S
```

1. plasma	6. hemoglobin	11. spleen	16. RES
2. thrombocytes	7. phagocytosis	12. hemostasis	17. Hemostasis
3. neutrophils	8. monocytes	13. fibrin	18. T cells
4. hematopoiesis	9. fibrinogen	14. lymphocytes	
5. bone marrow	10. albumin	15. erythrocyte	

II. Critical Thinking Questions and Exercises

DISCUSSION AND ANALYSIS

1. Refer to Table 33-2.
2. Refer to Chart 33-1.
3. Refer to Table 33-3 and chapter heading, "Hemolytic Anemias."
4. Refer to chapter heading, "Acute Lymphocytic Leukemia."
5. Refer to chapter heading, "Disseminated Intravascular Coagulation."
6. The INR is a standard method of reporting prothrombin times. The INR is needed to regulate the dosage of Coumadin.

CLINICAL SITUATIONS

CASE STUDY: SICKLE CELL CRISES

1. a
2. deformed, rigid, and sickle-shaped; 7 to 10 g/dL
3. bone marrow expansion to offset anemia
4. tissue hypoxia and necrosis due to inadequate blood flow to a specific organ or tissue
5. d
6. tachycardia, heart murmurs, and cardiomegaly
7. Answer may include stroke, infection, renal failure, heart failure, impotence, and pulmonary hypertension.
8. managing pain, preventing and managing infection, promoting coping skills, minimizing deficient knowledge, and monitoring/managing potential complications

CASE STUDY: LEUKEMIA

1. hematopoietic stem cell; age 60; 1
2. immature blast cells (greater than 30%)
3. d
4. b
5. b

CASE STUDY: HODGKIN DISEASE

1. a
2. b
3. c
4. d

CASE STUDY: TRANSFUSION

1. d
2. b
3. b
4. b

Chapter 34

I. Interpretation, Completion, and Comparison

MULTIPLE CHOICE

1. b	11. c	21. c
2. c	12. b	22. b
3. a	13. b	23. d
4. b	14. c	24. c
5. d	15. d	25. b
6. b	16. a	26. c
7. c	17. a	27. d
8. d	18. c	28. d
9. b	19. d	29. a
10. d	20. c	

MATCHING

1. f	4. c
2. a	5. b
3. e	6. d

FILL-IN

1. a. low-residue diet 1 to 2 days before test
   b. clear liquids the evening before
   c. a laxative the evening before
   d. NPO after midnight
   e. cleansing enemas until returns are clear in the morning
2. a. NPO 8 to 12 hours before the procedure
   b. no medications affecting gastric secretions 24 to 48 hours before test
   c. no smoking in the morning before test
3. a. NPO 6 to 12 hours before the procedure
   b. spraying or gargling with a local anesthetic
   c. administering intravenous Versed before the scope is introduced
4. a. liquids 24 to 72 hours before the examination
   b. laxative 48 hours before procedure
   c. laxatives until clear the morning of test, usually a polyethylene glycol electrolyte lavage solution (GoLYTELY)
   d. clear liquids starting at noon on the day before test

II. Critical Thinking Questions and Exercises

IDENTIFYING PATTERNS

1. Refer to Figures 34-3 and 34-5b.

Chapter 35

I. Interpretation, Completion, and Comparison

MULTIPLE CHOICE

1. c	9. b	16. a
2. d	10. c	17. a
3. b	11. d	18. a
4. a	12. c	19. a
5. d	13. b	20. c
6. b	14. a	21. a
7. b	15. a	22. a
8. b		

MATCHING

1. f	5. d
2. g	6. b
3. e	7. c
4. a	8. h

II. Critical Thinking Questions and Exercises

DISCUSSION AND ANALYSIS

1. Refer to Chart 35-2 and chapter heading, "Mouth Care."
2. Refer to chapter heading, "Dentoalveolar Abscess or Periapical Abscess."
3. Refer to chapter heading, "Disorders of the Salivary Glands."
4. Refer to Figure 35-4 and chapter heading, "Neck Dissection."
5. Refer to chapter heading, "Nursing Process: The Patient Undergoing Neck Dissection."

APPLYING CONCEPTS

1. local-regional metastasis
2. shoulder drop and poor cosmesis (visible neck depression)
3. pectoralis major
4. altered respiratory status, wound infection, and hemorrhage
5. hemorrhage and nerve injury
6. d
7. c
8. b
9. b
10. b

CLINICAL SITUATIONS

CASE STUDY: MANDIBULAR FRACTURE

1. The latest treatment for mandibular fractures involves rigid plate fixation or the placement of metal plates and screws into the bone to approximate and stabilize the bone.
2. b
3. b
4. Nasogastric suctioning is needed to remove stomach contents, thereby reducing the danger of aspiration.
5. c
6. b
7. c
8. a wire cutter

CASE STUDY: CANCER OF THE MOUTH

1. The typical lesion is a painless, indurated (hardened) ulcer with raised edges.
2. d
3. d
4. a
5. resectional surgery, radiation therapy, and chemotherapy

Chapter 36

I. Interpretation, Completion, and Comparison

MULTIPLE CHOICE

1. a	8. d	14. b
2. c	9. b	15. b
3. a	10. c	16. b
4. d	11. d	17. c
5. a	12. d	18. a
6. b	13. a	19. d
7. a		

MATCHING

1. e	4. a
2. b	5. c
3. d	

II. Critical Thinking Questions and Exercises

CLINICAL SITUATIONS

CASE STUDY: THE DUMPING SYNDROME

1. zinc deficiency, contaminated formula, malnutrition, and medication therapy
2. Medications that can increase the frequency of the dumping syndrome include Cleocin, digitalis, Inderal, Lincocin, theophylline, and quinidine.
3. a
4. d

CASE STUDY: TOTAL PARENTERAL NUTRITION

1. b	4. d
2. c	5. d
3. c	

APPLYING CONCEPTS

1. a. risk for impaired skin integrity at tube site
   b. risk for infection related to the presence of the wound and tube
   c. body image disturbance related to the presence of a tube
2. a. wound infection
   b. gastrointestinal bleeding
   c. premature removal of tube
3. leakage of fluid
4. seepage of gastric acid and spillage of feeding
5. 30 to 60 seconds
6. gently apply pressure with the bulb top of the syringe or elevate the syringe so the tubing is less curved
7. increasing the height increases the pressure of gravity, which could result in too much force on the incisional area and the outlet
8. An upright position facilitates digestion and decreases the risk for aspiration

Chapter 37

I. Interpretation, Completion, and Comparison

MULTIPLE CHOICE

1. d	8. b	15. d
2. b	9. d	16. b
3. a	10. c	17. d
4. b	11. a	18. c
5. d	12. a	19. c
6. c	13. d	20. b
7. a	14. d	

SHORT ANSWER

1. Dilute and neutralize the corrosive acid by using common antacids such as milk and aluminum hydroxide.
2. Patients with gastritis due to a vitamin deficiency exhibit antibodies against intrinsic factor, which interferes with vitamin B_{12} absorption.
3. Hypersecretion of acid pepsin and a weakened gastric mucosal barrier predispose to peptic ulcer development.
4. *Helicobacter pylori*
5. Answer may include hypersecretion of gastric juice, multiple duodenal ulcers, an increase in parietal cell mass, hypertrophied duodenal glands, and gastrinomas.
6. Stress ulcer refers to acute mucosal ulceration of the duodenal or gastric area that occurs after a stressful event.
7. Cushing's ulcers, which are common in patients with brain trauma, usually occur in the esophagus, stomach, or duodenum. Curling's ulcers occur most frequently after extensive burns and usually involve the antrum of the stomach and duodenum.
8. The objective of the ulcer diet is to avoid oversecretion and hypermotility in the gastrointestinal tract. Extremes of temperature should be avoided, as well as overstimulation by meat extractives, coffee, alcohol, and diets rich in milk and cream. Current therapy recommends three regular meals per day.
9. hemorrhage, perforation, and pyloric obstruction
10. When peptic ulcer perforation occurs, the patient experiences severe upper abdominal pain, vomiting, collapse, and an extremely tender abdomen that can be board-like in rigidity; signs of shock will be present.
11. 30 mL
12. adenocarcinoma

SCRAMBLEGRAM

1. achlorhydria
2. gastritis
3. hematemesis
4. melena
5. pylorus
6. pyrosis

II. Critical Thinking Questions and Exercises

DISCUSSION AND ANALYSIS

1. Refer to chapter heading, "Gastritis."
2. Gastritis occurs because the gastric mucous membrane becomes edematous and hyperemic. Superficial erosion occurs. Excess mucus is produced along with a scanty amount of gastric juice. Superficial ulceration can lead to hemorrhage.
3. H. pylori can be diagnosed by biopsy, serologic testing for antibodies, a 1-minute ultrarapid urease test, or a breath test.
4. Refer to Chart 37-4.
5. Refer to chapter heading, "Dumping Syndrome."

EXTRACTING INFERENCES

1. Refer to chapter heading, "Peptic Ulcer Disease."

CLINICAL SITUATIONS

CASE STUDY: GASTRIC CANCER

1. liver, pancreas, esophagus, and duodenum
2. ascites and hepatomegaly
3. esophagogastroduodenoscopy; computed tomography
4. b
5. 5-fluorouracil (5-FU)

Chapter 38

I. Interpretation, Completion, and Comparison

MULTIPLE CHOICE

1. d	5. c	9. b
2. b	6. a	10. d
3. c	7. d	11. b
4. c	8. b	12. d

13. a	17. a	21. d
14. d	18. c	22. b
15. d	19. c	23. c
16. d	20. d	24. b

CROSSWORD PUZZLE: TERMS ASSOCIATED WITH INTESTINAL AND RECTAL DISORDERS

Answers are found throughout chapter.

MATCHING

Column I	Column II
1-e	a-II
2-c	b-IV
3-f	c-V
4-a	d-I
5-b	e-III
6-d	f-VI

SHORT ANSWER

1. constipation, diarrhea, and fecal incontinence
2. irritable bowel syndrome (IBS) and diverticular disease
3. *Escherichia coli, Klebsiella, Proteus,* and *Pseudomonas*
4. adhesions; hernias and neoplasms
5. adenocarcinoid tumors
6. Refer to Chart 38-8.

II. Critical Thinking Questions and Exercises

DISCUSSION AND ANALYSIS

1. A series of neuromuscular actions are necessary for defecation. Rectal distention stimulates the inhibitory rectoanal reflex. This causes the internal and external sphincter, as well as the muscles in the pelvic region, to relax. Intra-abdominal pressure increases to propel the colon contents.

2. Straining at stool can cause the Valsalva maneuver (forcibly exhaling with the nose, mouth, and glottis closed), which results in increased intrathoracic pressure. This pressure tends to collapse the large veins in the chest. Cardiac output is decreased, and arterial pressure decreases. Almost immediately a rebound rise in arterial and venous pressure occurs. This can be dangerous for those with hypertension.

3. Pancreatic insufficiency causes reduced intraluminal pancreatic enzyme activity with maldigestion of lipids and proteins. Zollinger-Ellison syndrome causes hyperacidity in the duodenum that inactivates pancreatic enzymes. Celiac disease results in the destruction of the absorbing surface of epithelium as a toxic response to gluten fraction.

4. Refer to chapter heading, "Nursing Process: Management of the Patient with Inflammatory Bowel Disease."

5. Refer to Chart 38-4.

6. Refer to Chart 38-5.

7. Refer to Figures 38-7 and 38-8.

8. Refer to Table 38-5.

9. Refer to Table 38-6.

10. Refer to Chart 38-10.

RECOGNIZING CONTRADICTIONS

1. Diarrhea refers to more than three bowel movements per day, increased amount of stool, and looseness.

2. Appendicitis, the most common cause of emergency abdominal surgery, occurs in about 7% of the population.

3. The major complication of appendicitis is perforation, which occurs in 10% to 32% of cases.

4. The major cause of death from peritonitis is sepsis.

5. The distal ileum and colon are the most common areas affected by Crohn's disease.

6. More than 50% of patients with regional enteritis require surgery at some point.

7. Change in bowel habits is the most common symptom of colon cancer.

CLINICAL SITUATIONS

CASE STUDY: APPENDICITIS

1. c
2. c
3. d
4. d

CASE STUDY: PERITONITIS

1. d
2. a
3. a
4. a

IDENTIFYING PATTERNS

Refer to chapter heading, "Irritable Bowel Syndrome" and Figure 38-1.

Chapter 39

I. Interpretation, Completion, and Comparison

MULTIPLE CHOICE

1. d	11. a	21. c
2. c	12. d	22. d
3. d	13. c	23. d
4. c	14. b	24. d
5. b	15. c	25. b
6. d	16. d	26. d
7. d	17. a	27. d
8. d	18. b	28. d
9. b	19. a	29. d
10. b	20. d	30. d

MATCHING

1. c	5. d
2. e	6. g
3. b	7. f
4. a	

II. Critical Thinking Questions and Exercises

DISCUSSION AND ANALYSIS

1. Refer to Chart 39-1.

2. Hemolytic jaundice is the result of an increased destruction of red blood cells, which overloads the plasma with bilirubin so quickly that the liver cannot excrete the bilirubin as fast as it is formed. Hepatocellular jaundice is caused by the inability of damaged liver cells to clear normal amounts of bilirubin from the blood. Obstructive jaundice is usually caused by occlusion of the bile duct by a gallstone, an inflammatory process, a tumor, or pressure from an enlarged organ.

3. Refer to Figure 39-4 and chapter heading, "Ascites."

4. Refer to Figure 39-11 and chapter heading, "Surgical Bypass Procedures: Shunting."

5. Hepatic encephalopathy occurs when ammonia accumulates because damaged liver cells fail to detoxify and convert ammonia to urea. Elevated ammonia concentrations cause brain damage.

6. In alcoholic cirrhosis, necrotic liver cells are replaced by scar tissue, which gradually exceeds functioning liver tissue. Liver enlargement leads to obstruction of the portal circulation, which causes shunting of blood into vessels with lower pressures. Edema results from the concentration of plasma albumin. An overproduction of aldosterone causes sodium and water retention and potassium excretion. Anemia, gastritis, and vitamin deficiency lead to overall physical and mental deterioration.

CLINICAL SITUATIONS

CASE STUDY: LIVER BIOPSY

1. d
2. b
3. c

4. b
5. d

CASE STUDY: PARACENTESIS

1. c
2. d

3. a

CASE STUDY: ALCOHOLIC OR NUTRITIONAL CIRRHOSIS

1. c
2. d
3. c (2.2 lb = 1 kg)
4. c (normal protein intake is 0.8 to 1 g/kg)
5. c (normal sodium intake is 3 to 6 g/24 h without as
   cites; sodium restriction is minimal rather than severe)

CASE STUDY: LIVER TRANSPLANTATION

1. d
2. d

3. c
4. a

Chapter 40

I. Interpretation, Completion, and Comparison

MULTIPLE CHOICE

1. c	9. a	16. d
2. c	10. d	17. b
3. c	11. d	18. c
4. a	12. d	19. d
5. a	13. a	20. d
6. b	14. a	21. a
7. d	15. b	22. b
8. a		

SHORT ANSWER

1. 30 to 50 mL
2. insulin, glucagon, and somatostatin
3. amylase, trypsin, and lipase
4. calculous cholecystitis
5. Refer to Chart 40-4.

II. Critical Thinking Questions and Exercises

CLINICAL SITUATIONS

CASE STUDY: CHOLECYSTECTOMY

Brenda's Preoperative Situation

1. d
2. b

3. d

Brenda's Postoperative Situation

1. a
2. d

3. c

CASE STUDY: CHRONIC PANCREATITIS

1. long-term alcohol consumption
2. The inflammatory process causes the replacement of cells
   by fibrous tissues. This results in mechanical obstruction
   of the pancreatic and common bile ducts and the duodenum. Atrophy of the epithelium of the ducts causes
   destruction of the secreting cells of the pancreas.
3. diabetes mellitus
4. pancreaticojejunostomy
5. avoidance of alcohol and avoidance of foods found to
   cause abdominal pain and discomfort

Chapter 41

I. Interpretation, Completion, and Comparison

MULTIPLE CHOICE

1. c	15. d	31. d
2. b	16. d	32. d
3. c	17. a	33. c
4. c	18. c	34. a
5. c	19. d	35. d
6. d	20. d	36. c
7. a	21. d	37. d
8. d	22. d	38. c
9. d	23. a	
10. d	24. c	
11. c	25. a	
12. c	26. b	
13. a	27. d	
14. a (use 15 to	28. c	
20 kcal/kg of	29. d	
IBW)	30. d	

MATCHING

1. c	4. e
2. a	5. d
3. b	

SHORT ANSWER

1. nontraumatic amputations, blindness among working-
   age adults, and end-stage renal disease
2. 180 to 200 mg/dL
3. 14%

4. normalize insulin activity and blood glucose levels to reduce the development of vascular and neuropathic complications
5. nutrition management, exercise, monitoring, pharmacologic therapy, and education
6. 25 to 29; more than 30
7. 50% to 60% carbohydrate, 20% to 30% fat, and 10% to 20% protein
8. 25 to 30
9. Lispro (Humalog) and Aspart (NovoLog)
10. ketoacidosis
11. directly stimulating the pancreas to secrete insulin (cannot be used in patients with type 1 diabetes)
12. abdomen, posterior surface of the upper arms, anterior surface of the thighs, and the hips
13. hypoglycemia, diabetic ketoacidosis (DKA), and hyperglycemic hyperosmolar nonketotic syndrome
14. hypotension, profound dehydration, tachycardia, and altered neurologic status (seizures, hemiparesis)
15. cerebral edema, hyperglycemia and ketoacidosis, hypokalemia, hypoglycemia, and fluid overload (pulmonary edema, congestive heart failure)
16. Diabetic retinopathy

II. Critical Thinking Questions and Exercises

DISCUSSIONS AND ANALYSIS

1. Refer to Chart 41-1.
2. Insulin regulates the production and storage of glucose. In diabetes, either the pancreas stops producing insulin or the cells stop responding to insulin. Hyperglycemia results and can lead to acute metabolic complications such as diabetic ketoacidosis and hyperglycemic hyperosmolar nonketotic syndrome. Long-term complications can contribute to macrovascular or microvascular complications.
3. Type 1 diabetes is characterized by an absence of insulin production and secretion due to the autoimmune destruction of the beta cells of the islets of Langerhans. Type 2 diabetes is characterized by deficiency of insulin production and a decreased insulin action as well as increased insulin resistance.
4. Hyperglycemia develops during pregnancy because the secretion of placental hormones causes insulin resistance.
5. "Glycemic index" is used to describe how much a given food increases the blood glucose level compared with an equivalent amount of glucose.
6. Refer to chapter heading, "Complications of Insulin Therapy."
7. Refer to Table 41-5.

EXAMINING ASSOCIATIONS

1. 2
2. 2
3. 1
4. 1
5. 1
6. 2
7. 1
8. 2
9. 2
10. 1

IDENTIFYING PATTERNS

FLOW CHART: THE PATHOPHYSIOLOGIC SEQUENCE OF CHANGES THAT OCCUR WITH TYPE 1 DIABETES

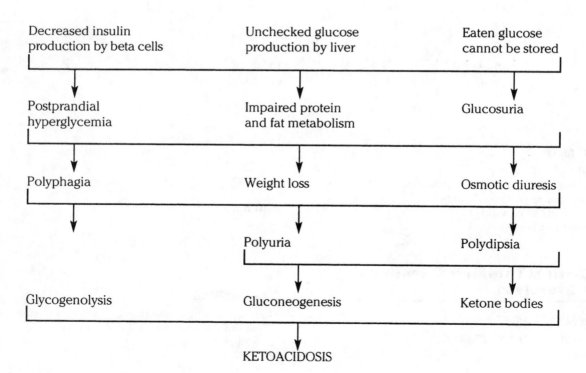

APPLYING CONCEPTS

1. Sensory neuropathy causes loss of sensation to pain and pressure; autonomic neuropathy causes an increase in skin dryness and the formation of skin fissures; motor neuropathy results in muscular atrophy.
2. 50%
3. Inadequate and compromised lower-extremity circulation interferes with the ability to get nutrients to the wound to promote healing and prevent the development of gangrene.
4. Hyperglycemia impairs the ability of specialized leukocytes to destroy bacteria, thus lowering the resistance to infection.
5. soft-tissue injury, formation of a fissure, and formation of a callus
6. bathe, dry, and lubricate the feet; inspect both feet; look for fissures on dry skin or between the toes; report any redness, swelling, or drainage; wear well-fitting, closed-toe shoes.
7. peripheral vascular disease may prevent oxygen, nutrients, and antibiotics from reaching the injured tissue.

CLINICAL SITUATIONS

CASE STUDY: TYPE 1 DIABETES

1. b	3. b
2. c	

CASE STUDY: HYPOGLYCEMIA

1. a	3. d
2. d	4. d

CASE STUDY: DIABETIC KETOACIDOSIS

1. d	4. a
2. a	5. b
3. d	6. d

Chapter 42

I. Interpretation, Completion, and Comparison

MULTIPLE CHOICE

1. d	11. a	21. d
2. b	12. d	22. a
3. a	13. d	23. d
4. d	14. b	24. c
5. a	15. d	25. d
6. d	16. a	26. d
7. a	17. d	27. c
8. d	18. a	28. a
9. b	19. c	29. a
10. b	20. d	

MATCHING

1. h		6. c	
2. g		7. f	
3. i		8. e	
4. d		9. j	
5. a		10. b	

SHORT ANSWER

1. negative feedback
2. steroid, protein or peptide, amine, and fatty acid derivatives
3. vasopressin; the excretion of water by the kidneys; oxytocin; milk ejection during lactation
4. Cushing's disease
5. diabetes insipidus; excessive thirst and large volumes of dilute urine
6. thyroxine (T_4), triiodothyronine (T_3), and calcitonin
7. autoimmune thyroiditis
8. diabetes mellitus
9. Graves' disease
10. Propacil and Tapazole
11. hypocalcemia and tetany
12. Trousseau's sign or Chvostek's sign
13. glucocorticoids, mineralocorticoids, and androgens

UNSCRAMBLED WORDS

1. pituitary
2. hypothalamus
3. somatotropin
4. SIADH (syndrome of inappropriate antidiuretic hormone)
5. iodine
6. exophthalmos
7. tetany

II. Critical Thinking Questions and Exercises

DISCUSSION AND ANALYSIS

1. Refer to chapter heading, "Diabetes Insipidus."
2. Refer to chapter heading, "Thyroid Tests."
3. Refer to Chart 42-3.
4. Refer to Chart 42-7.
5. Refer to chapter headings, "Addison's Disease" and "Cushing's Syndrome."

CLINICAL SITUATIONS

CASE STUDY: PRIMARY HYPOTHYROIDISM

1. d	4. d
2. d	5. b
3. b	

CASE STUDY: HYPERPARATHYROIDISM

1. a
2. a
3. apathy, fatigue, muscular weakness, nausea, vomiting, constipation, hypertension, and cardiac dysrhythmias
4. kidney stones
5. d
6. b
7. c

CASE STUDY: SUBTOTAL THYROIDECTOMY

1. d   4. a
2. d   5. b
3. d   6. a

Chapter 43

I. Interpretation, Completion, and Comparison

MULTIPLE CHOICE

1. b   3. c
2. b   4. a

5. b   10. b
6. c   11. d
7. d   12. d
8. a   13. d
9. a

SHORT ANSWER

1. nephron; cortex
2. 300 to 500 mL
3. aldosterone
4. 300 to 900 mOsm/kg
5. increased
6. antidiuretic hormone (ADH)
7. urea
8. creatine clearance

II. Critical Thinking Questions and Exercises

IDENTIFYING PATTERNS

FLOW CHART: PATHOPHYSIOLOGIC RESPONSES TO HYPOTENSION

Renal perfusion decreases

and

blood pressure decreases

↓

Kidneys release <u>renin</u>

↓

Liver manufactures <u>angiotensin I</u>

which converts to

↓

<u>angiotensin II</u> (a powerful vasoconstrictor)

↓

Adrenals release <u>aldosterone</u>

↓

<u>Increases sodium retention</u>

↓

Pituitary releases <u>ACTH</u>

↓

<u>Blood pressure increases</u>

↓   ↓

<u>Renal autoregulation occurs</u>   <u>Circulating blood volume increases</u>

Chapter 44

I. Interpretation, Completion, and Comparison

MULTIPLE CHOICE

1. d	11. c	21. d
2. d	12. a	22. d
3. a	13. d	23. d
4. d	14. b	24. b
5. b	15. a	25. b
6. b	16. a	26. b
7. a	17. b	27. d
8. c	18. d	28. d
9. c	19. a	29. b
10. b	20. a	

MATCHING

1. a	6. j
2. b	7. h
3. c	8. f
4. e	9. g
5. d	10. i

SHORT ANSWER

1. proteinuria, hematuria, decreased GFR, and altered sodium excretion
2. The urine in the early stages of acute glomerulonephritis is characteristically cola-colored.
3. creatinine and BUN
4. proteinuria, hypoalbuminemia, edema, and hypercholesterolemia
5. Prerenal conditions (hemorrhage, sepsis); intrarenal conditions (crush injuries, infections); postrenal conditions (obstruction distal to kidney)
6. Clinical manifestations seen in chronic renal failure include lethargy, headache, muscle twitching, seizures, nausea, vomiting, and diarrhea. There is also dehydration and the odor of urine on the breath
7. potassium levels greater than 5.5 mEq/L and T-wave elevations
8. arteriosclerotic cardiovascular disease
9. Answer may include hypotension, air embolism, chest pain, dysrhythmias, pruritus, dialysis disequilibrium, painful muscle cramping, nausea, vomiting, and exsanguination.
10. peritonitis
11. abdominal distention and paralytic ileus

II. Critical Thinking Questions and Exercises

DISCUSSION AND ANALYSIS

1. Refer to Figure 44-1.

2. Refer to Chart 44-2.
3. Refer to Chart 44-4.
4. Refer to chapter heading, "Dialysis."
5. Refer to chapter heading, "Dialysis."
6. Refer to chapter heading, "Peritoneal Dialysis."
7. Refer to chapter heading, "Renal Trauma."

APPLYING CONCEPTS

1. support arterial flow to the dialyzer
2. support reinfusion of the dialyzed blood
3. 2 weeks; time is needed for the venous segment of the fistula to dilate to accommodate the large-bore needles
4. squeeze a rubber ball for forearm fistulas
5. polytetrafluoroethylene; 10 days

CLINICAL SITUATIONS

CASE STUDY: CAPD

1. d	4. d
2. a	5. c
3. a	

CASE STUDY: ARF

1. c	4. b
2. d	5. b
3. b	6. d

Chapter 45

I. Interpretation, Completion, and Comparison

MULTIPLE CHOICE

1. a	10. b	18. c
2. c	11. a	19. d
3. a	12. c	20. a
4. d	13. b	21. d
5. b	14. b	22. c
6. b	15. d	23. b
7. b	16. d	24. a
8. d	17. d	25. d
9. d		

SHORT ANSWER

1. feelings of urgency, burning, and pain on urination; nocturia; incontinence; pelvic pain; and sometimes hematuria and back pain
2. chronic bacterial prostatitis
3. *Proteus, Klebsiella, Pseudomonas,* and *Staphylococcus*
4. anticholinergics, antispasmodics, and tricyclic antidepressants
5. to allow drainage in patients with neurogenic bladder dysfunction; to bypass an obstruction that blocks

urine flow; to provide postoperative drainage after urologic and other surgeries; and to monitor hourly urinary output in critically ill patients

6. *Escherichia coli, Klebsiella, Proteus, Pseudomonas, Enterobacteriaceae, Serratia,* and *Candida*
7. cloudy urine, hematuria, fever, chills, anorexia, and malaise
8. calcium oxalate, calcium phosphate, and uric acid

II. Critical Thinking Questions and Exercises

RECOGNIZING CONTRADICTIONS

1. The majority of nosocomial infections in the hospital are caused by <u>instrumentation of the urinary tract or catheterization.</u>
2. Urethrovesical reflux refers to the backward flow of urine <u>from the urethra into the bladder.</u>
3. Today, two diagnostic studies, <u>computerized tomography (CT) and ultrasonography,</u> are the preferred methods for diagnosing UTI.

DISCUSSION AND ANALYSIS

1. Refer to Chart 45-2.
2. Refer to Chart 45-3.
3. Refer to chapter heading, "Urinary Tract Infections."
4. Refer to Chart 45-6.
5. Refer to Chart 45-9.
6. Refer to Chart 45-12.

Chapter 46

I. Interpretation, Completion, and Comparison

MULTIPLE CHOICE

1. d	8. b	15. c
2. a	9. b	16. b
3. b	10. c	17. c
4. c	11. a	18. c
5. a	12. b	19. c
6. a	13. a	20. b
7. d	14. a	

SHORT ANSWER

1. 12 to 14 years; 10 years
2. follicle-stimulating; luteinizing hormone
3. 45 to 52 years; 51 years; 40
4. irregular or excessive vaginal bleeding, abnormal discharge, bleeding after menopause, painful intercourse (dyspareunia), bleeding after intercourse, urinary disturbances, and painful menstruation
5. 6 million
6. 20%
7. endometrial biopsy

8. atherosclerosis, angina, coronary artery disease, and osteoporosis
9. Answer may include headache, fatigue, low back pain, engorged or painful breasts, abdominal fullness, mood swings, general irritability, fear of loss of control, binge eating, and crying spells.
10. Lack of body fat and low caloric intake decrease hormonal function.
11. The pill blocks the stimulation of the ovary by preventing the release of follicle-stimulating hormone (FSH) from the anterior pituitary.
12. Absolute contraindications include a history of thromboembolic disorders, migraine headaches with visual auras, cerebrovascular disease, breast cancer, pregnancy, liver tumors, post–estrogen-dependent neoplasia, congenital hyperlipidemia, and abnormal vaginal bleeding.
13. Depo-Provera, a long-acting progestin that is injected intramuscularly, effectively inhibits ovulation for 3 months.
14. An emergency dose of estrogen or estrogen and progesterone, properly timed, can prevent pregnancy by inhibiting or delaying ovulation.
15. For in vitro fertilization, at an appropriate time, the egg is recovered by transvaginal ultrasound retrieval. Sperm and egg are coincubated for up to 36 hours so that fertilization can occur. Forty-eight hours after retrieval, the embryo is transferred to the uterine cavity by means of a transcervical catheter. Implantation should occur in 3 to 4 days.

MATCHING

1. f	5. e
2. d	6. g
3. h	7. c
4. a	8. b

II. Critical Thinking Questions and Exercises

DISCUSSION AND ANALYSIS

1. Refer to chapter heading, "Health History" and Chart 46-1.
2. Refer to chapter heading, "Female Genital Mutilation."
3. Refer to chapter heading, "Rape and Sexual Assault."
4. Refer to Chart 46-4.
5. Refer to chapter heading, "Endoscopic Examinations."
6. Refer to chapter heading, "Abnormal Uterine Bleeding."

RECOGNIZING CONTRADICTIONS

1. The WHI study was halted early because it found that hormone replacement therapy, after menopause, increased the risks of breast cancer, heart attack, stroke, and blood clots.

2. Women born to mothers who took DES during their pregnancy have a higher than average chance of developing cancer of the cervix.

3. A cervical cone biopsy is performed when a Pap smear is "suspicious"; it is always done with anesthesia.

4. Magnetic resonance imaging uses a magnetized field to produce an image; radiation is not necessary.

5. Progesterone is the most important hormone for preparing the endometrium for the fertilized ovum.

6. Painful cramps result from an excessive production of prostaglandins.

7. Mifepristone (RU-486) is approved for elective abortions up to 49 days from the last menstrual period.

8. The leading cause of a pregnancy-related death in the woman's first trimester is ectopic pregnancy.

EXTRACTING INFERENCES

1. A fertilized ovum implants in tissue other than the uterine area.

2. Possible causes are salpingitis, peritubal adhesions, structural abnormalities of the fallopian tube, previous ectopic pregnancy or tubal surgery, the presence of an IUD, and multiple previous abortions.

3. abdominal tenderness; sharp, colicky pain; some bleeding; gastrointestinal symptoms; and abnormal bleeding

4. The tube can be resected (salpingostomy) or removed (salpingectomy) along with an ovary (salpingo-oophorectomy).

5. determine whether any tissue remained

6. hemorrhage and shock

CASE STUDY: TOXIC SHOCK SYNDROME

1. c	4. d
2. a	5. c
3. b	

Chapter 47

I. Interpretation, Completion, and Comparison

MULTIPLE CHOICE

1. d	12. a	23. d
2. d	13. a	24. c
3. d	14. c	25. d
4. d	15. b	26. d
5. b	16. c	27. d
6. a	17. d	28. a
7. c	18. d	29. c
8. c	19. c	30. a
9. a	20. d	31. c
10. a	21. b	32. b
11. b	22. b	

SCRAMBLEGRAM

1. vulvodynia
2. Mycostatin
3. Flagyl
4. acyclovir
5. septic shock
6. cystocele
7. Pap smear
8. hysterectomy
9. menorrhagia
10. fibroids
11. DES
12. HRT
13. Kegel
14. fistula
15. prolapse
16. dermoid

II. Critical Thinking Questions and Exercises

DISCUSSION AND ANALYSIS

1. Estrogen breaks down glycogen into lactic acid, which is responsible for producing a low vaginal pH. A pH of 3.5 to 4.5 suppresses bacterial growth.
2. Refer to Chart 47-1.
3. Refer to chapter heading, "Human Papillomavirus."
4. Pelvic inflammatory disease (PID) is a condition of the pelvic cavity that may involve the uterus, fallopian tubes, ovaries, pelvic peritoneum, or pelvic vascular system.

CLINICAL SITUATIONS

CASE STUDY: BACTERIAL VAGINOSIS

1. a
2. b
3. c
4. a
5. a

CASE STUDY: HERPES GENITALIS

1. d
2. a
3. c
4. 50 million
5. mouth, oropharynx, mucosal surface, vagina, and cervix
6. Acyclovir, valacyclovir, and famciclovir
7. pain related to the presence of genital lesions, risk for recurrence of infections or spread of infection, anxiety and distress related to embarrassment, and insufficient knowledge about the disease and methods of avoiding spread and recurrences

CASE STUDY: PELVIC INFLAMMATORY DISEASE

1. uterus, fallopian tubes, ovaries, pelvic peritoneum, and pelvic vascular system

2. acute, subacute, recurrent, chronic, localized, and widespread
3. gonorrhea and chlamydia
4. ectopic pregnancy, infertility, recurrent pelvic pain, ovarian abscess, and recurrent disease
5. Localized symptoms are vaginal discharge, lower abdominal pain, dyspareunia, and tenderness after menses. Generalized symptoms are fever, general malaise, anorexia, nausea, headache, and vomiting.

Chapter 48

I. Interpretation, Completion, and Comparison

MULTIPLE CHOICE

1. b
2. b
3. a
4. a
5. c
6. d
7. a
8. b
9. d
10. b
11. d
12. c
13. d
14. c
15. d
16. b
17. b
18. b
19. b
20. c
21. b
22. d
23. c
24. c
25. a
26. d
27. c

MATCHING

1. e
2. g
3. a
4. c
5. b
6. d
7. f

II. Critical Thinking Questions and Exercises

CLINICAL SITUATIONS

CASE STUDY: SIMPLE MASTECTOMY

Preoperative Situation

1. c
2. d
3. b
4. c

Postoperative Situation

5. b
6. c
7. a

IDENTIFYING PATTERNS

FIGURE 1/Step 1: Stand in front of a mirror. Check both breasts for anything unusual. Look for a discharge from the nipples, puckering, dimpling, or scaling of the skin.

FIGURE 2/Step 2: Watch closely in the mirror as you clasp your hands behind your head and press your hands forward. Note any change in the contour of your breasts.

FIGURE 3/Step 3: Next, press your hands firmly on your hips and bow slightly toward the mirror as you pull your shoulders and elbows forward. Note any change in the contour of your breasts.

FIGURE 4/Step 4: Raise your left arm. Use 3 or 4 fingers of your right hand to feel your left breast firmly, carefully, and thoroughly. Beginning at the outer edge, press the flat part of your fingers in small circles, moving the circles slowly around the breast. Gradually work toward the nipple. Be sure to cover the whole breast. Pay special attention to the area between the breast and the underarm, including the underarm area itself. Feel for any unusual lump or mass under the skin. If you have any spontaneous discharge during the month—whether or not it is during your BSE—see your doctor. Repeat the examination on your right breast.

FIGURE 5/Step 5: Step 4 should be repeated lying down. Lie flat on your back, with your left arm over your head and a pillow or folded towel under your left shoulder. This position flattens the breast and makes it easier to check. Use the same circular motion described in Step 4. Repeat on your right breast.

Chapter 49

I. Interpretation, Completion, and Comparison

MULTIPLE CHOICE

1. b	8. d	14. d
2. d	9. d	15. a
3. b	10. a	16. c
4. b	11. c	17. b
5. a	12. b	18. a
6. a	13. a	19. c
7. c		

SHORT ANSWER

1. prostate-specific antigen (PSA) and digital rectal examination (DRE)
2. Answer should include 4 of 15 medications found in Chart 49-1.
3. *Escherichia coli*
4. burning, urgency, perineal discomfort, frequency, and pain with or after ejaculation
5. Symptoms of BPH include frequency of urination, nocturia, urgency, a sensation that the bladder has not emptied completely, hesitancy in starting urination, abdominal straining, a decrease in the volume and force of the urinary stream, recurring urinary tract infections, interruption of the urinary stream, and dribbling.
6. diethylstilbestrol (DES); Lupron, Zoladex, and Eulexin
7. Taxol and Taxotere
8. Heparin is given prophylactically because there is a high incidence of deep vein thrombosis and pulmonary embolism after prostatectomy.
9. Epididymitis is an infection of the epididymis that usually descends from an infected prostate or urinary tract. It passes upward through the urethra and ejaculatory duct and along the vas deferens to the epididymis.
10. human chorionic gonadotropin and alpha-fetoprotein

MATCHING

1. c
2. f
3. e
4. a
5. d
6. h
7. g
8. b

II. Critical Thinking Questions and Exercises

DISCUSSION AND ANALYSIS

1. Refer to chapter heading, "Erectile Dysfunction."
2. Refer to Chart 49-2.
3. Refer to Chart 49-3.
4. Refer to Table 49-1.
5. Refer to chapter heading, "Conditions Affecting the Testes and Adjacent Structures."

CLINICAL SITUATIONS

CASE STUDY: THE PATIENT UNDERGOING PROSTATECTOMY

1. assessment of general health status and establishment of optimum renal function
2. before acute urinary retention develops and damages the urinary tract and collecting system, or before cancer develops
3. d
4. stricture formation and retrograde ejaculation
5. hemorrhage, clot formation, catheter obstruction, and sexual dysfunction

6. Damage to the pudendal nerves may causes impotence.
7. anxiety related to the surgical procedure and its outcome, pain related to bladder distention, and knowledge deficit about factors related to the problem and the treatment protocol
8. warm compresses to the pubis and sitz baths
9. Prolonged sitting increases intra-abdominal pressure and increases the possibility of bleeding.
10. Teach the patient to tense the perineal muscles by pressing the buttocks together, holding the position for 15 to 20 seconds and then relaxing.

Chapter 50

I. Interpretation, Completion, and Comparison

MULTIPLE CHOICE

1. c	8. d	15. b
2. d	9. c	16. d
3. a	10. b	17. a
4. c	11. b	18. c
5. c	12. d	19. d
6. d	13. c	20. a
7. c	14. a	

MATCHING

Immunoglobulins

1. c	5. a
2. e	6. b
3. c	7. a
4. d	

Medications

1. d	5. b
2. b	6. a
3. a	7. e
4. c	

II. Critical Thinking Questions and Exercises

DISCUSSION AND ANALYSIS

1. Disorders arise from excesses or deficiencies of immunocompetent cells, alterations in cellular functioning, immunologic attack on self-antigens, and inappropriate or exaggerated responses to specific antigens.
2. Natural immunity, which is nonspecific, is present at birth. Acquired immunity is more specific and develops

throughout life. Passive acquired immunity is a temporary immunity transmitted from another source that has developed immunity through previous disease or immunization.

3. Complement is a term used to describe circulating plasma proteins that are made in the liver and activated when an antibody couples with an antigen.

4. Biologic response modifiers (BMRs) suppress antibody production and cellular immunity.

5. Stem cells continually replenish the body's supply of red and white cells. Once the immune system has been destroyed, stem cells can completely restore it with just a few cells.

SCRAMBLEGRAM

1. antibody
2. complement
3. antigen
4. helper T cells
5. phagocytes
6. interferons

Chapter 51

I. Interpretation, Completion, and Comparison

MULTIPLE CHOICE

1. d	6. d
2. d	7. a
3. d	8. b
4. b	9. b
5. b	10. d

II. Critical Thinking Questions and Exercises

IDENTIFYING PATTERNS

1. phagocytic dysfunction
2. B-cell deficiency, probably CVID
3. T-cell deficiency
4. ataxia-telangiectasia
5. a secondary immunodeficiency

EXAMINING ASSOCIATIONS

1. B-lymphocyte deficiency
2. CVID
3. progressive neurological deterioration
4. excess occurrences of lysis of erythrocytes

Chapter 52

I. Interpretation, Completion, and Comparison

MULTIPLE CHOICE

1. c	7. c	12. b
2. a	8. c	13. a
3. b	9. c	14. c
4. c	10. c	15. b
5. a	11. d	16. b
6. c		

SHORT ANSWER

1. California, Florida, and New York.
2. 1 million; African American; 72%
3. unprotected sex and the sharing of injection drug use equipment
4. blood, seminal fluid, vaginal secretions, amniotic fluid, and breast milk
5. retroviruses (viruses that carry their genetic material in the form of RNA rather than DNA)
6. HIV-RNA viral load, CD4 T-cell count levels, the clinical symptoms of the disease, and the patient's desire for compliance
7. maximum suppression of viral load, restoration/preservation of immunologic function, improved quality of life, and reduced HIV-related mortality and morbidity
8. anti-HIV drugs attempt to block viral replication within cells by inhibiting either reverse transcriptase or HIV protease
9. candidiasis
10. alpha-interferon

MATCHING

1. c		5. c
2. b		6. b
3. c		7. a
4. a		8. c

II. Critical Thinking Questions and Exercises

DISCUSSION AND ANALYSIS

1. Refer to Chart 52-2.
2. Refer to Chart 52-4.
3. Primary infection is that period from infection with HIV to the development of antibodies to HIV. It is the time during which the viral burden set point is achieved and includes the acute symptoms and early infection phases. During primary infection, a window period occurs, during which the person is infected but tests negative on the HIV antibody blood test.
4. Refer to chapter heading, "Vaccines."

5. The lesions are usually brownish pink to deep purple. They may be flat or raised and surrounded by hemorrhagic patches and edema.
6. Refer to chapter heading, "Nursing Process: The Patient with AIDS."

CLINICAL SITUATIONS

CASE STUDY: AIDS

1. Risky sexual practices and intravenous drug use
2. c
3. c
4. Answer may include opportunistic infections, impaired breathing or respiratory failure, wasting syndrome, fluid and electrolyte imbalance, and adverse reaction to medications.
5. d
6. d

Chapter 53

I. Interpretation, Completion, and Comparison

MULTIPLE CHOICE

1. d	8. b	15. b
2. c	9. b	16. d
3. c	10. d	17. d
4. d	11. d	18. b
5. a	12. a	19. c (0.1 mg/kg)
6. d	13. a	20. c
7. a	14. a	21. c

SHORT ANSWER

1. neutralizing toxic antigens, precipitating the antigens out of solution, and coating the surface of the antigens
2. an inappropriate or exaggerated antigen and antibody interaction or response causes tissue injury
3. the pain and fever seen with inflammatory responses
4. Type III hypersensitivity reactions are seen in systemic lupus erythematosus, rheumatoid arthritis, serum sickness, certain types of nephritis, and some types of bacterial endocarditis.
5. contact dermatitis and latex allergy
6. penicillin
7. 4 to 10 hours
8. avoidance of latex products

II. Critical Thinking Questions and Exercises

DISCUSSION AND ANALYSIS

1. An allergic reaction occurs when the body is invaded by an antigen, usually a protein that the body recognizes as foreign. The body responds in an effort to destroy the invading antigen. Antibodies (protein substances) are produced. When an interaction between the antigen and antibody results in tissue injury, an allergic reaction occurs and chemical mediators are released into the body.
2. Immunoglobulins are a group of serum proteins (antibodies formed by lymphocytes and plasma cells) that bind specifically with certain antigens to neutralize, agglutinate, and destroy various bacteria and foreign cellular material.
3. The systemic reactions of flushing, warmth, and itching rapidly progress to bronchospasm, laryngeal edema, severe dyspnea, cyanosis, and hypotension. Cardiac arrest and coma can occur.
4. Refer to chapter headings, "Skin Tests,"" "Provocative Testing,"" and "Radioallergosorbent Tests."
5. Refer to chapter heading, "Allergic Disorders."
6. Refer to chapter heading, "Anaphylaxis," and Chart 53-2.
7. Refer to chapter heading, "Pharmacologic Therapy."
8. Refer to Chart 53-7.
9. Refer to Table 53-4.

CLINICAL SITUATIONS

CASE STUDY: ALLERGIC RHINITIS

1. Possible nursing diagnoses include Potential ineffective breathing patterns, related to an allergic reaction; Knowledge deficit about allergy and recommended modifications in lifestyle; and Impaired adjustment, related to chronicity of condition and need for environmental modifications
2. restoration of a normal breathing pattern, knowledge about the causes and control of allergic symptoms, adjustment to alterations and modifications, and absence of complications
3. d
4. d
5. d
6. c

Chapter 54

I. Interpretation, Completion, and Comparison

MULTIPLE CHOICE

1. d	9. a	17. b
2. d	10. c	18. d
3. b	11. d	19. b
4. b	12. c	20. d
5. d	13. b	21. b
6. c	14. a	22. b
7. d	15. a	23. a
8. b	16. d	

MATCHING

1. c
2. d
3. e

4. a
5. f
6. b

II. Critical Thinking Questions and Exercises

DISCUSSION AND ANALYSIS

1. Refer to chapter heading, "Degeneration."
2. Exacerbation is a period of time when the symptoms of a disorder occur or increase in intensity and frequency. Remission is a period of time when symptoms are reduced or absent.
3. In inflammatory rheumatic disease, the inflammation occurs as the result of an immune response. Newly formed synovial tissue is infiltrated with inflammatory cells (pannus formation), and joint degeneration occurs as a secondary process. In degenerative rheumatic disease, synovitis results from mechanical irritation. A secondary inflammation occurs.
4. Refer to Table 54-2 and pages throughout the chapter for your answers.
5. Refer to Table 54-4.
6. Refer to chapter heading, "Persistent, Erosive Rheumatoid Arthritis."
7. Refer to chapter heading, "Polymyalgia Rheumatica."
8. Refer to chapter heading, "Degenerative Joint Disease."
9. Refer to chapter heading, "Metabolic and Endocrine Diseases Associated with Rheumatic Disorders."
10. Refer to chapter heading, "Fibromyalgia."

CLINICAL SITUATIONS

CASE STUDY: DIFFUSE CONNECTIVE TISSUE DISEASE

1. b
2. b
3. Answer may include weight loss, fever, anemia, fatigue, lymph node enlargement, and Raynaud's phenomenon.
4. d
5. c
6. COX-2 inhibitors
7. d

CASE STUDY: SYSTEMIC LUPUS ERYTHEMATOSUS (SLE)

1. chemical, hormonal, environmental, and genetic
2. an increase in autoantibody production that results from abnormal suppressor T-cell function, leading to immune complex deposition and tissue damage
3. pericardial friction rub, myocarditis, and pericarditis
4. severe anemia, thrombocytopenia, leukocytosis, leukopenia, and positive antinuclear antibodies
5. antimalarial
6. hypertension and atherosclerotic heart disease

INTERPRETING PATTERNS

Refer to Figures 54-1 and 54-3 as a framework for your outline.

Chapter 55

I. Interpretation, Completion, and Comparison

MULTIPLE CHOICE

1. b
2. a
3. b

4. a
5. b
6. c

II. Critical Thinking Questions and Exercises

ANALYZING COMPARISONS

1. skin coloring
2. jaundice
3. immune system
4. alopecia
5. scurvy
6. inspection
7. scales

IDENTIFYING PATTERNS

1. telangiectasis
2. syphilis
3. ecchymosis or petechia
4. urticaria
5. Kaposi's sarcoma

IDENTIFYING PATTERNS

Primary and secondary lesions: Answers to 1 to 8 should include any characteristics listed for each lesion in Chart 55-3.

APPLYING CONCEPTS

1. appearance of wrinkles, overlapping skin folds, appearance of sags, increased vulnerability to injury
2. diminished protection and cushioning of underlying organs and tissues, decreased muscle tone, decreased insulating properties
3. delayed wound healing, smaller vessels decrease in number and size
4. dry and scaly skin
5. decreased sebaceous gland functioning

Chapter 56

I. Comprehension and Interpretation

MULTIPLE CHOICE

1. d	12. a	23. d
2. d	13. b	24. b
3. c	14. d	25. a
4. d	15. a	26. a
5. d	16. d	27. d
6. b	17. d	28. c
7. d	18. c	29. d
8. c	19. c	30. d
9. b	20. a	31. c
10. b	21. c	32. d
11. b	22. d	

SHORT ANSWER

1. prevent additional damage, prevent secondary infection, revise the inflammatory process, and relieve symptoms
2. have a high moisture vapor transmission rate (some even have reservoirs to hold excessive exudate)
3. releasing increased amounts of growth factors into a wound (this process stimulates cell growth and granulation of skin)
4. Risk for impaired skin integrity related to changes in the barrier function of the skin
5. acne vulgaris
6. impetigo and folliculitis
7. *Staphylococcus aureus*
8. sepsis and keratoconjunctivitis; infection
9. skin cancer; basal cell carcinoma and squamous cell carcinoma; biopsy and histologic evaluation
10. more than 10 times/year

SCRAMBLEGRAM: TERMS USED TO DESCRIBE DERMATOLOGIC PROBLEMS

1. comedo
2. cheilitis
3. carbuncle
4. furuncle
5. tinea
6. pyodermas
7. liniments
8. xerosis
9. Santyl
10. gel
11. Lidex
12. Famvir
13. scabies
14. Eurax
15. TEN

II. Critical Thinking Questions and Exercises

DISCUSSIONS AND ANALYSIS

1. Moisture-retentive dressings result in reduced pain, fewer infections, less scar tissue, gentle autolytic débridement, decreased frequency of dressing changes, and increased efficiency at removing exudates.
2. Autolytic débridement is a process whereby the body's own digestive enzymes are used to break down necrotic tissue. A foul odor occurs when cellular debris is broken down. It is normal and expected.
3. Refer to chapter heading, "Folliculitis, Furuncles, and Carbuncles."

4. Refer to chapter heading, "Viral Skin Infections."
5. Refer to chapter heading, "Photochemotherapy."
6. Refer to chapter heading, "Toxic Epidermal Necrolysis and Stevens-Johnson Syndrome."
7. Refer to Chart 56-8.

CLINICAL SITUATIONS

CASE STUDY: ACNE VULGARIS

1. Open comedones, closed comedones, erythematous papules, inflammatory pustules, and inflammatory cysts
2. d
3. c
4. Benzoyl peroxide has an antibacterial effect because it suppresses *Propionibacterium acnes*, depresses sebum production, and helps breakdown comedo plugs.
5. Vitamin A clears up the keratin plugs from the pilosebaceous ducts by speeding up cellular turnover and forcing the comedo out of the skin.
6. c
7. a
8. scarring and infection

CASE STUDY: MALIGNANT MELANOMA

1. c
2. 20 to 45 years
3. lung cancer
4. d
5. c
6. c
7. a
8. 20% to 50%

Chapter 57

I. Interpretation, Completion, and Comparison

MULTIPLE CHOICE

1. b	10. c	19. c
2. b	11. a	20. c
3. d	12. a	21. d
4. c	13. a	22. b
5. c	14. b	23. c
6. d	15. a	24. b
7. b	16. a	25. c
8. b	17. d	26. c
9. c	18. b	27. c

28. b	31. a	34. d (3 g/kg)
29. b	32. c	35. b
30. c	33. b	

SHORT ANSWER

1. the very young (before age 4 years) and the elderly (after age 65 years)
2. in the home (usually in the kitchen)
3. 0.5%
4. the depth of the injury and the extent of injured body surface area
5. acute respiratory failure and acute respiratory distress syndrome (ARDS)
6. sepsis
7. injury to the rescuer
8. morphine sulfate
9. acute respiratory failure, distributive shock, acute renal failure, and compartment syndrome
10. *Staphylococcus, Proteus, Pseudomonas, Escherichia coli,* and *Klebsiella; Candida albicans*
11. hypertrophic scarring, keloid formation, and contractures

II. Critical Thinking Questions and Exercises

DISCUSSION AND ANALYSIS

1. Survival after large burn injury has significantly improved because of the following: research in fluid resuscitation, emergent burn treatment, inhalation injury treatment, and earlier débridement of wounds.
2. Carbon monoxide, a byproduct of the combustion of organic materials, combines with hemoglobin to form carboxyhemoglobin. Carboxyhemoglobin competes with oxygen for available hemoglobin-binding sites.
3. Refer to Chart 57-3.
4. Refer to chapter heading, "Emergency/Resuscitative Phase."
5. Refer to Chart 57-4.
6. Refer to Nursing Care Plan, Chart 57-7.
7. Fluid overload may occur when fluid is mobilized from the interstitial compartment back into the intravascular compartment. If the cardiac system cannot compensate for the excess volume, congestive heart failure may result.

IDENTIFYING PATTERNS

FLOW CHART: SYSTEMIC RESPONSE TO BURN INJURY

Major Burn Injury

Loss of <u>capillary integrity</u>

Fluid shift from <u>intravascular</u> space to <u>interstitial</u> space

due to a movement of <u>fluid, sodium, and protein</u>

Decreased <u>cardiac output</u>   Decreased <u>blood pressure</u>

Stimulation of <u>SNS</u>

which releases <u>catecholamines</u>

Increased <u>vasoconstriction</u>   Increased <u>heart rate</u>

Decreased <u>cardiac output</u>

CLINICAL SITUATIONS

See Plan of Nursing Care (Chart 57-7) for assistance with the completion of the assignment. A sample is shown here.

AIMEE'S SITUATION

Nursing diagnosis: Altered comfort, related to pain resulting from a burn injury
    Goals: Pain relief
    Nursing actions: Continue developmental growth patterns while providing for skin healing and grafting; maintain socialization patterns consistent with Aimee's peer group; assess Aimee's respiratory status
    Rationale: Airway compromise can occur rapidly in a significant burn injury as fluid shifts occur.
    Expected outcome: Aimee has a patient airway and does not exhibit any respiratory distress

Chapter 58

I. Interpretation, Completion, and Comparison

MULTIPLE CHOICE

1. c	7. c	13. c
2. d	8. d	14. c
3. c	9. c	15. a
4. d	10. d	16. c
5. d	11. b	17. b
6. d	12. a	

SHORT ANSWER

1. that the patient can see an object from 20 feet away that a person with 20/20 vision can see at 100 feet.
2. cataracts, diabetic retinopathy, glaucoma, and macular degeneration
3. glaucoma
4. pallor and cupping of the optic nerve disc
5. laser trabeculoplasty and laser iridotomy
6. cataracts
7. Patients report the sensation of a shade or curtain coming across the eye, cobwebs, bright flushing lights, or the onset of floaters. Pain is not reported.
8. irrigation with normal saline
9. *Streptococcus pneumoniae, Haemophilus influenzae,* and *Staphylococcus aureus*
10. "pink eye" (dilation of the conjunctival blood vessels)
11. diabetic retinopathy
12. cytomegalovirus (CMV)

MATCHING

1. b
2. c
3. f
4. j
5. a
6. e
7. g
8. d
9. h
10. I

CROSSWORD PUZZLE

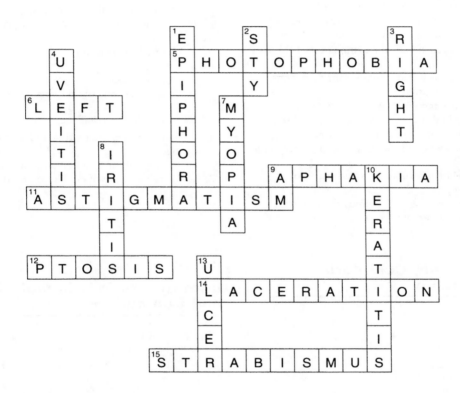

II. Critical Thinking Questions and Exercises

EXTRACTING INFERENCES

1. forms, stores and secretes tears in response to reflex or emotional stimuli
2. dilates and constricts in response to light
3. the highly vascularized, pigmented part of the eye that surrounds the pupil
4. the junction of the conjunctiva
5. protects the intraocular contents from trauma and helps maintain the shape of the eyeball
6. a mucous membrane that provides a barrier to the external environment and nourishes the eye
7. the angles at either end of the slits between the eyelids; no specific function
8. covers the uppermost portion of the iris and washes the cornea and conjunctiva with tears with every blink of the eyes
9. a small, fleshy projection of the lacrimal duct

DISCUSSION AND ANALYSIS

1. Refer to chapter heading "Cataracts."
2. Refer to chapter heading, "Refractive Surgeries."
3. Refer to chapter heading, "Infectious and Inflammatory Conditions."
4. Refer to chapter heading, "Surgical Procedures and Enucleation."

IDENTIFYING PATTERNS

1. blepharitis
2. sty (external hordeolum)

3. conjunctivitis
4. keratitis
5. cataract

CLINICAL SITUATIONS

CASE STUDY: CATARACT SURGERY

1. smoking, diabetes mellitus, alcohol abuse, and inadequate intake of antioxidant vitamins over time
2. painless blurring of vision, sensitivity to glare, and functional impairment due to reduced visual acuity
3. a grayish pearly haze in the pupil
4. d
5. extracapsular extraction
6. one to two nights

NURSING CARE PLAN: CATARACT SURGERY

Elise would have several immediate, intermediate, and long-term goals. An example is shown here. Refer to Chapter 58 for assistance with the completion of this care plan.

Nursing diagnosis: Altered visual sensory perception related to cataract formation

Goals: Make Elise familiar with her new environment; prepare the affected eye for surgery; encourage Elise to walk with her cane as independently as possible

Nursing action: Assess Elise's level of knowledge about her surgery

Rationale: Baseline information is necessary to determine teaching plan.

Expected outcome: Elise understands the purpose, process, and expected outcomes of her surgery.

Chapter 59

I. Interpretation, Completion, and Comparison

MULTIPLE CHOICE

1. a	8. d	15. d
2. b	9. b	16. d
3. d	10. d	17. c
4. a	11. c	18. c
5. b	12. d	19. a
6. c	13. a	20. d
7. b	14. c	

II. Critical Thinking Questions and Exercises

DISCUSSION AND ANALYSIS

1. Refer to chapter heading, "Evaluation of Gross Auditory Acuity."
2. Refer to Table 59-4.
3. Refer to Chart 59-3.

EXAMINING ASSOCIATION

Answers for questions 1 to 11 are related to Figure 59-1 and can be found in Chart 59-1.

CLINICAL SITUATIONS

CASE STUDY: MASTOID SURGERY

1. infection, otalgia, otorrhea, hearing loss, vertigo, erythema, edema, and odor of discharge
2. Answer may include reduction of anxiety, freedom from pain and discomfort, prevention of infection, stabilization/improvement of learning, absence of injury from vertigo, absence of or adjustment to altered sensory perception, return of skin integrity, and knowledge about the disease process and surgical intervention.
3. a sense of aural fullness or pressure (intermittent pain may last for 2 to 3 weeks after surgery)
4. c
5. an elevated temperature and purulent drainage
6. d
7. c
8. straining, exertion, and moving or lifting heavy objects

CASE STUDY: MÉNIÈRE'S DISEASE

1. vertigo, tinnitus, fluctuating and progressive sensorineural hearing loss, a feeling of pressure or fullness in the ear, and nausea and vomiting.
2. an overabundance of circulating fluid
3. vertigo
4. b
5. a
6. a

Chapter 60

I. Interpretation, Completion, and Comparison

MULTIPLE CHOICE

1. d	8. d	15. a
2. b	9. d	16. a
3. a	10. a	17. c
4. d	11. b	18. b
5. a	12. c	19. b
6. a	13. a	20. c
7. b	14. c	21. c

MATCHING

1. e	4. c
2. f	5. a
3. d	6. b

II. Critical Thinking Questions and Exercises

EXAMINING ASSOCIATIONS

AUTONOMIC NERVOUS SYSTEM

Organ or Tissue	Parasympathetic Effect	Sympathetic Effect
a. bronchi	constriction	dilation
b. cerebral vessels	dilation	constriction
c. coronary vessels	constriction	dilation
d. heart	inhibition	acceleration
e. iris	constriction	dilation
f. salivary glands	secretion	secretion
g. smooth muscle of bladder wall	constriction	inhibition
h. smooth muscle of large intestine	increased motility	inhibition
i. smooth muscle of small intestine	increased motility	inhibition

CRANIAL NERVES

Nerve no.	Column I	Column II
I	olfactory	smell
II	optic	vision
III	oculomotor	eye movement
IV	trochlear	eye movement
V	trigeminal	facial sensation
VI	abducens	eye movement
VII	facial	taste and expression
VIII	vestibulocochlear	hearing and equilibrium
IX	glossopharyngeal	taste
X	vagus	swallowing, gastric motility, and secretion
XI	spinal accessory	trapezius and sternomastoid muscles
XII	hypoglossal	tongue movement

DIAGRAM OF THE BRAIN

THALAMUS

1. Receives, synthesizes, and relays all stimuli except for olfactory stimuli; all memory, sensation, and pain impulses pass through here.
2. Relays impulses to visceral and somatic effectors

HYPOTHALAMUS

1. Maintains sugar and fat metabolism
2. Regulates water balance and metabolism
3. Regulates body temperature
4. Regulates blood pressure
5. Influences the body's response to stress
6. Maintains the sleep-wake cycle
7. Controls the autonomic nervous system
8. Regulates aggressive and sexual behavior

PITUITARY

1. Regulates growth and reproduction
2. Controls various metabolic activities

Chapter 61

I. Interpretation, Completion, and Comparison

MULTIPLE CHOICE

1. d	9. a	17. c
2. d	10. d	18. a
3. a	11. d	19. c
4. c	12. c	20. b
5. b	13. d	21. b
6. d	14. a	22. c
7. c	15. d	23. a
8. c	16. d	24. b

SHORT ANSWER

1. respiratory distress, pneumonia, aspiration, pressure ulcer, deep vein thrombosis, and contractures
2. pneumonia, aspiration, and respiratory failure
3. a change in the level of consciousness (LOC)
4. brain stem herniation, diabetes insipidus, and syndrome of inappropriate antidiuretic hormone (SIADH)
5. administer osmotic diuretics and corticosteroids, restrict fluids, drain cerebrospinal fluid, hyperventilate the patient, control fever, and reduce cellular metabolic demands
6. intraventricular catheter, subarachnoid bolt, epidural or subdural catheter, and fiberoptic transducer-tipped catheter
7. brain herniation
8. increased ICP, infection, and neurologic deficits
9. cerebrovascular disease
10. status epilepticus
11. Answer may include bright lights; stress; depression; sleep deprivation; fatigue; foods containing tyramine, monosodium glutamate, or nitrates; aged cheese; and oral contraceptives.

MATCHING

1. a and f		4. a
2. c and e		5. c
3. b		

II. Critical Thinking Questions

DISCUSSION AND ANALYSIS

1. Airway management is a vital nursing function for a patient with altered level of consciousness. The nurse should put the patient in the lateral or semiprone position with the head elevated about 30 degrees, remove secretions from the posterior pharynx and upper trachea by suctioning, perform frequent oral hygiene, auscultate the lungs every 8 hours, and initiate postural drainage and chest physiotherapy.
2. Refer to chapter heading, "Nursing Process: The Patient with an Altered Level of Consciousness."
3. Refer to chapter heading, "New Trends in Neurologic Monitoring."
4. Refer to chapter heading, "Detecting Early Indications of Increasing ICP."
5. It is believed that reducing body temperature helps decrease cerebral edema, reduce the oxygen and metabolic requirements of the brain, and protect the brain from continued ischemia.
6. Refer to chapter heading, "Nursing Management: Seizure," and Chart 61-4.

IDENTIFYING PATTERNS

1. surgery involving removal of a portion of the skull
2. increased blood pressure and decreased heart rate and respirations in response to increased pressure on the medulla oblongata
3. decortication
4. unrelenting pain accompanied by nausea, vomiting, and visual disturbances
5. rhythmic waxing and waning of the rate and depth of respirations alternating with brief periods of apnea

CLINICAL SITUATIONS

PLAN OF NURSING CARE: UNCONSCIOUS PATIENT

Refer to Chapter heading, "Nursing Process: The Patient with an Altered Level of Consciousness," and Table 61-1.

APPLYING CONCEPTS

Refer to chapter heading, "Nursing Assessment of the Unconscious Patient," and Table 61-1.

Chapter 62

I. Interpretation, Completion, and Comparison

MULTIPLE CHOICE

1. b	7. d	13. a
2. a	8. a	14. b
3. a	9. c	15. d
4. b	10. d	16. c
5. a	11. c	17. d
6. b	12. a	

SHORT ANSWER

1. stroke; brain attack
2. age, sex, race, and ethnicity
3. transient ischemic attack, reversible ischemic neurologic deficit, stroke in evolution, and completed stroke
4. A bruit is an abnormal sound heard on auscultation resulting from interference with normal blood flow. A patient with a TIA may have a bruit over the carotid artery.
5. carotid endarterectomy
6. decreased cerebral blood flow and inadequate oxygen delivery to the brain
7. stroke, cranial nerve injuries, infection or hematoma at the incision, and carotid artery disruption
8. brain tissue, the ventricles, or the subarachnoid space
9. the development of cerebral vasospasm
10. cerebral hypoxia, decreased cerebral blood flow, and extension of the area of injury

MATCHING

1. d	5. b
2. h	6. g
3. e	7. c
4. a	8. f

II. Critical Thinking Questions and Exercises

DISCUSSION AND ANALYSIS

1. A brain attack is a disruption of cerebral blood flow caused either by an obstruction or by rupture of a blood vessel. Blood alteration initiates a series of cellular metabolic events called an ischemic cascade. Initially, low cerebral blood flow (a penumbra region) exists. Intervention needs to occur at this time, before calcium influx and increased glutamate activate a number of damaging pathways.
2. Refer to Table 62-2.
3. Based on the major nursing diagnoses, the nurse would focus her care on the following interventions, which are not all-inclusive: improving mobility and preventing joint deformities, preventing shoulder pain, enhancing self-care, managing sensory-perceptual difficulties, managing dysphagia, attaining bladder and bowel control, improving communication, maintaining skin integrity, and helping with family coping.

CLINICAL SITUATIONS

Refer to chapter heading, "Nursing Process: The Patient Recovering from an Ischemic Stroke," and Charts 62-3 and 62-4.

Chapter 63

I. Interpretation, Completion, and Comparison

MULTIPLE CHOICE

1. d	8. c	14. b
2. c	9. d	15. b
3. b	10. a	16. d
4. d	11. b	17. a
5. d	12. d	18. b
6. d	13. c	19. b
7. d		

SHORT ANSWER

1. leakage of cerebrospinal fluid from the ears and the nose
2. obstructed blood flow can decrease tissue perfusion, causing cellular death and brain damage
3. headache, dizziness, lethargy, irritability, and anxiety
4. difficulty in awakening, difficulty in speaking, confusion, severe headache, vomiting, and weakness on one side of the body
5. hematoma (either epidural, subdural, or intracerebral)
6. coma, hypertension, bradycardia, and bradypnea
7. coma, absence of brain stem reflexes, and apnea
8. decreased cerebral perfusion; cerebral edema and herniation; impaired oxygenation and ventilation; impaired fluid, electrolyte, and nutritional balance; and risk of posttraumatic seizures
9. eye opening, verbal responses, and motor responses to verbal commands or painful stimuli
10. systemic infections, neurosurgical infections, and heterotrophic ossification
11. 5th cervical, 6th cervical, 7th cervical, 12th thoracic, and 1st lumbar
12. pleuritic chest pain, anxiety, shortness of breath, and abnormal blood gas values
13. deep vein thrombosis, orthostatic hypotension, and autonomic dysreflexia
14. the urinary tract, respiratory tract and pressure ulcers.

II. Critical Thinking Questions and Exercises

DISCUSSION AND ANALYSIS

1. Head injuries, the most common cause of death from trauma in the United States, affect about 1.4 million people annually. Of these victims, about 50,000 die. Males between the ages of 15 and 24 years are at highest risk.
2. Refer to Chart 63-2.
3. Refer to chapter heading, "Types of Brain Injury."
4. Brain injury can cause significant brain damage because of obstructed blood flow and decreased tissue perfusion. The brain cannot store oxygen and glucose to any significant degree. Irreversible brain damage and cell death occurs when the blood supply is interrupted for even a few minutes.
5. The Act regulates acceptable medical standards for defining death—the irreversible loss of all brain function.
6. Refer to Chart 63-5 for a list of activities.
7. Refer to chapter heading, "Autonomic Dysreflexia."

CLINICAL SITUATIONS

PLAN OF NURSING CARE: CERVICAL SPINE INJURY

Refer to chapter heading, "Nursing Process: The Patient with Acute Spinal Cord Injury," for assistance with the development of a nursing care plan for Katie.

PLAN OF NURSING CARE: PARAPLEGIA

Refer to chapter heading, " Nursing Process: The Patient with Tetraplegia or Paraplegia," for assistance with the development of a nursing care plan for Matthew.

Chapter 64

I. Interpretation, Completion, and Comparison

MULTIPLE CHOICE

1. a	7. c
2. a	8. c
3. d	9. b
4. d	10. c
5. c	11. c
6. a	

SHORT ANSWER

1. meningitis, brain abscesses, various types of encephalitis, Creutzfeldt-Jakob disease, and variant Creutzfeldt-Jacob disease
2. severe headache, high fever, a stiff neck (nuchal rigidity), photophobia, a positive Kernig sign, and a positive Brudzinski sign
3. herpes simplex virus (HSV); acyclovir (Zovirax)
4. a polyclonal antibody (protein 14-3-3) in cerebrospinal fluid
5. myelin material that surrounds the nerve fibers in the brain and spinal cord
6. relapsing-remitting, secondary progressive, and primary progressive
7. acetylcholine receptors
8. diabetes, alcoholism, and occlusive vascular disease

MATCHING

1. b	6. f
2. b	7. g
3. e	8. h
4. d	9. h
5. f	10. d

II. Critical Thinking Questions and Exercises

DISCUSSION AND ANALYSIS

1. To assess for Kernig's sign, the nurse would ask the patient to extend one leg while the opposite thigh is flexed on the abdomen. Inability to do this is considered positive for bacterial meningitis. To assess for Brudzinski's sign, the nurse would ask the patient to flex his neck. If flexion of the knees and hips occurs at the same time, the test is considered positive for bacterial meningitis.
2. Demyelination refers to the destruction of myelin, the fatty and protein material that surrounds nerve fibers in the brain and spinal cord. This destruction results in impaired transmission of nerve impulses.
3. Refer to chapter heading, "Multiple Sclerosis: Medical Management."
4. Refer to chapter heading, "Myasthenic Crisis."

CLINICAL SITUATIONS

CASE STUDY: MULTIPLE SCLEROSIS

1. d	3. a
2. d	4. d

Chapter 65

I. Interpretation, Completion, and Comparison

MULTIPLE CHOICE

1. d	6. d	11. b
2. c	7. a	12. b
3. d	8. b	13. d
4. c	9. a	14. a
5. c	10. b	15. c

SHORT ANSWER

1. lung, breast, lower gastrointestinal tract, pancreas, kidney, and skin
2. headache, nausea and vomiting, and papilledema
3. hemiparesis, seizures, and mental status changes
4. intramedullary
5. Answer should include five of the following: Parkinson's disease, Huntington's disease, Alzheimer's

disease, amyotrophic lateral sclerosis, muscular dystrophies, degenerative disc disease, and postpolio syndrome.
6. tremor, rigidity, bradykinesia, and postural instability
7. fatigue, progressive muscle weakness, cramps, fasciculations (twitching), and incoordination
8. muscle wasting and weakness, abnormal elevation in blood muscle enzymes, and myopathic findings on EMG and muscle biopsy
9. C5–C6 or C6–C7
10. hematoma at the surgical site, causing cord compression and neurologic deficit; recurrent or persistent pain after surgery

MATCHING

1. d	5. h
2. c	6. f
3. g	7. b
4. a	8. e

II. Critical Thinking Questions and Exercises

DISCUSSION AND ANALYSIS

1. A variety of physiologic changes can occur, such as increased ICP and cerebral edema, seizure activity and focal neurologic signs, hydrocephalus, and altered pituitary function.
2. Brain tumors are classified according to origin: those arising from the covering of the brain, those developing in or on the cranial nerves, those originating within brain tissue, and metastatic lesions originating elsewhere in the body.
3. Refer to chapter heading, "Nursing Process: The Patient with Cerebral Metastasis or Incurable Brain Tumor."
4. Refer to chapter heading, "Stereotactic Procedures."
5. Refer to chapter heading, "Huntington's Disease."
6. Refer to chapter heading, "Surgical Management: Degenerative Disk Disease."

CASE STUDY: PARKINSON'S DISEASE

1. d	3. d
2. c	4. b

CASE STUDY: HUNTINGTON'S DISEASE

Refer to Chart 65-5 for assistance with the development of a nursing care plan for Mike.

EXTRACTING INFERENCES

Use chapter headings relevant to tumors as a reference.

Chapter 66

I. Interpretation, Completion, and Comparison

MULTIPLE CHOICE

1. b	6. a
2. a	7. d
3. a	8. b
4. c	9. b
5. a	10. b

MATCHING

1. h	6. e
2. i	7. d
3. b	8. c
4. j	9. a
5. g	10. f

SHORT ANSWER

1. arthritis
2. hip fractures
3. 98%
4. 206
5. 150 mg
6. sternum, ileum, vertebrae, ribs
7. parathyroid hormone and calcitonin
8. 4 months
9. crepitus

SCRAMBLEGRAM

1. periosteum
2. ligaments
3. sarcomere
4. tendons
5. osteoporosis
6. scoliosis
7. effusion
8. arthrocentesis

II. Critical Thinking Questions and Exercises

DISCUSSION AND ANALYSIS

1. General functions of the musculoskeletal system include protection, support, locomotion, mineral storage, hematopoiesis, and heat production.
2. Refer to chapter heading, "Structure and Function of the Skeletal System."
3. Refer to chapter heading, "Bone Formation (Osteogenesis)."
4. Vitamin D increases calcium in the blood by promoting calcium absorption from the gastrointestinal tract and by accelerating the mobilization of calcium from the bone.
5. Refer to chapter heading, "Bone Maintenance."
6. Refer to chapter heading, "Bone Healing."
7. Refer to chapter heading, "Skeletal Muscle Contraction."
8. Refer to Table 66-1.
9. Refer to Figure 66-3.
10. Refer to chapter heading, Diagnostic Evaluation."

EXTRACTING INFERENCES

Refer to chapter headings, "Structure and Function of the Articular System" and "Structure and Function of the Skeletal System."

Chapter 67

I. Interpretation, Completion, and Comparison

MULTIPLE CHOICE

1. c	10. c	18. a
2. b	11. b	19. a
3. b	12. b	20. c
4. d	13. d	21. c
5. a	14. b	22. c
6. d	15. c	23. a
7. b	16. a	24. d
8. d	17. d	25. d
9. b		

SHORT ANSWER

1. reduce a fracture, correct a deformity, apply uniform pressure to underlying soft tissue, and provide support and stability for weak joints
2. A fiberglass cast is light in weight and water resistant; it does not soften when wet.
3. necrosis, impaired tissue perfusion, pressure ulcer formation, and possible paralysis
4. The toes or fingers should be pink, warm, and easily moved (wiggled). There should be minimal swelling and discomfort. The blanch test should be carried out to determine rapid capillary refill.
5. pain, pallor, pulselessness, paresthesia, and paralysis
6. Answer may include unrelieved pain, swelling, discoloration, tingling, numbness, inability to move fingers or toes, and any temperature changes.
7. compartment syndrome, pressure ulcers, and disuse syndrome
8. to minimize muscle spasms; to reduce, align, and immobilize fractures; to lessen deformities; and to increase space between opposing surfaces within a joint
9. chlorhexidine solution
10. osteomyelitis

11. pressure ulcer, atelectasis, pneumonia, constipation, anorexia, urinary stasis and infection, and venous thromboemboli with PE or DVT
12. unilateral calf tenderness, warmth, redness, and swelling (increased calf circumference)
13. 70%; 5 to 7 days; 20%; 1% to 3%
14. thromboembolism, peroneal nerve palsy, infection, and limited range of motion

II. Critical Thinking Questions and Exercises

DISCUSSION AND ANALYSIS

1. Answer may include compartment syndrome, pressure ulcer, disuse syndrome, and delayed union or nonunion of the fracture.
2. Answer should include knowledge of the treatment regimen, relief of pain, improved physical mobility, achievement of maximum level of self-care, healing of lacerations and abrasions, maintenance of adequate neurovascular function, and absence of complications.
3. Compartment syndrome occurs when the circulation and function of tissue within a confined area (casted area) is compromised. Treatment requires that the cast be bivalved; a fasciotomy may be necessary. See Figure 67-2.
4. Volkmann's contracture is a serious complication of impaired circulation in the arm. Contracture of the fingers and wrist occurs as the result of obstructed arterial blood flow to the forearm and the hand. The patient is unable to extend the fingers, describes abnormal sensation, and exhibits signs of diminished circulation to the hand. Permanent damage develops within a few hours if action is not taken.
5. Refer to chapter heading, "Long Casts."
6. The major nursing goals for a patient in traction may include understanding of the treatment regimen, reduced anxiety, maximum comfort, maximum level of self-care, maximum mobility within therapeutic limits of traction, and absence of complications.
7. Refer to Chart 67-7.
8. Refer to Chart 67-8.
9. Refer to Chart 67-9.
10. Refer to chapter headings, "Nursing Process: Preoperative Care of the Patient Undergoing Orthopedic Surgery" and "Nursing Process: Postoperative Care of the Patient Undergoing Orthopedic Surgery."

CLINICAL SITUATIONS

CASE STUDY: BUCK'S TRACTION

1. a
2. the patient's body weight and the bed position adjustments
3. inspect the skin for abrasions and circulatory disturbances; make certain the skin is clean and dry before any tape or foam boot is applied.
4. d

5. skin color, skin temperature, capillary refill, edema, pulses, sensations, and ability to move
6. A positive Homans' sign indicates deep vein thrombosis.

CASE STUDY: TOTAL HIP REPLACEMENT

1. deep vein thrombosis and pulmonary embolism
2. dislocation of the hip prosthesis, excessive wound drainage, thromboembolism, and infection
3. c
4. d
5. leg shortening, inability to move the leg, malalignment, abnormal rotation, and increased localized discomfort
6. b
7. b

Chapter 68

I. Interpretation, Completion, and Comparison

MULTIPLE CHOICE

1. d	7. d	13. d
2. b	8. c	14. b
3. b	9. c	15. d
4. c	10. c	16. c
5. a	11. d	17. a
6. c	12. b	18. b

SHORT ANSWER

1. Answer should include five of these conditions: acute lumbosacral strain, unstable lumbosacral ligaments, weak lumbosacral muscles, osteoarthritis of the spine, spinal stenosis, intervertebral disk problems, and unequal leg length.
2. Risk for ineffective tissue perfusion, peripheral, related to swelling; Acute pain related to surgery, inflammation, and swelling; Impaired physical mobility related to foot-immobilizing device; Risk for infection related to the surgical procedure/surgical incision
3. reduced bone density and altered bone structure
4. third
5. Calcitonin, which inhibits bone resorption and promotes bone formation, is decreased. Estrogen, which inhibits bone breakdown, is decreased. Parathyroid hormone, which increases with age, enhances bone turnover and resorption.
6. 2.5; 1.0 to 2.5
7. a deficiency in activated vitamin D (calcitriol), which promotes calcium absorption from the gastrointestinal tract
8. calcitonin, bisphosphonates, and plicamycin

II. Critical Thinking Questions and Exercises

DISCUSSION AND ANALYSIS

1. Refer to chapter heading, "Bursitis and Tendinitis."
2. Refer to chapter headings, "Carpal Tunnel Syndrome" and "Dupuytren's Disease."
3. Refer to chapter heading, "Common Foot Problems."
4. Refer to chapter heading, "Paget's Disease."

APPLYING CONCEPTS

Refer to Figure 68-6 as a reference and chapter heading, "Common Foot Problems."

CLINICAL SITUATIONS

CASE STUDY: OSTEOPOROSIS

1. the rate of bone resorption is greater than the rate of bone formation.
2. Women have a lower peak bone mass than men, and estrogen loss affects the development of the disorder.
3. c
4. a
5. c
6. d

Chapter 69

I. Interpretation, Completion, and Comparison

MULTIPLE CHOICE

1. d	9. d	16. d
2. b	10. a	17. a
3. d	11. b	18. c
4. b	12. b	19. a
5. c	13. a	20. d
6. d	14. d	21. c
7. a	15. b	22. d
8. b		

MATCHING

PART I

1. c	3. b
2. a	4. e

PART II

1. c	3. a
2. b	4. d

SHORT ANSWER

1. tissue death caused by anoxia and diminished blood supply
2. the rubbing of bone fragments against each other
3. osteomyelitis, tetanus, and gas gangrene
4. Early complications are shock, fat embolism, compartment syndrome, deep vein thrombosis, thromboembolism, DIC, and infection. Delayed complications are delayed union and nonunion, avascular necrosis of bone, reaction to internal fixation devices, complex regional pain syndrome (CRPS), and heterotrophic ossification.
5. restoring blood volume and circulation, relieving the patient's pain, providing adequate splinting, protecting against further injury
6. deep vein thrombosis, thromboembolism, and pulmonary embolus
7. Colles' fracture
8. deep vein thrombosis
9. atelectasis and pneumonia

II. Critical Thinking Questions and Exercises

EXAMINING ASSOCIATIONS

1. an injury to the ligaments around a joint
2. subluxation
3. surgical repair
4. failure of the fractured bone ends to unite
5. allograft
6. trochanteric region

DISCUSSION AND ANALYSIS

1. Refer to chapter heading, "Contusions, Strains and Sprains."
2. Refer to chapter heading, "Types of Fractures."
3. Refer to chapter heading, "Types of Fractures."
4. Refer to Chart 69-3.
5. Refer to chapter heading, "Fat Embolism Syndrome."
6. Refer to chapter heading, "Compartment Syndrome."
7. Refer to chapter heading, "Fractures of Specific Sites: Femur."

EXTRACTING INFERENCES

1. medial collateral ligament; acute onset of pain, point tenderness, and joint stability; hemarthrosis
2. anterior cruciate ligament (ACL); near-normal ROM has returned; 6 to 12 months
3. meniscal injury; MRI; an effusion into the knee joint; 1 to 2 weeks

CLINICAL SITUATIONS

CASE STUDY: ABOVE-THE-KNEE AMPUTATION

1. d	5. a
2. d	6. d
3. d	7. b
4. d	8. d

Chapter 70

I. Interpretation, Completion, and Comparison

MULTIPLE CHOICE

1. c	8. c	15. d
2. d	9. d	16. d
3. d	10. d	17. d
4. c	11. c	18. d
5. a	12. a	19. d
6. d	13. c	20. a
7. d	14. d	

SHORT ANSWER

1. Colonization is used to describe microorganisms that remain present without host interference or interaction.
2. Infection indicates a host interaction with an organism.
3. smear and stain, the culture and organism identification, and the antimicrobial susceptibility
4. The World Health Organization and the Centers for Disease Control and Prevention
5. *Clostridium difficile,* methicillin-resistant *Staphylococcus aureus,* and vancomycin-resistant *Enterococcus*
6. Answer may include smallpox, measles, mumps, rubella, chickenpox, polio, diphtheria, pertussis, and tetanus.
7. pneumococcus, meningococcus, and *Haemophilus influenzae*
8. West Nile virus, Legionnaire's disease, Lyme disease, Hanta virus, and Ebola virus
9. sexually transmitted diseases; 19
10. Ebola and Marburg viruses

MATCHING

1. a	5. f
2. d	6. c
3. b	7. g
4. e	8. h

II. Critical Thinking Questions and Exercises

EXAMINING ASSOCIATIONS

Use Figure 70-1 to fill in each blank. Use terms on the perimeter of each link as a guide for choosing a nursing intervention.

DISCUSSION AND ANALYSIS

1. Refer to chapter heading, "Disease."
2. Refer to chapter heading, "Isolation Precautions."
3. Refer to Table 70-4.
4. Refer to chapter heading, "Nursing Process: The Patient with an Infectious Disease."
5. Refer to chapter heading, "Diarrheal Diseases."

Chapter 71

I. Interpretation, Completion, and Comparison

MULTIPLE CHOICE

1. d	8. b	14. d
2. c	9. a	15. c
3. c	10. c	16. d
4. b	11. d	17. d
5. b	12. d	18. d
6. b	13. c	19. a
7. a		

SHORT ANSWER

1. hepatitis B and human immunodeficiency virus (HIV)
2. speak, breathe, or cough
3. A hematoma is a tumor-like mass of blood trapped under the skin
4. liver
5. drowning
6. between 1 and 9 years
7. syrup of ipecac
8. Variola (smallpox) and *B. anthracis* (anthrax)

II. Critical Thinking Questions and Exercises

DISCUSSION AND ANALYSIS

1. Refer to chapter heading, "Triage."
2. Refer to chapter heading, "Endotracheal Intubation," and Figure 71-1.
3. Refer to chapter heading, "Hypovolemic Shock."
4. Lactated Ringer's solution is initially useful because it approximates plasma electrolyte composition and osmolality, allows time for blood typing and screening, restores circulation, and serves as an adjunct to blood component therapy.
5. Refer to chapter heading, "Heat Stroke."
6. Refer to chapter heading, "Ingested (Swallowed) Poisons."
7. Refer to chapter heading, "Inhaled Poisons: Carbon Monoxide Poisoning."
8. Refer to chapter heading, "Alcohol Withdrawal Syndrome/Delirium Tremens."
9. Refer to chapter heading, "Posttraumatic Stress Disorder."

APPLYING CONCEPTS

Refer to Chart 71-3.

CLINICAL SITUATIONS

1. Refer to chapter heading, "Intra-abdominal Injuries."
2. Refer to Chapter heading, "Anaphylactic Reaction."
3. Refer to Chart 71-11.
4. Refer to Table 71-1.
5. Refer to chapter heading, "Psychiatric Emergencies."

Chapter 72

I. Interpretation, Completion and Comparison

MULTIPLE CHOICE

1. c	6. d	11. b
2. d	7. b	12. d
3. c	8. c	13. a
4. b	9. b	14. b
5. b	10. a	

SHORT ANSWER

1. anthrax; chlorine
2. Department of Health and Human Services; Department of Justice; Department of Homeland Security
3. California; Colorado; Washington, D.C.; and North Carolina
4. The Incident Command System is a management tool for organizing personnel, facilities, equipment, and communication for any emergency. Its activation during emergencies is mandated by the federal government.
5. the degree and nature of the exposure to disaster, loss of loved ones, existing coping strategies, available resources and support, and personal meaning attached to the event
6. Defusing is a process by which an individual receives education about recognition of stress reactions and management strategies for handling stress. Debriefing is a more complicated intervention; it involves 2- to 3-hour processes during which participants are asked about their emotions, symptoms, and any other psychological ramifications.
7. anthrax and smallpox
8. ciprofloxacin or doxycycline; 100%
9. 30%
10. Pulmonary chemical agents act by destroying the pulmonary membrane that separates the alveolus from the capillary bed. When this happens, the individual cannot release carbon dioxide or acquire oxygen.

II. Critical Thinking Questions and Exercises

DISCUSSION AND ANALYSIS

1. Refer to Chart 72-1.
2. Refer to chapter heading, "Components of the Emergency Operations Plan."
3. A critically ill individual with a high mortality rate would be assigned a low triage priority because it would be unethical to use limited resources on those with a low chance of survival. Others who are seriously ill and have a greater chance of survival should be treated.
4. Cultural considerations include language differences, religious preferences (e.g., hygiene, diet, medical treatment), rituals of prayer, traditions for burying the dead, and the timing of funeral services.
5. Some common behavioral responses are depression, anxiety, somatization (fatigue, malaise), posttraumatic stress disorder, substance abuse, interpersonal conflicts, and impaired performance.
6. Refer to chapter heading, "The Incident Command System," and Chapter 3.
7. Refer to chapter heading, "Smallpox."
8. Refer to chapter heading, "Nerve Agents."
9. Refer to chapter heading, "Types of Radiation."
10. Refer to chapter heading, "Acute Radiation Syndrome."